Pattern Analysis for Histopathologic Diagnosis of Melanocytic Lesions

Almut Böer-Auer • Harald Kittler
Philipp Tschandl

Pattern Analysis for Histopathologic Diagnosis of Melanocytic Lesions

A Guide to Practical Dermatopathology

Springer

Almut Böer-Auer
Department of Dermatopathology
Dermatologikum Hamburg
Hamburg, Germany

Department of Dermatology
Münster University
Münster, Germany

Philipp Tschandl
Department of Dermatology
Medical University of Vienna
Vienna, Austria

Harald Kittler
Department of Dermatology
Medical University of Vienna
Vienna, Austria

ISBN 978-3-031-07665-7 ISBN 978-3-031-07666-4 (eBook)
https://doi.org/10.1007/978-3-031-07666-4

This Springer imprint is published by the registered company Springer Nature Switzerland AG
The registered company address is: Gewerbestrasse 11, 6330 Cham, Switzerland

To my teachers and my students, with gratitude

Almut Böer-Auer

To my wife Elisabeth, my greatest mentor

Harald Kittler

To Sophie

Philipp Tschandl

Foreword

Visual patterns can be defined as morphological features that follow a repeatable scheme, allowing predictions to be made according to a given pattern. In dermatology and dermatopathology, the predictions consist of clinical and histopathological diagnoses. In our approach to patients with pigmented skin tumors, we constantly use pattern analysis, even when we don't realize we are doing so; these patterns reflect our experience, both clinicopathological (i.e., experience acquired by working as physicians) and theoretical (i.e., experience acquired by reading pertinent literature or listening to presentations).

On the other hand, a precise knowledge of various diagnostic patterns is paramount in order to allow us to recognize them properly. In this book, Böer-Auer, Kittler, and Tschandl use pattern analysis as the main approach to histopathological diagnosis of benign and malignant melanocytic tumors, showing how this method can be effectively used in order to classify cases correctly. Pattern analysis in dermatopathology is widely used for the classification of inflammatory dermatoses and was developed mostly by one of the giants of this field, A. Bernard Ackerman. Ackerman's book on inflammatory dermatoses diagnosed by pattern analysis is a masterpiece, and one of the rare examples of a medical book still useful almost 50 years after its first publication.

In this volume, Böer-Auer, Kittler, and Tschandl show that the same method can be successfully applied to the histopathological diagnosis of melanocytic tumors, allowing to classify cases by an integration of different patterns and of other histopathological features. This book adds a new dimension to the histopathological diagnosis of melanocytic tumors, by providing a detailed and precise analysis of different patterns that can be recognized under the microscope. As a former student and co-worker of A. Bernard Ackerman, Almut Böer-Auer very well knows the importance of rational approach and pattern analysis for dermatopathological diagnosis of skin diseases; Harald Kittler and Philipp Tschandl add their year-long experience in dermatopathology and in pattern recognition, turning this publication a very valuable source for all those who are interested in dermatopathological diagnosis of melanocytic tumors.

Graz, Austria Lorenzo Cerroni

Acknowledgments

We especially want to thank Danijela Dobrosavljevic Vukojevic, Gerardo Ferrara, and Lorenzo Cerroni for providing us with first-rate images, which are a much valued addition to the contents.

Contents

About the Authors

Almut Böer-Auer is Dermatologist, Dermatopathologist, and Director of Academics at the Dermatologikum Hamburg, Germany, and Associate Professor at the Department of Dermatology at Münster University in Germany. She has been interested in histopathologic pattern diagnosis of skin diseases for almost two decades. One of her research focuses is identification and validation of diagnostic patterns by correlation with ancillary methods like molecular diagnostics. She has authored and co-authored many scientific articles and textbook chapters and is devoted to teaching dermatopathology nationally and internationally.

Harald Kittler is Associate Professor of Dermatology at the Department of Dermatology, Medical University of Vienna, in Vienna/Austria with a subspecialization in dermatopathology. His special clinical interest resides in the diagnosis of melanocytic skin lesions. His main research interest is digital dermoscopy, follow-up of pigmented skin lesions, computer-assisted digital dermoscopy, and dermatopathology. Dr. Kittler has been working for over 20 years in the field of dermoscopy and dermatopathology and has been lecturing and publishing a large number of scientific articles.

Philipp Tschandl is Associate Professor of Dermatology with a subspecialization in dermatopathology and managing director of the dermatopathology laboratory at the Department of Dermatology of the Medical University of Vienna in Austria. He has published research on growth dynamics of melanoma, melanoma association with pre-existing nevi, as well as early detection of melanoma with dermatoscopy. His work also includes the application of artificial intelligence alone and in collaboration with physicians for improving medical diagnoses and decision-making.

Introduction

1

Why do we need another textbook of dermatopathology dedicated to the diagnosis of melanocytic lesions? The answer is simple and surprising. Currently, there is no pathology textbook of melanocytic lesions rooted in pattern analysis. This is surprising because pattern analysis revolutionized the way dermatopathologists approach inflammatory and non-melanocytic neoplastic lesions. When A. Bernard Ackerman introduced pattern analysis in 1970, his ambitions were higher than the title of the book, "Histologic diagnosis of inflammatory skin diseases", suggested. His aim was to cover all skin diseases, inflammatory and neoplastic, in a single book, but he soon realized that this was too large a task to complete in a reasonable timeframe. Holding a signed publisher contract with an explicit dead line in his hand, he decided to restrict the book to inflammatory diseases. Later, he and his coworkers applied pattern analysis to neoplastic skin lesions, most notably to adnexal neoplasms with apocrine, follicular, and sebaceous differentiation. Together with his co-authors Lorenzo Cerroni and Helmut Kerl, he published "Pitfalls in the histopathologic diagnosis of malignant melanoma" in 1994, a book which, in his own words, "uses repeatable criteria for the histopathologic diagnosis of melanocytic neoplasms of all types". We owe important suggestions and ideas to this influential work, which are also reflected in the present book. However, A. Bernard Ackerman, the intellectual father of pattern analysis, never wrote a book on pattern analysis of melanocytic lesions. It is true that not all of his ideas and views have withstood the test of time, but pattern analysis certainly has, and so we have taken it upon ourselves to fill this gap.

What is pattern analysis? Pattern analysis is based on deductive reasoning and consists of two parts, a descriptive and an analytic part. It starts with a description and ends with the diagnosis. Because it commences with the description and not with the diagnosis, it is a bottom-up approach. Top-down approaches, on the other hand, start with the diagnosis. In general, patterns are composed of basic elements like mosaics are composed of individual tiles. The basic element of pattern analysis for the histopathologic diagnosis of melanocytic lesions is the neoplastic melanocyte. The morphology, arrangement, and distribution of melanocytes form the main patterns that typify nevi and melanoma. Additional criteria, such as stromal or epidermal changes, complete and refine these patterns.

In a first step, pattern analysis provides a tool that allows the observer to describe melanocytic lesions in a meaningful and repeatable fashion. In a second step, pattern analysis offers a rule-based algorithm to deduce the diagnosis, which, if applied consistently, should be as robust and repeatable as the description. We are aware that morphologic methods such as dermatopathology always contain an observer dependent, subjective, part, which is one of the main reasons for the

A. Böer-Auer et al., *Pattern Analysis for Histopathologic Diagnosis of Melanocytic Lesions*,
https://doi.org/10.1007/978-3-031-07666-4_1

low inter-rater agreement of the pathologic diagnosis of melanocytic skin lesions [1]. Other reasons include a confusing multitude of classifications and terms, lack of training or experience, and lack of a structured method. If pattern analysis is applied consistently, the inter-rater agreement will improve, at least with regard to the descriptive part of pattern analysis. The second, analytic, part of pattern analysis, will always be influenced by the personal style and the individual threshold of the reporting pathologist. We believe that this subjectivity is not harmful, provided that the final interpretation is in line with the description.

Usually, there are two main reasons for consulting a medical textbook. The first is that the reader wants to learn more about the subject at hand, for example, because of a genuine interest. The second reason is that the reader seeks advice on a specific case, for which the diagnosis is not obvious. Traditional textbooks will be perfectly suited for those who want to learn but will not be exceedingly helpful for those who seek advice on a specific case. The reason for this is that most textbooks are organized in a top-down fashion with tables of content that contain lists of diagnoses. To extract specific information, you will have to search for diagnoses. This will not be helpful if you do not know the diagnosis. This book, on the other hand, is organized in a bottom-up fashion and the reader can search for patterns and diagnoses alike. With the possibility to search for patterns, we want to support the reader in classifying unknown cases. Our book is not an atlas of melanocytic proliferations where you can look up examples for given diagnoses. It is intended to be more like a map that gives you directions if you lose your way. If you want to acquire a general knowledge of this field, you can read it page by page from the beginning to the end. If, however, you want to find guidance for a specific case you can consult only Chap. 7. Does this sound too abstract? Let us consider a use case.

Take, for example, the complex melanocytic neoplasm shown in Fig. 1.1. The diagnosis is not obvious. Which page would you open in a traditional textbook of dermatopathology? Would you look in the chapters of melanoma, combined nevi, deep penetrating nevi, Spitz nevus, atypical

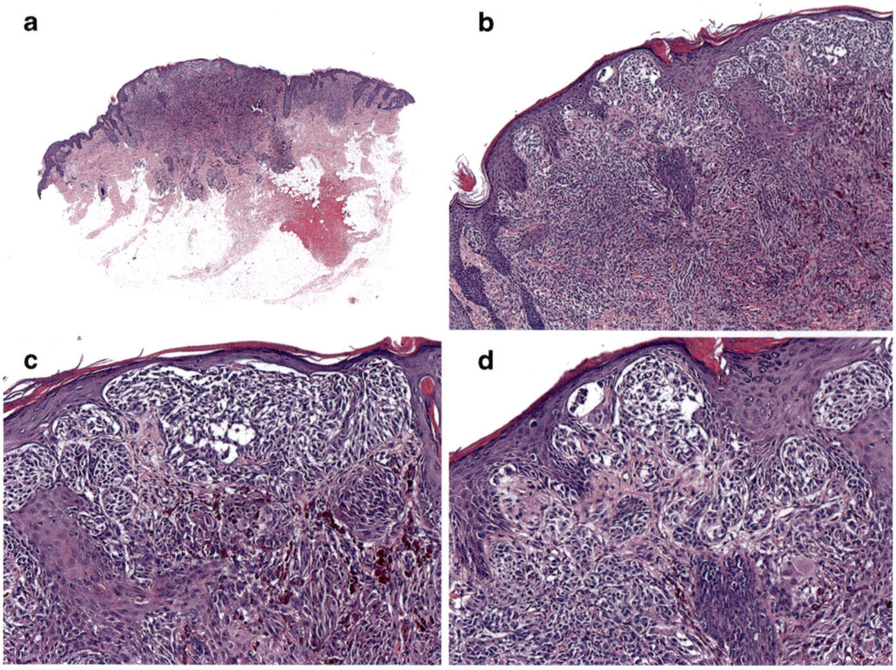

Fig. 1.1 (**a**–**l**) A complex melanocytic neoplasm of a prepubescent child (see text for a detailed description). (Courtesy of the Department of Dermatology, Medical University of Vienna)

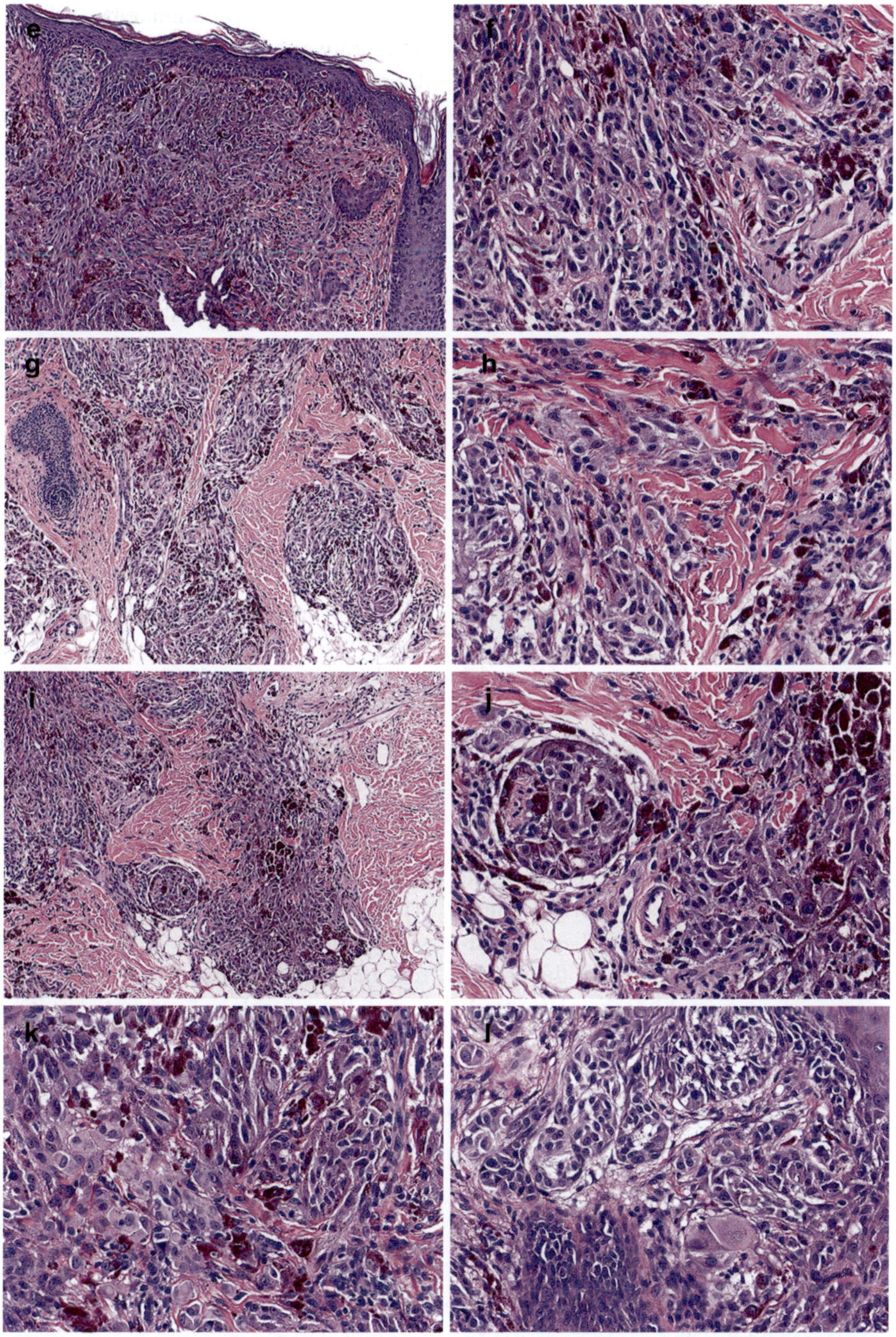

Fig. 1.1 (continued)

Spitz tumor, congenital nevi, or in all of the mentioned chapters?

It would be much easier to search by pattern first and not by diagnosis. Studying the pattern, you find a fairly asymmetric melanocytic neoplasm that involves the epidermis, the dermis, and superficial parts of the subcutis. The melanocytes in the epidermis are mainly arranged in nests with some pagetoid spread. The nests vary in size and shape and are irregularly distributed. The melanocytes in the dermis are plump, spindle, and epithelioid, and a significant proportion of dermal melanocytes is heavily pigmented. There are abundant melanophages and no obvious maturation. After scanning the lesion in higher magnification for minutes, you find one mitosis in the deeper portions of the lesion. Given this description, pattern analysis would lead to two, maximal three differential diagnoses, possibly *deep penetrating nevus* versus *Spitz nevus* versus *melanoma*. Next, you seek additional information. After contacting the referring clinician, you learn that this lesion comes from the cheek of a prepubescent boy (Fig. 1.2a). You also learn that this boy has Xeroderma pigmentosum, a genetic condition that predisposes for UV-induced skin malignancies such as keratinocyte cancer and melanoma. You ask yourself if this information should change your assessment. The clinician also offers you to have a look at the dermatoscopic image of this case (Fig. 1.2b) but you have no experience in dermatoscopy and you decline.

However, you ask yourself if it would be useful to have some basic knowledge in clinical dermatology and in dermatoscopy, especially for the diagnosis of melanocytic neoplasms. An experienced colleague tells you that clinical information is mostly useless and occasionally misleading. The answer is always in the slide, and if it is not in the slide, it is nowhere, he says and, having a short glimpse at your slide, he would call it a melanoma. Because you still hesitate to call this lesion a melanoma, you do immunohistochemistry studies, which do not help you. You heard that it is possible to perform molecular studies such as comparative genomic hybridization (CGH) or fluorescence in situ hybridization (FISH) but they are not available at your site. You will have to send tissue to another laboratory and the results will not be available within the next 3 weeks. Another colleague tells you that her experience with CGH is that it does not remove doubts, sometimes it even creates new ones. Finally, you will need to file a report taking everything into account including the consequences the patient and you will have to face if your diagnosis is wrong. You will have to weigh the consequences of calling a nevus a melanoma against the consequences of calling a melanoma a nevus in a 3-year-old. You realize that you are not sure what these consequences are either way. Adding everything up, you feel that you cannot exclude the diagnosis of melanoma in this context, but you want to convey your uncertainty in your report, but how?

The point is that the answers to most of these questions that came up during the study of this case will not be found in traditional textbooks. We do not claim, of course, that you will find all the answers in this book, but we are at least aware of the questions and will not ignore them. According to our experience, pattern analysis will provide you with a framework that will allow you to manage complex and uncertain cases in a repeatable and meaningful fashion. Pattern analysis will not resolve uncertainty but it will reduce confusion.

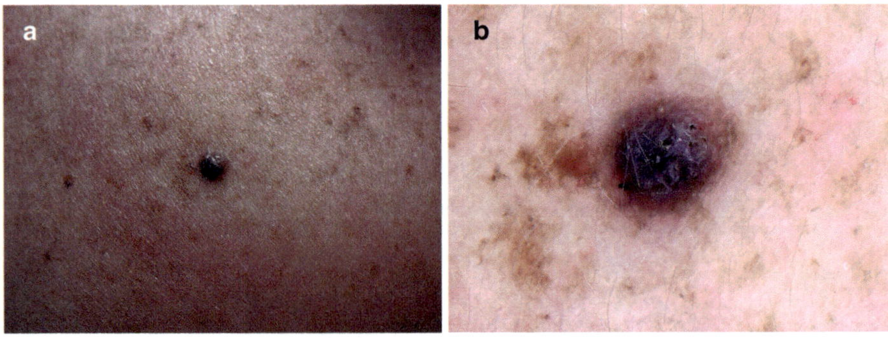

Fig. 1.2 Close-up clinical image (**a**; left) and dermatoscopy (**b**; right) of the lesion on the cheek shown in Fig. 1.1. Although the patient is a prepubescent child, there is severe chronic sun damage in the surrounding skin. The child suffers from Xeroderma pigmentosum, a hereditary condition that is typified by UV-sensitivity and susceptibility to UV-induced skin neoplasms such as squamous cell carcinoma and basal cell carcinoma but also melanoma. (Courtesy of the Department of Dermatology, Medical University of Vienna)

Diagnostic categories with uncertain prognosis such as atypical Spitz tumor (AST), superficial atypical melanocytic proliferation of uncertain malignant significance (SAMPUS), or melanocytic tumor with uncertain malignant potential (MELTUMP) represent a constant source of confusion. There is certainly a need for such categories in practice because some melanocytic neoplasms can be diagnosed neither as benign (nevus) nor as malignant (melanoma) with confidence. There are, however, different points of view about the best way to express this ambiguity. One school of thought will blame the lesion ("the lesion does not know what it is"), the other the ignorance of the reporting pathologist ("I do not know what it is"). The authors of this book are proponents of the latter school of thought, but throughout this book we will try to reconcile both approaches.

Is it still appropriate to write a textbook on the histologic diagnosis of melanocytic skin lesions that is centered on morphology? Is it not expected that a purely morphologic diagnosis will be outdated soon and replaced by molecular methods that categorize and diagnose melanocytic skin lesions more precisely? We do not think so. Although we acknowledge that molecular methods provide useful additional information in selected cases, we predict that even 10 years from now the vast majority of melanocytic neoplasms will be diagnosed by microscopic examination of pieces of tissue stained by hematoxylin and eosin. The reasons for our bold claim are manifold but can be condensed to one single argument. Conventional light microscopy is a relatively cheap examination technique that combines high accuracy with broad availability. If, however, this textbook is outdated in 10 years and the final diagnosis of melanocytic neoplasms is based only on molecular findings, we will happily put our microscopes in the basement and spend our time more wisely.

2 Historical Perspective

The following historical summary is not meant to be complete. Many important figures and events are not mentioned. To avoid exhaustion of readers and authors alike, the summary provides only as much information as necessary to deliver the narrative and to help the interested reader understand the big picture. For a more detailed review of the history of the clinical and histopathologic diagnosis of melanoma we refer to recent review articles by Kittler [2] and Weyers [3].

Although from the current point of view it seems that most of what has been published about the pathology of melanocytic proliferations pre-1970s is outdated, the study of historic books and manuscripts is not futile. It teaches us three important lessons. ***First***, that scientific knowledge is embedded in a specific historic context, which shapes the beliefs and concepts of scientists, who live at that time. If we study medical publications from the past, no matter how brilliantly they were written, we cannot help to be amused about the lack of scope and depth, outdated concepts, and primitive techniques. We easily feel superior to the physician-scientists of the past but we should not. Looking back should make us more humble, because most of our current concepts and techniques, no matter how sophisticated they seem to us today, will be equally outdated in the future. ***Second***, we learn that we cannot easily shake off the past. The current classification of nevi and melanoma as set forth by the World Health Organization (WHO) for example is replete with historic ballast. The bulky terminology of nevi, which differs from textbook to textbook, is illogical because it grew historically. Nevi have been named according to different ordering principles, such as anatomic site (acral nevus), time of appearance (congenital nevus/acquired nevus), clinical criteria (eclipse nevus, blue nevus), or in an eponymic way (Spitz nevus). The result is an incoherent hodgepodge of terms that complicate the study of melanocytic proliferations. The ***third*** and probably most important lesson is that evolving concepts in dermatopathology are tightly linked to other specialities and influenced by general trends. Changing paradigms in the standard of care outside the field of dermatopathology had a significant impact on the concepts inside the field of dermatopathology. The shift of focus towards early recognition in the 1980s, the invention of the handheld dermatoscope, the increased awareness and melanoma-related anxiety of the public, and the increased vulnerability of pathologists to malpractice lawsuits created a pull towards lowering thresholds for the diagnosis of melanoma, especially for melanoma in situ. In a few decades, the landscape shifted from underdiagnosis to overdiagnosis of melanomas, a development that is now met with increased criticism. By overdiagnosis we mainly refer to the inflation of the diagnosis of in situ or microinvasive melanomas with unknown prognostic significance. The undesired consequences of overdiagnosis are manifold.

A. Böer-Auer et al., *Pattern Analysis for Histopathologic Diagnosis of Melanocytic Lesions*,
https://doi.org/10.1007/978-3-031-07666-4_2

Apart from putting a significant financial burden on health care systems, overdiagnosis is associated with increased anxiety and morbidity of affected individuals. All these developments are difficult to comprehend without a basic understanding of their historical evolution. Studying the past will also allow us to look into the future. As of the time of the first edition of this book, the incidence of melanoma seems to have peaked, which might indicate that melanoma overdiagnosis reached a zenith. It is quite likely that the pendulum swings back in the other direction. It is our task to make sure that the pendulum levels off at a desirable position.

2.1 Melanoma

As pointed out recently in a more comprehensive historical outline, a good starting point for a historical summary on the histopathologic diagnosis of melanoma is the work of L. V. Ackerman in the late 1940s [2]. He was one of the first to describe the pathology of "melanocarcinoma," as it was called then, in a systematic way. The clinical photos and micrographs of his original publications demonstrate how advanced typical cases of melanoma were in 1948 [4]. The concept of L.V. Ackerman was that melanoma usually starts in a nevus and that "*it is most unusual to find the changes of malignant melanoma entirely within the epidermis with no change in the dermis.*" This statement demonstrates that the concept of melanoma in situ did not exist in 1948.

A few years later in 1953, Arthur Allen and Sophie Spitz co-authored an article, in which they set forth their belief that all melanomas start in a preexisting mole, especially in an "*active junctional nevus*" [5]. The micrograph of the "*activated junctional nevus immediately preceding the development of infiltrating melanocarcinoma*" shown in Fig. 9 of their article of 1953 clearly shows a melanoma in situ. What has been called a precursor by Allen and Spitz, would be called a melanoma today.

In the late 1960s and early 1970s, Clark in the USA and McGovern in Australia propagated a "*histogenetic*" classification of melanoma, which continues to be relevant until today [6–8]. In its original form the classification included three subtypes: nodular melanoma, superficial spreading melanoma, and lentigo maligna melanoma. Nodular melanoma was typified by pure vertical growth, while superficial spreading melanoma expands along the epidermis (radial or horizontal growth phase). The fourth subtype, acral lentiginous melanoma, was added later. In the early 1970s, Clark and his coworkers also established the anatomic levels of invasion, and at the same time Arthur Breslow introduced the invasion thickness as a prognostic marker for primary melanoma of the skin [9, 10]. In the mid-1970s, A. Bernard Ackerman and his coworkers set forth histopathologic criteria for the diagnosis of melanoma that are still widely used by dermatopathologists (Table 2.1) [11]. Ackerman also popularized the concept of melanoma in situ, clinically and pathologically, and negated the concept of precursor lesions such as "Allen's active junctional nevus," "Hutchinson's melanotic freckle," "Kossard's lentiginous dysplastic nevus of the elderly," and "precancerous melanosis of Dubreuilh," which, according to his opinion, were evasions from the correct diagnosis of melanoma in situ.

Pre-1980s, melanoma in situ was not widely accepted as authentic melanoma but rather viewed as a precursor. The clinical diagnosis of

Table 2.1 Significant histopathologic features of superficial spreading melanoma according to Price, Rywlin, and Ackermann 1976

Poor circumscription of the intraepidermal melanocytic component of the lesion with lateral extension of individual melanocytes
Increased number of melanocytes, solitary and in nests, within and **above the epidermal basal-cell layer** and within adnexal epithelium (Pagetoid appearance)
Marked **variation in size and shape** of the melanocytic nests
Confluence of melanocytic nests rather than discrete nests
Absence of maturation of melanocytes with descent into the dermis
Melanocytes with **nuclear atypia**
Melanocytes in **mitosis**
Necrosis or degeneration of melanocytes

melanoma was based on gross features such as ulceration or bleeding. In the mid-1980s, however, education campaigns such as the propagation of the ABCD criteria, which addressed health care professionals and the public alike, shifted the focus towards early recognition. Dermatoscopy, which became increasingly popular in the 1990s, improved the accuracy for the diagnosis of melanoma in comparison to inspection with the unaided eye, especially for flat and small lesions lacking ABCD criteria. Finally, in January 1992, the National Institutes of Health (NIH) held a consensus conference to discuss the clinical and histological characteristics of early melanoma [12]. The consensus panel agreed that melanoma in situ is a distinct entity. With this official acceptance of "melanoma in situ" as authentic melanoma, the stage was finally set for early recognition to lift off. Increased public awareness, the availability of a new and affordable in vivo examination technique (i.e., dermatoscopy), and the lower hesitancy of pathologists to diagnose melanoma in situ acted in accordance: The incidence for melanoma skyrocketed and increased more than for any other type of cancer.

In the following years it was discovered that dermatopathologists tend to disagree, not only on concepts and terminology, but also whether a given melanocytic proliferation is benign or malignant [1, 13–15]. Problems commonly occur in lesions that are small or flat or have a spitzoid morphology. For these "borderline" lesions, the community invented terms with uncertain prognosis such as atypical Spitz tumor (AST) [16] and superficial atypical melanocytic proliferation of uncertain malignant significance (SAMPUS) [17].

Since the discovery of the S100 protein in melanoma in the 1980s [18–20], a considerable number of other immunohistochemical markers have been used to assist in the differentiation of melanocytic proliferations from other neoplasms. Despite initial enthusiasm that some markers could also be used in the assessment of challenging melanocytic neoplasms, and despite some encouraging results with the melanoma-associated antigen PRAME (PReferentially expressed Antigen in MElanoma), examination of conventional slides stained with hematoxylin and eosin still remain the gold standard for the diagnosis of melanocytic proliferations. There was, however, a certain hope that these difficulties in diagnosis will vanish with more sophisticated molecular techniques. In the early 2000s the molecular revolution in medicine gained momentum and new observations challenged our concepts of melanoma biology. The first turning point was the discovery of the significance of BRAF mutations in melanoma and in nevi [21], which was soon followed by the detection of other tumorigenic mutations in other oncogenes [22] and climaxed in the description of the genomic landscape of melanoma [23, 24]. While some of these discoveries translated into identification of "druggable" biologic targets [25], the new insights into the genetic landscape of melanoma did not translate into reliable diagnostic methods for "borderline lesions." Although molecular techniques such as fluorescence in situ hybridization (FISH) [26] or comparative genomic hybridization (CGH) [27, 28] have been used to better classify borderline lesions such as Spitz tumors, they remain auxiliary techniques, which need to be integrated with clinical and dermatoscopic observations as well as with conventional pathology [29]. The importance of genetic alterations for the classification of melanoma has been increased dramatically by the introduction of the new WHO classification of melanocytic neoplasms in 2018 [30]. The WHO classification tried to integrate the complex and ever evolving genetic landscape of melanoma with the classic histogenetic classification and with UVR-exposure. At present, even with the best will, this undertaking can only be described as a piecemeal effort, which has a certain theoretical but hardly any practical value. Some of the implicit and explicit hypotheses that form the theoretical backbone of the new WHO classification look like ad hoc assumptions invented to save the classic histogenetic model from falsification. Furthermore, it can be expected that more sophisticated genomic analyses such as whole genome sequencing, methylation studies, and high resolution spatial transcriptomics will become more widely available in the future and will provide new insights into the interaction of germline mutations, somatic mutations, and UV-signature mutations [31]. It is likely that these new insights will make it necessary to adjust and revise the theoretical framework of the current classification and add new ad hoc assumptions.

The recent hype associated with artificial intelligence (AI) and deep learning in image-based diagnostic medicine did not leave dermatopathology untouched [32]. It is, however, currently unknown how such algorithms will be used in clinical routine. Beyond fully automatic diagnosis, which is the least likely use case, potential roles of AI range from filters for triage, quality control, predictive models, quality assurance, and decision support to the discovery of new knowledge.

2.2 Melanocytic Nevi

There is no coherent history of the histopathology of melanocytic nevi. It is a fragmented landscape of individual observations with repeated attempts to integrate them into a general classification of nevi, all of which have failed in one way or another. If the history of melanocytic nevi would be a movie, it would have a non-linear narrative replete with broken up chronologies, spirals, meanders, parallel developments, and story lines that go nowhere. Fascinating and open to interpretation, like David Lynch's acclaimed movie "Mulholland Drive," but difficult to follow and full of riddles.

In the past, many nevi were eponymously named after their first descriptors, such as Meyerson, Spitz, Reed, Clark, Unna, and Miescher nevus. We welcome the recent attempts to abolish eponyms in dermatology and restrict ourselves to those eponyms that are part of the latest WHO classification. These are mainly the two terms Spitz and Reed nevus and, with limitation, Meyerson nevus. In this book we will not use the term "Clark nevus," which has been used as a synonym for "dysplastic nevus" by those who reject the term "dysplastic." We will also not use the terms Miescher and Unna nevus, which refer to nevi with a dermal pattern that differ mainly by anatomic location (Miescher nevus is a dermal nevus on the face and Unna nevus on the trunk).

Historically, there is a long-lasting controversy about the origin of cells that make up a nevus and whether they should be called nevus cells, nevocytes, nevomelanocytes, or melanocytes. In the 1950s, Arthur Allen still believed that melanocytes in the epidermis develop from keratinocytes despite convincing evidence that they derive from the neural crest, which was suggested by Masson already in the 1920s [33]. Masson also proposed that nevi originate in the dendritic melanocytes of the dermoepidermal junction. The root of this concept can be traced back to Unna, who suggested that epidermal cells move into the dermis to give rise to intradermal nevus cells ("Abtropfung") in 1893 [34]. Although most students of the subject concluded that Unna referred to melanocytes, he did not specify which cells move into the dermis. It was not possible to differentiate melanocytes from keratinocytes with certainty until Bloch in 1917 was able to localize melanocytes in the epidermis through identification of tyrosinase via the DOPA reaction [35]. In contrast to Unna's concept of "Abtropfung," Cramer's concept of "Hochsteigerung" is based on the idea that "nevus cells" ascend from the dermis into the epidermis.

The current concept oof melanocyte precursor migration is based on experimental studies in zebrafish, mice, and chicken. This work identified two pathways of melanocyte migration, both located in the neural crest. One is the dorsolateral pathway, in which melanoblasts originating from the neural crest migrate into the epidermis along the evolving somites and the axons of the spinal nerves. The other, more recently identified pathway, is the dorsoventral pathway, in which melanocytes derive from Schwann cell precursors. Kinsler et al. recently suggested a third pathway that occurs around the time of gastrulation, presumably located within the mesoderm [36]. All three migration patterns are important to understand the patterns of congenital pigmentary disorders including those of congenital nevi. While the first two pathways explain segmental patterns like in macular nevus spilus, the latter pathway may be responsible for the non-segmental patterns of large congenital nevi with satellite lesions.

Like all nevi, congenital melanocytic nevi are regarded as clonal disorders that harbor somatic mutations, which in the case of large congenital nevi occur most commonly in the NRAS-gene [37]. Congenital nevi are usually contrasted with "acquired" nevi. However, this distinction, as simple as it may seem, is problematic because the term "congenital nevus" is not used consistently. If "congenital" is defined strictly as "visible at birth," many, mostly small congenital nevi, would be labeled as acquired. This led to the concept of "tardive congenital nevi," which are not visible at birth, but can still be identified as congenital because of specific clinical, dermatoscopic, or histopathologic features. Acquired nevi, on the other hand, have been classified according to different criteria, which resulted in a hodgepodge of terms that is difficult to grasp because of the lack of any consistent ordering principle. There is, however, general agreement that different types of nevi are typified by different sets of mutations. The most common activating mutations found in acquired nevi occur in the BRAF- and, albeit less often, in the NRAS-oncogene [38]. BRAF or NRAS mutations are commonly found in so-called "dysplastic" nevi, which, according to some authors, have gained additional genetic alterations that differentiate them from common nevi (junctional, compound, and dermal nevi). Spitz nevi, on the other hand, are acquired nevi typified by a different set of somatic mutations such as ALK fusions or mutation of HRAS [39], whereas blue nevi are characterized by GNAQ mutations [40]. Other acquired nevi such as halo nevi, Meyerson nevi, or nevi on special sites do not have a distinct set of genetic alterations but are characterized by other criteria such as inflammatory reactions or anatomic site.

Apart from somatic mutations, germline mutations will also have an impact on the number, and also on the morphology of nevi. Germline mutations of the tumor suppressor gene CDKN2A, for example, are associated with the phenotype of the familial atypical multiple mole melanoma (FAMMM) syndrome [41, 42], which is typified by multiple "atypical" nevi and a family history of melanoma. The term "atypical" here has been used to indicate that these nevi are larger and more irregular than "typical" nevi. The terms "dysplastic nevus" and "dysplastic nevus syndrome" have been used in a similar but not identical way. Another, albeit rare, germline mutation that has an impact on nevus counts and appearance occurs in the BAP-1 tumor suppressor gene. Individuals with this mutation are prone to a specific type of nevus characterized by large dermal melanocytes with abundant cytoplasm [43]. These are just two prominent examples of a multitude of genes that influence both, the number and appearance of nevi and melanoma risk. In reality, multiple genes interact leading to a complicated inheritance of nevus and melanoma traits, which is further complicated by environmental factors such as UVR-exposure and by simple chance. The result is a complex relationship between nevi and melanoma that has been responsible for many misunderstandings and misconceptions regarding the evolution of melanocytic neoplasms in the past.

2.3 The Relationship Between Melanocytic Nevi and Melanoma

Historically, nevi were regarded as precursors and simulators of melanoma as well as indicators of melanoma risk. This three-fold relationship between melanoma and nevi has confused generations of clinicians and pathologists alike. The confusion is so great because all three potential roles are grounded in fact, but each role has its own rules that cannot be carried over to the other. If, for example, a nevus simulates a melanoma, it does not necessarily mean that the very same nevus has a higher chance to transform into a melanoma. Or if, by chance, a melanoma develops in a nevus, it does not mean that this nevus has to be atypical or "dysplastic." The confusion arose because the three potential roles of nevi, i.e., precursor, imitator, and indicator, were mixed together in the general model of "stepwise tumor progression," which became a paradigm in the field of melanoma biology. Key concepts of this tumor model were the stepwise progression of normal melanocytes, via a common nevus, towards a "dysplastic" nevus, into in situ and finally invasive melanoma, on one hand, and the phenotype of multiple "atypical" nevi ("dysplastic nevi") as indicator of melanoma risk, on the other. "Dysplastic nevi" were generally regarded as an intermediate step between a common nevus and a melanoma. Although parts of this model are useful, it fails to cover all aspects of the complex relationship between nevi and melanoma. There is no doubt that stepwise accumulations of somatic mutations are drivers of the evolution of melanoma. However, whether this stepwise accumulation of mutations is visible by light microscopy in the form of a gradual increase in "architectural disorder" and "cellular atypia" is less certain, although this link between genetic changes and morphology has always been tacitly accepted as fact by proponents of the prevailing model of stepwise tumor progression.

Current evidence suggests that only 20–25% of all melanomas develop in a pre-existing nevus [44]. The majority of melanomas develop de novo and not in pre-existing nevi of any type. If a melanoma develops in a nevus, it may be any type of nevus including "dysplastic" and "non-dysplastic" nevi [45, 46]. Furthermore, the relationship between the number of nevi and melanoma is more easily explained by correlation and not by a causal connection, meaning that the number of nevi and the risk of developing melanoma are linked via common factors such as germline mutations or environmental factors. In the 2018 WHO classification of melanocytic neoplasms, which we will discuss later in greater detail, the unidimensional progression model from nevi to melanoma has been replaced by a more garnished model that allows for nine different pathways to melanoma. Although this model is more complex, it is based on the same principles and suffers from the same contradictions.

3 Classifications

Every textbook of dermatology or dermatopathology has a different way to classify melanocytic neoplasms and we have no intention of adding a new one. Classifications come and go. The current WHO classification of melanocytic tumors, for example, will be refined, reworked, and finally replaced by a more fashionable one. Pattern analysis, on the other hand, is timeless; it can be mapped to every classification, current and future. However, we acknowledge the need to follow the rules of the prevailing orthodoxy when it comes to issuing pathologic reports. For this reason, we will discuss the 2018 WHO classification in greater detail and establish its relation to other classifications and to pattern analysis. We will also briefly focus on the MPATH-Dx reporting scheme, which is an attempt to improve the consistency and comparability of pathologic reports by classifying melanocytic proliferations according to suggested treatment rather than specific diagnoses.

3.1 The WHO Classification of Melanocytic Tumors[1]

In spring 2022, when these lines were written, the currently valid WHO classification 2018 for melanocytic tumors was already 4 years old, and it is possible that it had already been revised at the time of printing. However, this is irrelevant in that much of what we say here specifically about the 2018 WHO classification will also apply to upcoming classifications. In general, the WHO Classification 2018 is more of an ontology than a classification. Unlike simple classifications, ontologies are more complex and provide a set of concepts that creates classes and taxonomies. The main ordering principle of the WHO classification is the pathway concept which attempts to integrate *etiology* (UVR exposure), *pathogenesis* (sequence of "causal" events), and *genomic* alterations. It also involves other attributes such as anatomic site (e.g., acral nevi and acral melanoma) or histomorphology (e.g., nodular and nevoid melanoma), albeit less consistently and

[1]To be consistent with the WHO publications we use the expression "melanocytic tumors" in this chapter although we prefer to use the terms "lesions," "proliferations," or "neoplasms" in combination with the attribute melanocytic. The reason for our preference is that some melanocytic proliferations, such as lentigo simplex or macular nevus spilus, do not form "tumors."

A. Böer-Auer et al., *Pattern Analysis for Histopathologic Diagnosis of Melanocytic Lesions*,
https://doi.org/10.1007/978-3-031-07666-4_3

not as explicitly as the pathway concept. Because more than one attribute is involved, the creators refer to it as a multidimensional classification. It is important to note that the histogenetic classification by Clark and McGovern [8], which preceded the current WHO classification of melanoma, was already multidimensional because it included histomorphologic criteria ("superficial spreading melanoma") as well as anatomic site ("acral lentiginous melanoma"). Although it is considerably more complex, the current WHO classification builds on the old histogenetic classification, but unlike the old one, which had no general ordering principle for nevi, it tries to integrate nevi and melanoma under the pathway concept. The current WHO classification has been repeatedly criticized, most eloquently by Weyers [47]. One point of critique was that the creators of the classification have not been able to bring themselves to get rid of historical ballast. This critique, however justified it may be, fails to take into account the enormous difficulties that arise by the admirable attempt to integrate complex new data and old concepts into a new paradigm. We have enormous respect for the domain-specific knowledge of the experts of the classification. The WHO classification has great explanatory power just like the cosmological work by Ptolemy. Ptolemy was a genius and one of the greatest scientists of all time. His complex theory of the laws that govern celestial motion was definitely wrong, but he still made impressive predictions.

The first surprise for anyone studying the WHO classification is that the basic principle for classifying melanocytic neoplasms is not the distinction between melanoma (malignant) and nevi (benign), but the distinction of nine pathways (Table 3.1). This contradicts the structure of almost all textbooks of dermatology and dermatopathology, where melanoma and nevi are usually separate chapters. The pathway concept further demands that each pathway, at least in theory, consists of benign, intermediate, and malignant neoplasms although it is generally accepted [44] that most melanomas develop de novo and not in a precursor lesion. It is therefore not surprising that there is no logical benign or intermediate precursor lesion in many of the nine pathways, or that some of the intermediate categories contain generic descriptions such as "intraepidermal atypical melanocytic proliferation" instead of diagnoses (Table 3.1).

The nine pathways are divided into three major groups that differ according to UVR exposure. The first group includes only a single path-

Table 3.1 Nine pathways to melanoma according to the WHO classification 2018

Pathway	Benign	Intermediate/low grade	Intermediate/high grade	Malignant
1	Nevus	Low-grade dysplasia, BAP-1 inactivated nevus, deep penetrating nevus	High-grade dysplasia, BAP-1 inactivated melanocytoma, deep penetrating melanocytoma, primary epithelioid melanocytoma	Superficial spreading melanoma, melanoma arising in one of the melanocytomas
2	?	?	Lentigo maligna/melanoma in situ	Lentigo maligna melanoma
3	?	?	Lentigo maligna/melanoma in situ	Desmoplastic melanoma
4	Spitz nevus	Atypical Spitz tumor	Spitzoid tumor of uncertain malignant potential	Spitz melanoma
5	?	Intraepidermal atypical melanocytic proliferation of uncertain significance	Acral melanoma in situ	Acral melanoma
6	?	Intraepidermal atypical melanocytic proliferation	Mucosal melanoma in situ	Mucosal melanoma
7	Congenital nevus	Nodule in congenital nevus	Melanoma in situ in congenital nevus	Melanoma in congenital nevus
8	Blue nevus	Cellular blue nevus	Atypical cellular blue nevus	Melanoma in blue nevus
9	?	?	?	Uveal melanoma

way, which is associated with low or intermediate cumulative sun damage. This pathway starts with a nevus that progresses either into low-grade and high-grade dysplasia or into a melanocytoma and then finally into melanoma, either superficial spreading melanoma (which arises in high-grade dysplasia) or melanoma arising in one of the melanocytomas, either BAP-1 inactivated melanocytoma, deep penetrating melanocytoma, or primary pigmented melanocytoma. The term melanocytoma is used as a generic term for the intermediate category except for low-grade and high-grade dysplasias. The key driver mutations of this pathway are the BRAF V600E mutation or NRAS mutations either in association with TERT mutations (high-grade dysplasias and superficial spreading melanoma), BAP-1 inactivation (BAP-1 inactivated melanocytoma), CTNNB1 or APC mutations (deep penetrating melanocytoma), or PRKAR1A and PRKCA mutations (pigmented epithelioid melanocytoma). The second group of pathways includes two pathways that are both related to high cumulative sun damage. One gives rise to lentigo maligna melanoma, the other to desmoplastic melanoma. No convincing benign or low-grade intermediate precursor is offered for both pathways. Lentigo maligna is the non-invasive precursor lesion of this pathway. The main driver mutations in this pathway are NRAS, BRAF, and KIT mutations for lentigo maligna melanoma and NF1 for desmoplastic melanoma. The remaining six pathways are not related to UV exposure and chronic sun damage. Three of the six remaining pathways are related to anatomic site (acral, mucosal, and uveal melanoma), and the other three have specific nevus precursors (Spitz nevus, blue nevus, and congenital nevus). The pathways are typified by specific mutations such as the Spitz pathway by HRAS mutations, the acral and mucosal pathway by KIT mutations, the blue nevus and uveal pathway by GNAQ or GNA11 mutations, and the congenital nevus pathway by NRAS mutations, although other mutations also play a role. Nodular melanoma and nevoid melanoma can occur in any of the nine pathways.

Apart from the difficulty to find precursor lesions for some pathways, other inconsistencies complicate the understanding. Melanoma in situ is the immediate precursor of invasive melanomas in most but not in all pathways. Melanocytomas, atypical Spitz tumor, MELTUMP, or STUMP, which are all dermal proliferations, play the role of the precursor in other pathways. In the Spitz pathway, for example, there is no in situ precursor lesion. Spitz melanoma in situ does not exist, only atypical Spitz tumor and STUMP. Furthermore, in the congenital nevus pathway a proliferative nodule is the low-grade intermediate, and melanoma in situ the high-grade intermediate, precursor lesion. This contradicts the original stepwise progression model, where we have a continuum from low-grade dysplasia to high-grade dysplasia to melanoma in situ. Proliferative nodules and melanoma in situ in a congenital nevus are obviously not a continuum, but two different entities. The pathway concept is also incomplete, since melanoma of the conjunctiva is not included in the pathway concept although it is mentioned as a specific subtype of melanoma. According to a study published in 2021, which demonstrated by whole genome sequencing that melanoma of the conjunctiva is typified by a predominance of UVR-induced DNA damage, conjunctival melanoma should be included in one of the intermediate or high UVR-exposure pathways, and not in the mucosal pathway [48].

Another difficulty is the integration of nevi. Blue nevi, Spitz nevi, BAP-1 inactivated nevi, deep penetrating nevi, and congenital nevi are integrated in the pathway concept but all other nevus types that are listed in the WHO classification are not. The classification of nevi is still a disjointed list of various entities that do not fit into the "multidimensional pathway classification" and are only loosely linked by improvised assumptions. Examples of the difficulties encountered in integrating nevi into the pathway concept are that junctional, compound, or dermal nevi are listed in the category of melanocytic tumors in intermittently sun-exposed skin, even though these nevi can occur at any anatomic site, including the face (high chronic sun exposure) and acral (no or low chronic sun exposure). The same is true for other nevi, such as recurrent nevi or congenital nevi, for example. Another logical difficulty is that categories are not exclusive. Acral nevi are nevi on a special site but are not included in special site nevi. Congenital nevi may appear on any site, including special sites and acral. Does congenital trump acral if a congenital nevus appears on the sole? These are just a few examples of logical inconsistencies that arise if an ontology is created without consulting experts in the field of knowledge representation.

The best way to digest the WHO classification of melanocytic tumors is to leave aside the pathway concept entirely. This leads to a list of entities that can, in the spirit of the WHO classification, be categorized into benign lesions (nevi), "intermediate" lesions, and melanoma (Table 3.2). This list of entities is very similar to what can be found in most textbooks of dermatology and dermatopathology. Although we do not use some terms and categories in the list, we still consider it useful. All the entities of this list will be covered in this book, but discussed from the point of view of pattern analysis.

The WHO classification of melanocytic tumors is a model developed by individuals who have been directly involved in cutting-edge research on melanocyte pathology and biology. The disadvantage of this approach is that the resulting classification, however sophisticated from a research perspective, is impractical for daily routine. As a result, the current classification is rarely used in practice. The WHO classification is ambitious but fails to reach its main purpose, to integrate all melanocytic neoplasms under the multidimensional pathway concept in a meaningful way. It seems that the uncompromising adherence to the precursor concept forced the experts to compromise on consistency and practicability. It is currently unclear if the

Table 3.2 Leaving aside the pathway concept of the WHO classifications of melanocytic tumors leads to a list of entities similar to most textbooks of dermatology and dermatopathology

Nevus	Intermediate category	Melanoma
Junctional, compound, and dermal nevus	Melanocytoma	Melanoma in situ including lentigo maligna
Nevus spilus	Atypical Spitz tumor	Superficial spreading melanoma
Halo nevus	SAMPUS	Nodular melanoma
Nevus of special sites	MELTUMP	Acral melanoma
"Dysplastic nevus"	High-grade dysplastic nevus	Desmoplastic melanoma
Simple lentigo	IAMPUS	Mucosal melanoma
Lentiginous melanocytic nevus	IAMP	Uveal melanoma
Meyerson nevus		Nevoid melanoma
Recurrent nevus		Lentigo maligna melanoma
Deep penetrating nevus		Spitz melanoma
Combined nevus		Melanoma arising in a nevus
BAP-1 inactivated nevus		Metastatic melanoma
Spitz nevus		Conjunctival melanoma
Reed nevus		
Acral nevus		
Genital nevus		
Blue nevus		
Cellular blue nevus		
Ito and Ota nevus		
Dermal melanocytosis		
Congenital nevus		
Conjunctival nevus		
Proliferative nodule		

SAMPUS superficial atypical melanocytic proliferation of uncertain significance, *MELTUMP* melanocytic tumor of uncertain malignant potential, *IAMPUS* intraepidermal atypical melanocytic proliferation of uncertain significance, *IAMP* intraepidermal atypical melanocytic proliferation approach failed because of our incomplete knowledge of the proposed pathways or because the pathway concept in its current form is flawed in principle.

3.2 Other Classifications

All classifications are arbitrary; there is no single true classification. Classifications are models and we know that "all models are wrong but some are useful." Classification is useful if it serves the intended purpose, and to achieve this, model creators must make choices. They have to determine the domain and the scope of the classification and define terms, attributes, and classes. For hierarchical classifications the creators have to decide on whether to build it bottom-up, starting from the most specific class and then group similar classes into more generic concepts, or top-down, starting with the most general concepts. Basically, the current WHO classification is a top-down approach starting with the presumed etiology (low, intermediate, and high chronic sun damage) as the most general concept and branches out further based on histomorphology, anatomic site, and involved driver mutations. The main purpose of the WHO classification was to integrate new research data with the old histogenetic classification and the classic model of stepwise tumor progression, but not to serve pathologists and clinicians. From the point of view of practicing pathologists and clinicians, a classification should be simple, consistent, and based on well-defined, exclusive categories. Ideally, it should also reduce noise (inter- and intraobserver variability) and support clinical decision making. In contrast to the WHO classification, the Melanocytic Pathology Assessment Tool and Hierarchy for Diagnosis (MPATH-Dx) reporting scheme [49] tries to address all these issues.

3.2.1 The MPATH-Dx Reporting Scheme

Motivations for the creation of the MPATH-Dx reporting scheme included the lack of standardized diagnostic terminology and the disagreement among pathologists in diagnostic thresholds. Because the creators of the MPATH-Dx reporting scheme observed that pathologists tend to agree more on treatments, they decided to center their classification on suggested treatments and not on specific diagnosis. Furthermore, treatment suggestions can be expressed in simple and clear language avoiding the usual confusion created by ambiguous diagnostic terminology such as "superficial atypical melanocytic proliferation of uncertain significance." Finally, in the case of uncertainty, appropriate treatment decisions may compensate for diagnostic ignorance, especially from a patient perspective: "They may not know what it is but at least they know what to do." Like the BI-RADS scoring system that is used for the interpretation of mammograms in breast cancer screening, the MPATH-Dx reporting scheme has categories stratified by the degree of observed abnormality and the corresponding level of intervention (Table 3.3).

The five categories span from class I (no apparent risk for continued local proliferation and adverse outcome, no further treatment required) to class V (greater risk for regional or distant metastasis, wide excision with >1 cm safety margin recommended). In their original publication, the authors mapped specific diagnoses to each class (Table 3.4). Classes I and II included nevi and classes IV and V the invasive

Table 3.3 Skeleton of the MPATH-Dx reporting scheme. Adopted according to Piepkorn et al. [49]

Class	Risk of progression	Suggested management
I	Melanocytic lesions with very low risk of progression	No further treatment recommended
II	Melanocytic lesions with low risk of progression	Narrow but complete excision <5 mm
III	Melanocytic lesions with higher risk of progression	Complete excision with >5 mm but <10 mm margins
IV	AJCC pT1a and pT1b invasive melanomas	Complete excision with 10 mm margins
V	AJCC pT2 and higher invasive melanomas	Complete excision with >10 mm margins and sentinel lymph node biopsy

Table 3.4 Mapping of diagnoses to the MPATH-Dx reporting according to Piepkorn et al. [49]

MPATH-Dx class	Specific diagnoses and terms
I	Common nevus—junctional, compound, intradermal, combined, congenital pattern
	Lentiginous nevus, junctional or compound
	Common blue nevus
	Ephelis
	Mildly dysplastic nevus (nevus with architectural disorder and cytological atypia; Clark's nevus, junctional or compound), mild
	Congenital melanocytic nevus: junctional, compound, or intradermal
	Solar lentigo
	Lentigo simplex
	Ito/Ota/Mongolian spot
	Halo nevus
	Persistent (recurrent) nevus
	Lentiginous melanocytic proliferation (of sun-damaged OR non-sun-damaged skin) with mild atypia
	Nevus of special anatomic site: acral, genital, flexural, milkline and breast, scalp
	Atypical nevus NOS including mildly atypical nevus of special anatomic site (acral, genital, flexural, milkline/breast, etc.)
II	Moderately dysplastic nevus (nevus with architectural disorder and cytological atypia; Clark's nevus, junctional or compound)
	Moderately atypical nevus NOS, including atypical nevus of special anatomic site: acral, genital, flexural, milkline and breast, scalp
	Pigmented spindle cell nevus: junctional or compound
	Spitz nevus conventional: junctional, compound, or intradermal
	Lentiginous melanocytic proliferation with moderate atypia (of sun-damaged OR non-sun-damaged skin)
	Blue nevus: cellular or epithelioid
	Deep penetrating nevus/plexiform spindle cell nevus
III	Severely dysplastic nevus (nevus with architectural disorder and cytological atypia; Clark's nevus, junctional or compound)
	Melanoma, in situ (common/pagetoid/superficial spreading melanoma)
	Melanoma, in situ, lentiginous, sun-damaged skin (lentigo maligna)
	Melanoma, in situ, lentiginous non-solar (i.e., acral or other)
	Melanoma, in situ, not otherwise specified (NOS)
	Lentiginous melanocytic proliferation with severe atypia (of sun-damaged OR non-sun-damaged skin)
	Atypical/dysplastic/Spitz tumor (junctional, compound, or dermal)
	Atypical pigmented spindle cell tumor (junctional or compound)
	Severely atypical nevus NOS including atypical nevus of special anatomic site (acral, genital, flexural, milkline/breast, scalp, etc.)
	Proliferative nodules in congenital melanocytic nevi (moderate/severe atypia and/or mitotic activity)
	Melanocytic lesion of uncertain malignant potential
	Pagetoid intraepidermal melanocytic proliferation (PIMP)

Table 3.4 (continued)

MPATH-Dx class	Specific diagnoses and terms
IV + V[a]	Acral lentiginous melanoma
	Blue nevus-like, a melanoma resembling or originating from a blue nevus
	Desmoplastic melanoma
	Heavily pigmented melanoma, a melanoma resembling epithelioid blue nevi or melanomas developing in animals
	Invasive melanoma, unclassifiable
	Lentigo maligna melanoma
	Melanoma arising in a congenital nevus
	Nevoid melanoma (a melanoma resembling a common nevus)
	Nodular melanoma
	Persistent melanoma
	Pigmented spindle cell-like, a melanoma resembling pigmented spindle cell nevus or plexiform spindle cell nevus
	Spitz-like, a melanoma that resembles a Spitz nevus/tumor
	Superficial spreading melanoma

[a] Class depends on invasion thickness of invasive melanoma: class IV: AJCC stage pT1a and pT1b; class V: AJCC stage pT2 or higher

melanomas. Invasion thickness was used to differentiate between class IV and V invasive melanomas, mirroring the 7th edition of the AJCC staging system [50]. AJCC stage pT1a and pT1b invasive melanomas were included in class IV, AJCC stage pT2 or higher in class V. The intermediate class III contains melanoma in situ but also, among others, severely atypical ("dysplastic") nevi or atypical Spitz tumor. Although this makes sense from the management perspective, because "severely dysplastic nevi" and melanoma in situ are usually treated alike (complete excision with 5 mm margin), it is confusing because melanomas and nevi should not belong to the same category from a biological point of view. Furthermore, the MPATH-Dx reporting scheme leaves it open whether terms of the intermediate category such as "severely dysplastic nevi" or "atypical Spitz nevi" pertain to the imitator or the precursor role of nevi.

As already mentioned, the prevailing school of thought will blame the lesion ("the lesion does not know what it is") focusing on the precursor role, while others, including the authors of this book, will blame the ignorance of the reporting pathologist ("I do not know what it is") focusing on the imitator role. The pragmatic solution suggested by the creators of the MPATH-Dx reporting scheme is that it does not matter which line of thought is true, because the management is the same. In other words, the MPATH-Dx reporting schema does not solve the controversies surrounding intermediate categories like "severely dysplastic nevus" or "atypical Spitz tumor"; it deems them irrelevant. This strategy will not eliminate diagnostic uncertainty, but it may decrease ambiguity and noise in clinical practice. All intermediate terms have been stuffed into a single category together with melanoma in situ, the MPATH-Dx class III. Such a generic class for "unknown and uncertain" lesions has the potential advantage of mitigating unnecessary overreactions following the diagnosis of melanoma in situ or "atypical Spitz tumor." As a euphemistic paraphrase for "melanoma in situ," MPATH-Dx class III may counteract the inflation of the incidence of melanoma. The tendency to overcall junctional melanocytic proliferations as in situ or microinvasive melanoma has been identified as one of the main drivers of the rising incidence of melanoma in light skin individuals in the past decades [51]. The diagnosis of "atypical Spitz tumor," on the other hand, has often been accompanied by unnecessary invasive procedures such as sentinel node biopsies, especially in prepubescent children, although sentinel node biopsies are neither informative nor beneficial in this scenario [52]. In practice, however, we experience the worrisome trend that the MPATH-Dx class III is increasingly used to upgrade benign lesions that would otherwise have been diagnosed as mildly or moderately "dysplastic" nevi instead of downgrading melanoma in situ. This exposes the weakness of pragmatic and practical approaches like the MPATH-Dx reporting scheme, which offer little theoretical background. They can be used to serve any purpose, even one that contradicts the original intent. Another disadvantage of the management-based solution of the MPATH-Dx reporting system is that it is short-sighted. It does not take into account potential differences in long-term management. A history of melanoma increases the lifetime risk of a second melanoma, but a history of "atypical spindle cell tumor" or similar diagnoses mixed together in MPATH-Dx Class III does not.

The MPATH-Dx reporting scheme has not been the only attempt to standardize reporting of melanocytic lesions. In 2021 Katz et al. proposed the MOLEM (Management of Lesion to Exclude Melanoma) reporting scheme. According to the authors it "*better reflects clinical practice than the MPATH-Dx schema in lesions excised to exclude melanoma by combining diagnoses with similar prognostic outcomes for melanocytic and non-melanocytic lesions into standardized classification categories*" [53]. Like the MPATH-Dx reporting scheme it has five classes. The major difference is that MOLEM also includes non-melanocytic lesions (Table 3.5). It has been validated and proved to be clinically useful in a cohort of 217 lesions. It suffers, however, from the same difficulties as the MPATH-Dx reporting scheme and probably even more so because it had to integrate non-melanocytic lesions. This resulted in classes that contain entities as dissimilar as nevi, cysts, and seborrheic keratosis. The integration of keratinocyte cancer (squamous cell carcinoma and basal cell carcinoma) also led to the counterintuitive result that the highest class (class V) does not contain the diagnoses with the highest risk.

Table 3.5 The MOLEM reporting scheme according to Katz et al. [53]

MOLEM	Risk of progression	Suggested management	Examples
I	Very low risk	No further treatment or topical	Benign nevus, mildly atypical nevus, seborrheic keratosis, lichenoid keratosis, cyst
II	Low risk	Narrow but complete excision <5 mm	Moderately atypical nevus, Spitz nevus, deep penetrating nevus
III	Higher risk	Complete excision with >5 mm but <10 mm margins	Melanoma in situ, severely atypical nevus
IV	Highest risk	Complete excision with >10 mm margins	Invasive melanoma
V	High risk	Definitive excision and malignant non-melanoma management pathway	Basal cell carcinoma, squamous cell carcinoma in situ

3.2.2 AJCC and TNM Melanoma Staging

At the time of writing, the applicable melanoma staging system is the 8th edition of the American Joint Committee on Cancer (AJCC) Melanoma Staging System, launched in January 2018 [50]. The AJCC staging of melanoma is a prognostic classification based on the TNM stages. For the patient it is the most meaningful classification because it will impact personal choices and medical decisions. The T categories T1–T4 stratify the primary tumor according to only two attributes, invasion thickness and presence of ulceration (Table 3.6). Besides invasion thickness and

Table 3.6 Melanoma T categories according to the 8th edition of the American Joint Committee on Cancer (AJCC) Melanoma Staging System [50]

T category	Invasion thickness	Ulceration
Tis	Not applicable	Not applicable
T1		
T1a	<0.8 mm	Without ulceration
T1b	<0.8 mm	With ulceration
T1b	0.8–1.0 mm	With or without ulceration
T2		
T2a	>1.0–2.0 mm	Without ulceration
T2b	>1.0–2.0 mm	With ulceration
T3		
T3a	>2.0–4.0 mm	Without ulceration
T3b	>2.0–4.0 mm	With ulceration
T4		
T4a	>4.0 mm	Without ulceration
T4b	>4.0 mm	With ulceration

Adapted from the American Joint Committee on Cancer (AJCC), Chicago, Illinois. The original and primary source for this information is the AJCC Cancer Staging Manual, 8th Edition (2017), published by Springer International Publishing (Gershenwald JE, Scolyer RA, Hess KR, et al. Melanoma of the Skin. In: Amin AB, Edge SB, Greene, FL, et al. (Eds). AJCC Cancer Staging Manual. 8th Ed. New York: Springer; 2017:563–585) [50, 54]

ulceration, pathologists are encouraged to report additional attributes such as the number of mitoses, the Clark level of invasion, or the presence or absence of tumor-infiltrating lymphocytes, although they will not alter the tumor stage. We consider this good advice because the attributes used to stratify the T-categories are subject to change. Some of the attributes mentioned above were included in former editions of the AJCC staging system and may be reinstalled again in future versions, depending on the updated results of survival data. The AJCC melanoma classification is fact-based and relies on large amounts of data, and unlike the classifications discussed previously, it has a purpose with a clear outcome: predicting survival. Patients who have only the primary tumor but no metastases fall into either stage I or II, depending on the T category of the primary tumor (Table 3.7). Stage III is the stage of lymph node metastasis and stage IV of distant metastasis. The AJCC staging system is very useful for predicting survival on a population level,

Table 3.7 Melanoma clinical stage groups according to TNM

Clinical stage	T	N	M
0	**Tis**	N0	M0
IA	**T1a**	N0	M0
IB	**T1b**	N0	M0
	T2a	N0	M0
IIA	**T2b**	N0	M0
	T3a	N0	M0
IIB	**T3b**	N0	M0
	T4a	N0	M0
IIC	**T4b**	N0	M0
III	Any T	**≥N1**	M0
IV	Any T	Any N	**M1**

Adapted from the American Joint Committee on Cancer (AJCC), Chicago, Illinois. The original and primary source for this information is the AJCC Cancer Staging Manual, 8th Edition (2017), published by Springer International Publishing (Gershenwald JE, Scolyer RA, Hess KR, et al. Melanoma of the Skin. In: Amin AB, Edge SB, Greene, FL, et al. (Eds). AJCC Cancer Staging Manual. 8th Ed. New York: Springer; 2017:563–585) [50, 54]

but the utility for the individual patient is questionable. We predict that the era of precision medicine demands more personalized approaches including molecular data and other specific health data that may influence individual outcome irrespective of tumor stage.

3.2.3 ICD-11 and ICD-O Codes

The International Statistical Classification of Diseases and Related Health Problems (ICD) coding system meets criteria of a hierarchical classification and of a simple thesaurus, which is more or less a list of applicable terms. It is a legally mandated health data standard created and managed by the WHO. The latest version, ICD-11, is officially in effect from January 2022, but experience shows that implementation in practice takes longer, so older ICD versions are still in use at the same time. The ICD-11 code offers semantic interoperability independent of language and is distributed under a permissive license. It also includes histologic extension codes that are relevant for the practicing dermatopathologist (Table 3.8).

Table 3.8 Selected ICD-11 histologic extension codes of nevus and melanoma

Nevus	Melanoma
Spindle cell nevus/Reed nevus (XH2P88/XH9QV1)	Melanoma (XH4846)
Spitz/Epithelioid cell nevus (XH79G6)	Acral melanoma (XH9L11)
Spitz nevus, atypical (XH9WF4)	Amelanotic melanoma (XH3TK1)
Blue nevus, NOS (XH7QJ7)	Desmoplastic melanoma, NOS (XH1Z15/XH1P36)
Cellular blue nevus (XH3X84)	Lentigo maligna melanoma (XH9NL4)
Balloon cell nevus (XH8RN4)	Nodular melanoma (XH4QG5)
Simple lentigo/Lentigo simplex (XH88L0)	Superficial spreading melanoma (XH08X7)
Lentiginous melanocytic nevus (XH9QC8)	Spindle cell melanoma (XH25M1)
Junctional nevus (XH1M79)	Spitzoid/Epithelioid cell melanoma (XH0QL5)
Compound nevus (XH27A6)	
Dermal nevus (XH2MQ5)	
Combined nevus (XH0DU8)	
Deep penetrating nevus (XH81Y1)	
Special site Nevus (Genital, Conjunctival; XH5EL4/XH8FS8)	
Acral nevus (XH9DB2)	
Meyerson nevus (XH8NP4)	
Meningeal melanocytosis (XH8974)	
Halo nevus (XH5971)	
Diffuse melanocytosis (XH6DN3)	
Nevus spilus (XH40S8)	
Congenital melanocytic nevus (XH5YN0)	

The International Classification of Diseases for Oncology (ICD-O) is a domain-specific extension of the ICD-code for neoplastic diseases (Table 3.9), which has been adopted by SNOMED (Systematized Nomenclature of Medicine), another important computer-readable ontology of medical terms. As you can see from Table 3.9, the ICD-O list of melanocytic lesions is the usual hodgepodge of terms that includes paradoxes such as “juvenile melanoma” as a subset of “epithelioid and spindle cell nevus” and “malignant blue nevus.” The 5th digit of the ICD-O codes is the “behavior code,” indicating the biology of the tumor. The extension 0 stands for “benign,” 1 for “intermediate,” 2 for “in situ,” 3 for “malignant, primary,” 6 for “malignant metastatic,” and 9 for “malignant uncertain whether primary or metastatic,” respectively. The ICD-O code is widely used by cancer registries and compatible with the pathway concept of the current WHO classification of melanocytic tumors, to which it can be mapped.

Table 3.9 List of ICD-O codes of melanocytic lesions

M8720/0 Pigmented nevus, NOS
Melanocytic nevus
Nevus, NOS
Hairy nevus
M8720/2 Melanoma in situ
M8720/3 Malignant melanoma, NOS (except juvenile melanoma M8770/0)
Melanoma, NOS
M8721/3 Nodular melanoma
M8722/0 Balloon cell nevus
M8722/3 Balloon cell melanoma
M8723/0 Halo nevus
Regressing nevus
M8723/3 Malignant melanoma, regressing
M8725/0 Neuronevus
M8726/0 Magnocellular nevus (C69.4)
Melanocytoma, eyeball
Melanocytoma, NOS
M8727/0 Dysplastic nevus
M8728/0 Diffuse melanocytosis
M8728/1 Meningeal melanocytoma
M8728/3 Meningeal melanomatosis
M8730/0 Nonpigmented nevus

Table 3.9 (continued)

Achromic nevus
M8740/0 Junctional nevus, NOS
Intraepidermal nevus
M8740/3 Malignant melanoma in junctional nevus
M8741/2 Precancerous melanosis, NOS
M8741/3 Malignant melanoma in precancerous melanosis
M8742/3 Lentigo maligna melanoma
Hutchinson melanotic freckle
M8743/3 Superficial spreading melanoma
M8744/3 Acral lentiginous melanoma, malignant
M8745/3 Desmoplastic melanoma, malignant
Neurotropic melanoma, malignant
Melanoma, desmoplastic, amelanotic
M8746/3 Mucosal lentiginous melanoma
M8750/0 Intradermal nevus
Dermal nevus
M8760/0 compound nevus
Dermal and epidermal nevus
M8761/0 Small congenital nevus
M8761/1 Giant pigmented nevus, NOS
Intermediate and giant congenital nevus
M8761/3 Malignant melanoma in giant pigmented nevus/congenital melanocytic nevus
M78762/1 Proliferative dermal lesion in congenital nevus
M8770/0 Epithelioid and spindle cell nevus
Juvenile nevus
Juvenile melanoma
Spitz nevus
Pigmented spindle cell nevus of Reed
M8770/3 Mixed epithelioid and spindle cell melanoma
M8771/0 Epithelioid cell nevus
M8771/3 Epithelioid cell melanoma
M8772/0 spindle cell nevus, NOS
M8772/3 Spindle cell melanoma, NOS
M8773/3 Spindle cell melanoma, type A
M8774/3 Spindle cell melanoma, type B
M8780/0 Blue nevus, NOS
Jadassohn blue nevus
M8780/3 blue nevus, malignant
M8790/0 Cellular blue nevus

3.3 The Relationship Between Pattern Analysis and Classifications

Classifications are about general concepts that create prototypes or universals, pattern analysis is about interpreting particular instances histomorphologically with a consistent method. When applying pattern analysis, we classify a lesion according to its pattern first and then assign a diagnosis. These are two different tasks. Most classifications discussed so far contain elements of pattern analysis. The diagnosis of "common blue nevus," for example, is characterized by a dermal pattern of monomorphic spindle melanocytes arranged in fascicles. As we will see later in more detail, this is pure pattern analysis. The term "blue nevus," however, already points to another dimension: clinical appearance. "Blue nevi" are only blue if you look at them in vivo with the unaided eye or with dermatoscopy but they are anything but blue when viewed ex vivo in sections stained with hematoxylin and eosin. There is no classification based solely on pattern analysis. The classifications mentioned so far add other attributes, such as anatomic site (e.g., acral nevus and acral melanoma), history (e.g., congenital nevus, acquired nevus, recurrent nevus), molecular findings (e.g., BAP-1-deficient nevus), clinical appearance (e.g., halo nevus, blue nevus), and more recently, UVR exposure as in the current WHO classification. The incoherent mixing of attributes renders these classifications fuzzy and difficult to apply. Some "blue nevi" are not blue, and some nevi that are blue, are not "blue nevi." Furthermore, some features such as the history and clinical presentation cannot be observed under the microscope. The inability to observe all dimensions at once is a major disadvantage of most multidimensional classifications. A unidimensional classification based on the examination of histomorphologic patterns alone would be more consistent and easier to apply but incomplete, in the same way as a purely molecular or purely clinical classification of melanocytic lesions would be incomplete. It seems that classifications can achieve either completeness or consistency, but not both. An entity or disease is usually a multidimensional concept, and although it is an important part of the puzzle, the microscopic examination of a small piece of tissue alone is usually not sufficient to describe all its aspects. In pattern analysis we apply an assessment by pattern first, which is unidimensional in the sense that it only uses attributes observable under the microscope, and in a next step we map our observation to the multidimensional concept we call diagnosis. Making a diagnosis using one of the multidimensional classifications mentioned before is a top-down procedure; the diagnostic categories are predefined by convention, usually by some kind of authority like the WHO. Classifying a lesion according to pattern is a bottom-up procedure, the authority is the person behind the microscope who has to describe and interpret the histomorphologic attributes of a specific lesion.

Pattern analysis should also be differentiated from pattern recognition. Pattern recognition is the "blink" approach, while "pattern analysis" is the "think" approach. With experience, pathologists tend to eyeball a lesion in low power and then make a diagnosis in milliseconds, usually the correct one. It seems that they skip the time consuming task of assigning a pattern, but they do not, they recognize patterns quickly and efficiently. While stereotypic cases can be easily diagnosed by pattern recognition, it can be misleading with more complex cases as we will discuss in Chap. 8, "bias, noise, and error." Ideally, the pathologist who applies pattern analysis is aware that, especially in complex cases, the final diagnosis also involves other aspects beyond what is observable under the microscope. Mapping patterns to diagnoses can be extremely difficult, especially if the information is incomplete, which is virtually always the case.

4 Pattern Analysis

Pattern analysis is well developed in the realm of microscopic diagnosis of inflammatory skin diseases, where it brings together patterns of infiltrates, patterns of epidermal changes, and composition of infiltrates in a stepwise process to specific diagnosis [55]. However, in diagnosis of melanocytic lesions it is established only in rough categories, mostly for assessment at scanning magnification, e.g., symmetry/asymmetry and circumscription [56–59]. Yet melanocytic proliferations also assume highly characteristic patterns at intermediate and high magnifications. These can be defined and recognized morphologically.

Melanocytic lesions can affect solely the epidermis, the dermis, or the subcutis, or they may involve a combination of them. By far the most lesions involve epidermis and dermis. Traditionally, the term "junctional" is used for benign intraepidermal melanocytic proliferations and "in situ" for malignant intraepidermal melanocytic proliferations while "compound" designates a benign melanocytic lesion involving epidermis and dermis, and "dermal" a benign melanocytic lesion involving only the dermis. In contrast, dermal involvement of a malignant melanocytic proliferation is called "invasive" when primary and "metastatic" when secondary [1]. Essentially, such terminology implies a diagnosis prior to the description of the morphology, which is violating the orderly stepwise process of morphological observation and decision making. Moreover, it is impossible to be used in challenging lesions, in which a diagnosis relies on weighting the numerous observations made at each magnification. Therefore, we seek here to describe patterns of melanocytes in skin and subcutaneous tissue in a purely descriptive language and without any premature assumption about diagnosis and biological behavior. For the purpose of clarity we use the term "pattern" exclusively for arrangement of melanocytes, whereas we refer to accompanying characteristics of epidermis, connective tissue, vessels, and infiltrates as "changes."

4.1 Architecture and Silhouette

At scanning magnification, a melanocytic lesion can be well circumscribed meaning that the outline of the lesion can be identified easily, or it can be ill-defined meaning that the lesion intermingles with the surrounding tissue so that the outline cannot be determined straightforwardly (Fig. 4.1a–f). The proliferation is also assessed at scanning magnification in regard to its mainly involved histologic compartments: epidermis,

A. Böer-Auer et al., *Pattern Analysis for Histopathologic Diagnosis of Melanocytic Lesions*,
https://doi.org/10.1007/978-3-031-07666-4_4

papillary dermis, reticular dermis, and/or subcutis. Epidermal, dermal, and subcutaneous proliferations should also be studied for axial symmetry, the axis being a vertical line in the middle of the lesion [56]. If the architecture and arrangement on one side of the axis is very similar to that on the other side, the lesion is called symmetric (Fig. 4.1a–c), if it is different it is called asymmetric (Fig. 4.1d–f). In general, poor circumscription and asymmetry are seen more often in malignant proliferations, whereas symmetry and good circumscription are seen in benign lesions. However, a lesion can be well circumscribed and asymmetric (Fig. 4.1d), or can be poorly circumscribed and symmetric (Fig. 4.1c), thereby not immediately implying the biological nature of the lesion. Hence, assessment of these two architectural features needs to be made independently prior to interpretation of the findings.

In some cases, circumscription and symmetry are difficult to assess, because the lesion is not clearly visible in routine H&E staining (Fig. 4.1e, f). In this situation, immunostaining with melanocytic markers such as MelanA staining can be of great help, because it highlights the architecture and silhouette of the lesion (see also Sect. 6.4).

It always has to be kept in mind that a microscopic section presents the silhouette only in a two-dimensional image in which the right side can be compared to the left side of the lesion. In reality, however, the lesion is a three-dimensional proliferation and while it may seem symmetrical in one section it may actually be asymmetrical in the third dimension. When more than one section through a lesion is available, a three-dimensional imagination of the lesion can be developed in the brain and must also be assessed carefully for symmetry (Fig. 4.1g–i). If just one cut through the center of the lesion is available, this exercise is not possible, and a clinical or dermatoscopic image may be the only option to assess the lesion for asymmetry in the third dimension which is not seen in the section (Fig. 4.1g–i).

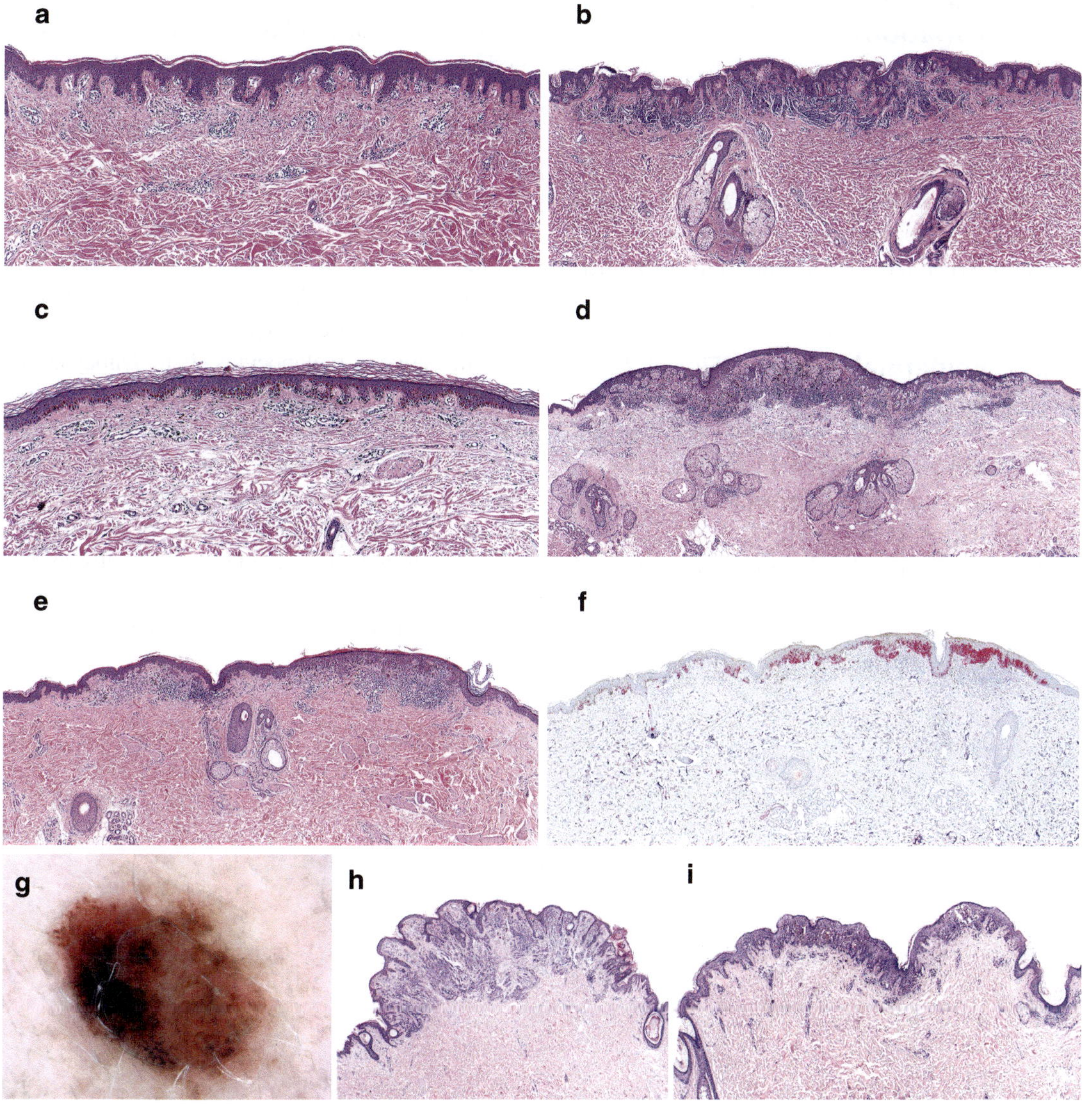

Fig. 4.1 (**a**–**i**) Symmetry and circumscription. (**a**) Well-circumscribed melanocytic proliferation, symmetric, intraepidermal: junctional nevus. (**b**) Well-circumscribed melanocytic proliferation, symmetric, epidermal and dermal: superficial congenital nevus. (**c**) Poorly circumscribed but symmetric, intraepidermal: lentiginous junctional nevus. (**d**) Well-circumscribed melanocytic proliferation, but strikingly asymmetric, epidermal and dermal: melanoma (Note the blue-gray color of the superficial dermis caused by extensive solar elastosis). (**e**) Poorly circumscribed and asymmetric, intraepidermal: melanoma in situ. (**f**) MelanA staining of the lesion shown in (**e**) highlights the poor circumscription and asymmetry. (**g**) Dermatoscopic image of a melanoma associated with a dermal nevus with asymmetry mainly in one axis. (**h**) Symmetric, well circumscribed, dermal: the nevus part of the lesion is shown in (**g**), hiding asymmetry in the third dimension. (**i**) Poorly circumscribed, asymmetric, intraepidermal: melanoma in situ part of the lesion shown in (**g**). (Courtesy of the Dermatologikum Hamburg, except (**g**–**i**) courtesy of the Department of Dermatology, Medical University of Vienna)

4.2 Main Patterns and Their Variations

Scanning magnification usually suffices to determine whether a melanocytic lesion involves the epidermis, dermis, subcutis, or a combination of these. If a lesion is present in more than one of these compartments, the arrangement of cells in each part is examined separately and in contrast to each other.

4.2.1 Epidermal Patterns (Figs. 4.2, 4.3, 4.4, and 4.5)

4.2.1.1 Pigmented Keratinocytes, No Increase in Melanocytes (Fig. 4.2a, b)

In the epidermis, the keratinocytes show an increased deposition of melanin, but the number of melanocytes is not increased. Pigmented keratinocytes may be present in the basal layer only or also in suprabasal layers including the cornified layer.

4.2.1.2 Increased Single Melanocytes: Regular/Irregular (Fig. 4.2c, d)

The number of melanocytes in the basal layer is increased. The distribution of melanocytes may be regular (equidistant, Fig. 4.2c) or irregular (not equidistant, Fig. 4.2d). Regular distribution of melanocytes requires at least one keratinocyte to be present between melanocytes. If melanocytes are attached closely (no keratinocyte between them), this is referred to as "back-to-back"-melanocytes and represents an irregular arrangement of melanocytes. In nevi single melanocytes increased in number are mostly seen at the base of rete ridges, whereas suprapapillary epidermis is usually spared. Single melanocytes increased in number in suprapapillary zones are a hint to melanoma.

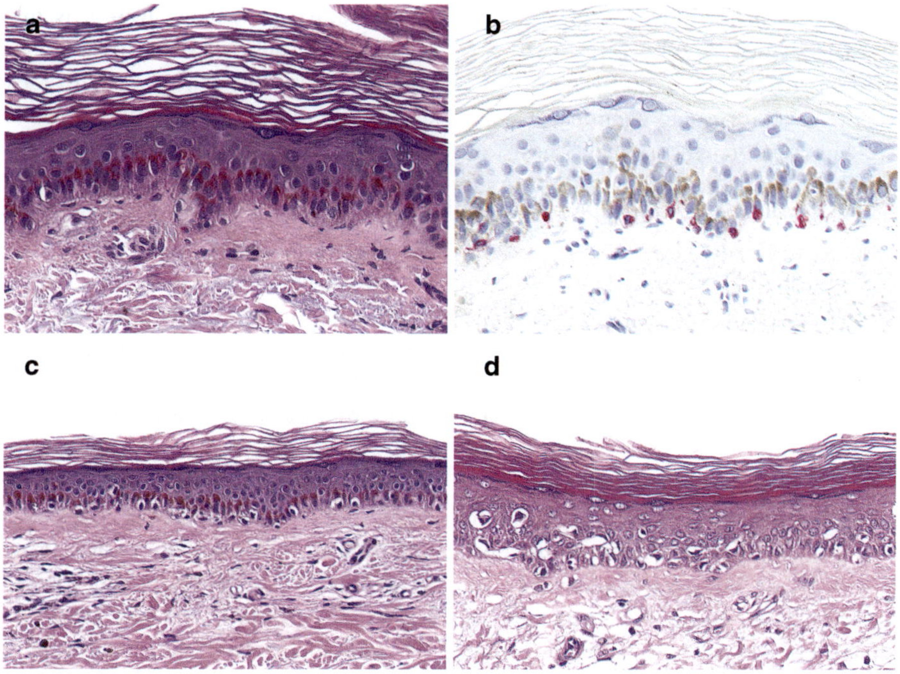

Fig. 4.2 (**a**–**d**) Epidermal patterns: single melanocytes. (**a**) Pigmentation of the epidermal basal layer and regularly distributed single melanocytes in the basal layer, not increased in number: incipient solar lentigo (note also the prominent hyperkeratosis and solar elastosis in the dermis). (**b**) MelanA staining of the lesion shown in (**a**): regularly distributed single melanocytes in the basal layer, not increased in number. (**c**) Pigmentation of the epidermal basal layer and regularly distributed single melanocytes in the basal layer, increased in number in a simple lentigo. (**d**) Irregularly distributed single melanocytes in the basal layer, increased in number in a melanoma in situ. (Courtesy of the Dermatologikum Hamburg)

4.2.1.3 Nests of Melanocytes: Arrangement, Size, Shape, and Number (Fig. 4.3a–h)

Melanocytes tend to form aggregations of cells which have historically been termed "nests of melanocytes." By strict definition, at least three melanocytes in immediate juxtaposition are required to apply the term "nest."

Nests of melanocytes are assessed in several ways: arrangement, size, shape, microanatomic localization and number compared with single melanocytes. Nests can be distributed regularly (equidistant) (Fig. 4.3a, b) throughout a lesion or they show variation in distance (irregular arrangement) (Fig. 4.3c, e) and they can be situated at the base of rete ridges (Fig. 4.3a, b, d) or anywhere in the epidermis (Fig. 4.3c, e). The size of nests may be even (Fig. 4.3a, b), meaning that nests share a similar diameter, or uneven, meaning that nests vary in size (Fig. 4.3c, e). In regard to the outline of nests, it is not only the size but also the shape that is assessed. Nests may assume a round shape (Fig. 4.3a–c) or they may show confluence to form irregular outlines (Fig. 4.3e, f) including elongated bands or polycyclic shapes.

In the assessment of nests, it is important to compare the number of nests to the number of single melanocytes in a lesion to decide (1) which of the patterns is the predominant one (e.g., nests in Fig. 4.3a, b, c, e versus single cells in Fig. 4.3d, f), and (2) whether the arrangement of both patterns to each other is overall symmetrical or asymmetrical.

The observation of nested vs. single melanocytes in the epidermis is also substantial in the assessment of circumscription of a lesion. In general, a lesion that ends with nests at both sides is well circumscribed, a lesion that ends on one or both sides with single melanocytes is poorly circumscribed. That means that circumscription cannot always be assessed solely at scanning magnification. It requires at least intermediate magnification to confirm the circumscription identified at scanning magnification.

Epidermal nests of melanocytes may be separated from surrounding epithelium by a narrow space, which is called cleft. Such a cleft is an artifact that typically occurs in Spitz nevi (Fig. 4.3g) but clefts may also form between intraepidermal aggregations of melanocytes and the underlying dermis (Fig. 4.3h), a feature seen more commonly in melanoma.

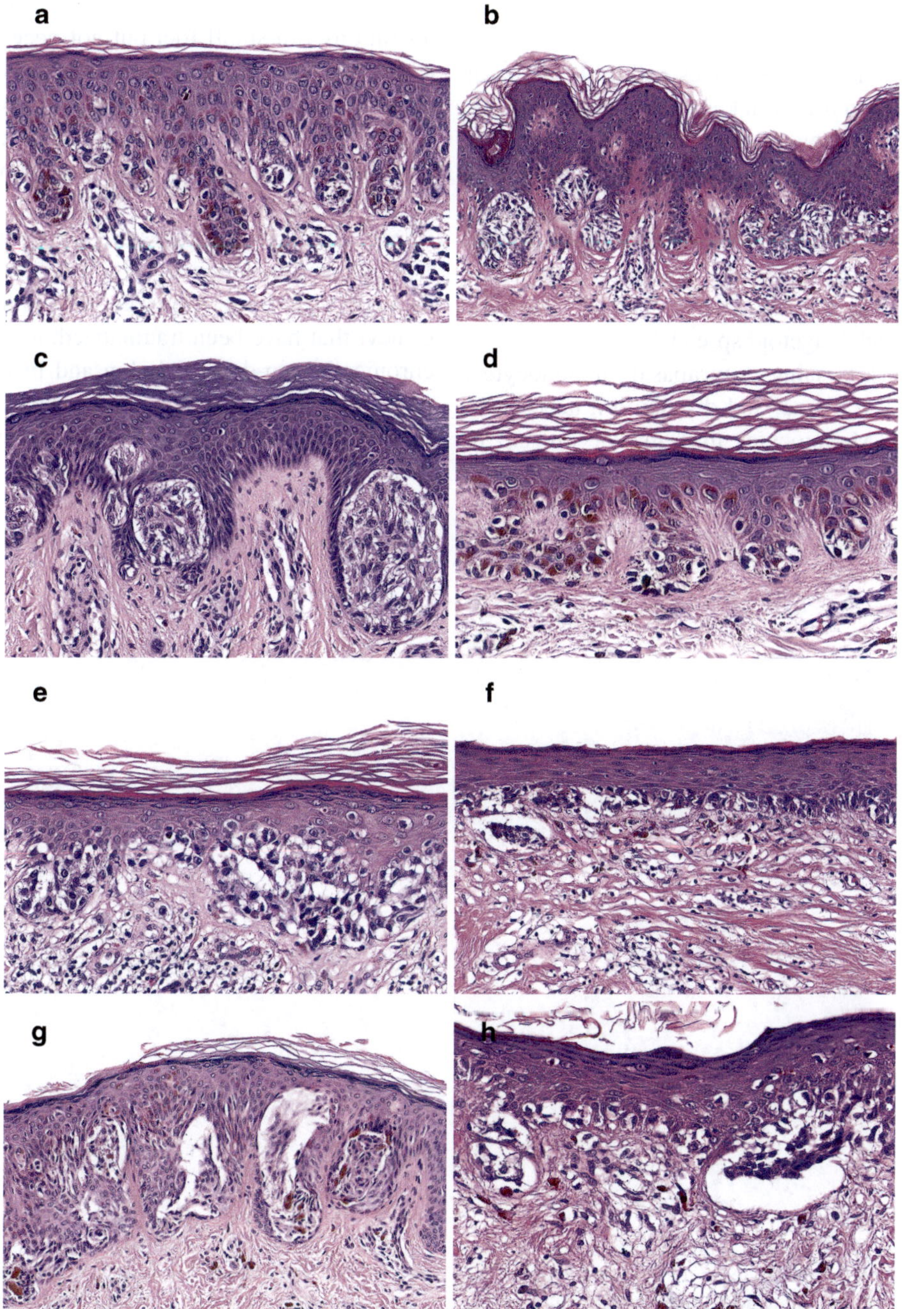

Fig. 4.3 (**a**–**h**) Epidermal patterns: nests of melanocytes. (**a**) Small nests, even in size, at the base of rete ridges, regularly distributed in a junctional nevus. (**b**) Large nests, even in size, at the base of rete ridges, regularly distributed in a superficial congenital nevus. (**c**) Nests varying in size, located mostly at the base of rete ridges in a Spitz nevus. (**d**) Small nests at the base of elongated rete ridges on the right and single melanocytes on the left in a junctional nevus. (**e**) Nests at the base of elongated rete ridges, irregular in size and shape and confluent to larger aggregations in a melanoma in situ. (**f**) Few nests and numerous single melanocytes in irregular distribution, and flattened rete ridges, in a melanoma in situ. (**g**) Clefts between intraepidermal nests and surrounding epidermis in a Spitz nevus. (**h**) Cleft between intraepidermal nests and underlying dermis in a melanoma in situ. (Courtesy of the Dermatologikum Hamburg)

4.2.1.4 Suprabasal Melanocytes (Fig. 4.4a–d)

In normal skin, melanocytes reside in the basal layer between the basal keratinocytes. In melanocytic proliferations, melanocytes can be present in the basal layer or in suprabasal layers including the granular and the cornified layer, as single melanocytes or in the form of nests. A variety of terms has been used to designate suprabasal melanocytes, among them "scatter," "upward spread," and "pagetoid spread."

When assessing suprabasal melanocytes, number, level, size, and distribution need to be observed. Melanocytes may just be present in the spinous zone, or they may also be in the granular and cornified layer. The suprabasal melanocytes may be present in the center of the lesion only, in small foci but not necessarily in the center, or involving broader zones or even the entire lesion. If suprabasal melanocytes are found in the entire lesion, the arrangement of them still can be regular (equidistant) or irregular (not equidistant).

Suprabasal melanocytes are a prominent feature in many melanomas (Fig. 4.4b–d), but they also appear in Spitz and Reed nevi, in acral nevi or nevi that have been traumatized, as well as in chronically sun-damaged skin and in epidermis next to fresh excision scars. Moreover, some melanomas may not show prominent suprabasal melanocytes, e.g., some melanomas on sun-damaged skin.

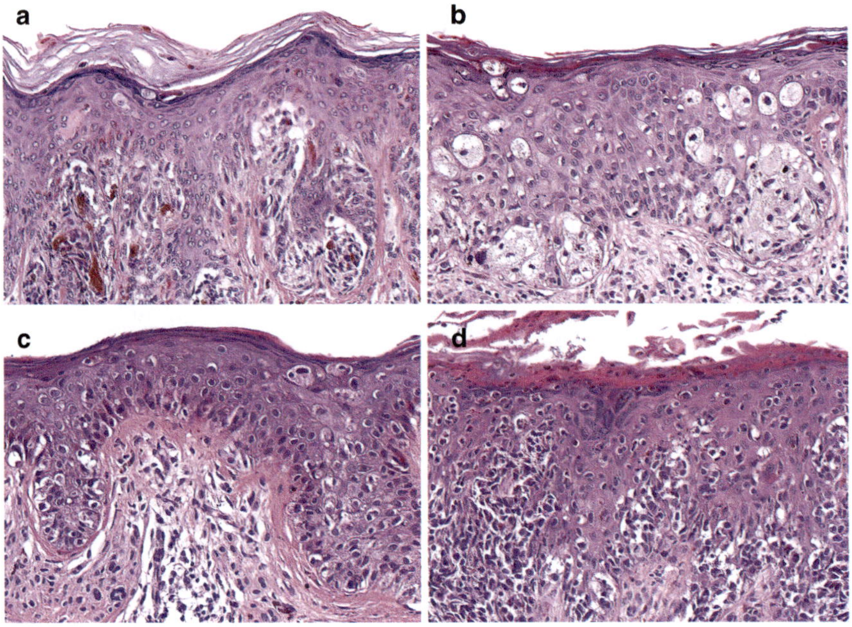

Fig. 4.4 (**a**–**d**) Epidermal patterns: suprabasal melanocytes. (**a**) Single melanocytes in the spinous, granular, and cornified layer in a Spitz nevus. (**b**) Large melanocytes in the spinous, granular, and cornified layer in a melanoma. (**c**) Few small nests of melanocytes in the spinous and granular layer in a melanoma. (**d**) Numerous single melanocytes and irregularly formed nests in the spinous, granular, and cornified layer in a melanoma. (Courtesy of the Dermatologikum Hamburg)

4.2.1.5 Epithelial Adnexal Involvement (Fig. 4.5a–d)

Epithelium of adnexal structures may also show melanocytic proliferations in the form of single melanocytes and/or nests of melanocytes. Most commonly involved are openings of hair follicles (infundibula) in melanoma in situ on facial skin (Fig. 4.5a, b), but eccrine structures, too, may show proliferations of melanocytes in ductal and rarely glandular epithelium (Fig. 4.5c, d). This finding has been termed "syringotropism" by some authors [60, 61]. Within adnexal epithelia, melanocytic proliferations are assessed in the very same way as they are in the epidermis: dominance of single cells or nests, regular versus irregular distribution, confluence of nests, suprabasal melanocytes. Single melanocytes in eccrine ductal or eccrine glandular epithelium are a clue to melanoma (See Fig. 4.5c, d), if not seen in the context of a deep congenital nevus.

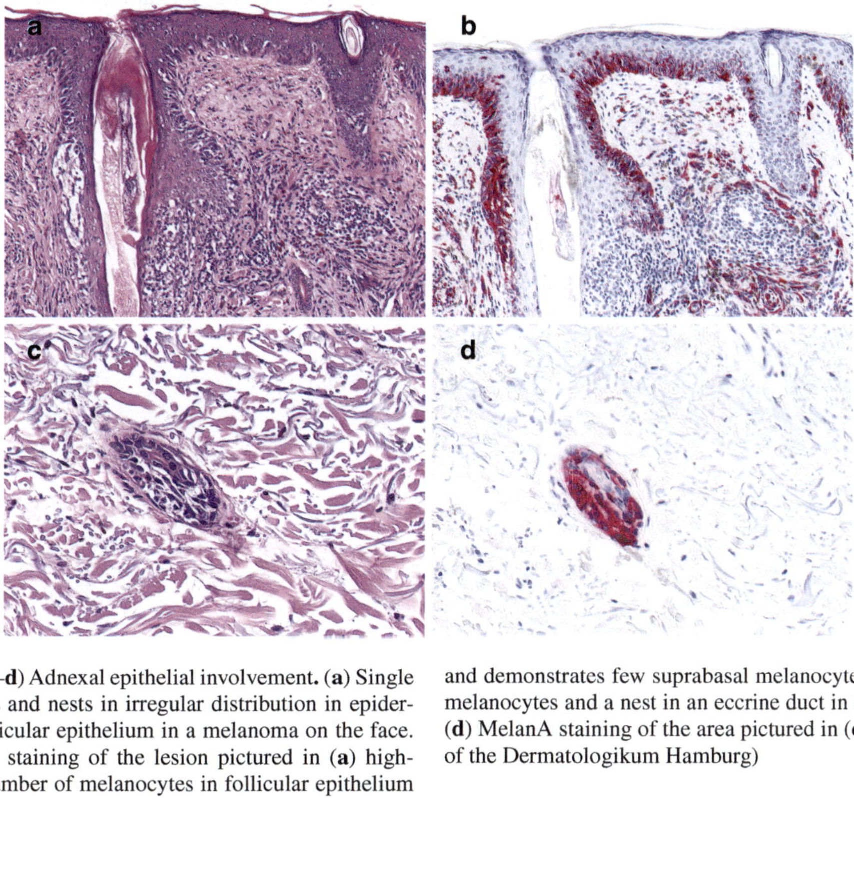

Fig. 4.5 (**a**–**d**) Adnexal epithelial involvement. (**a**) Single melanocytes and nests in irregular distribution in epidermis and follicular epithelium in a melanoma on the face. (**b**) MelanA staining of the lesion pictured in (**a**) highlights the number of melanocytes in follicular epithelium and demonstrates few suprabasal melanocytes. (**c**) Single melanocytes and a nest in an eccrine duct in a melanoma. (**d**) MelanA staining of the area pictured in (**c**). (Courtesy of the Dermatologikum Hamburg)

4.2.2 Dermal Patterns (Figs. 4.6, 4.7, and 4.8)

In the dermis, melanocytes may be found in the papillary dermis, in the reticular dermis, or both. Melanocytes may be present as single melanocytes, in nests or forming larger aggregations such as nodules or sheets.

4.2.2.1 Single Melanocytes (Fig. 4.6a, b)

Solitary melanocytes may be found in the papillary and/or reticular dermis and they can be regularly distributed (equidistant) or irregularly distributed (not equidistant).

4.2.2.2 Nests (Fig. 4.6c–e)

When melanocytes form collections of more than three, they are referred to as nests. Just like in the epidermis, nests can be distributed regularly or irregularly, the size may be even or uneven and the outline may assume a round shape or nests may show confluence to form irregular elongated bands or polycyclic shapes.

4.2.2.3 Nodules and Sheets (Fig. 4.6e)

Nodules are round aggregations which are larger than nests. When aggregations of melanocytes are even larger, with irregular outlines and involve huge parts of a tissue compartment, they are designated "sheets."

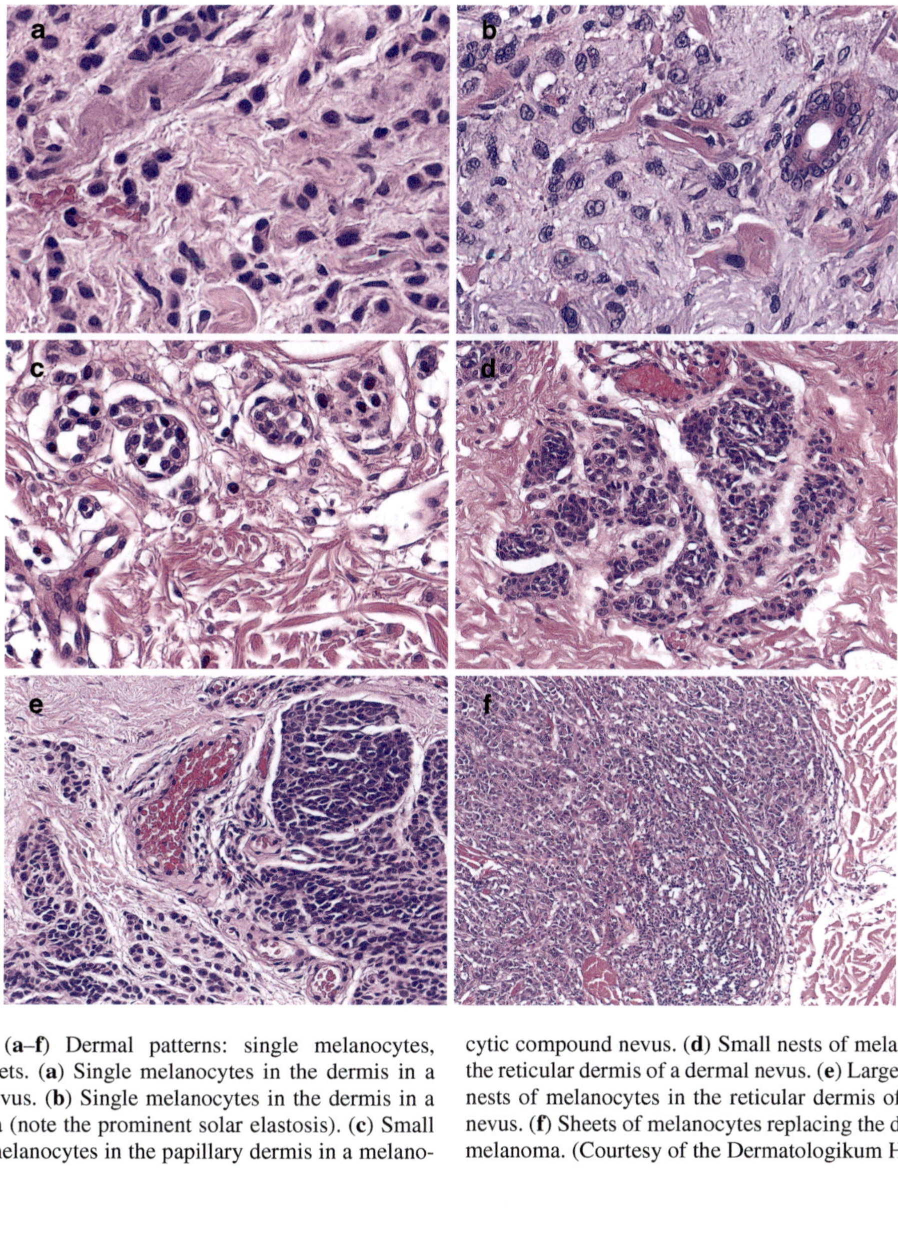

Fig. 4.6 (**a**–**f**) Dermal patterns: single melanocytes, nests, sheets. (**a**) Single melanocytes in the dermis in a dermal nevus. (**b**) Single melanocytes in the dermis in a melanoma (note the prominent solar elastosis). (**c**) Small nests of melanocytes in the papillary dermis in a melanocytic compound nevus. (**d**) Small nests of melanocytes in the reticular dermis of a dermal nevus. (**e**) Large and small nests of melanocytes in the reticular dermis of a dermal nevus. (**f**) Sheets of melanocytes replacing the dermis in a melanoma. (Courtesy of the Dermatologikum Hamburg)

4.2.2.4 Interstitial Strands/Fascicles (Fig. 4.7a, b)

The space between collagen bundles in the reticular dermis has been designated *interstice*. When single melanocytes are present between collagen bundles, they can be arranged closely, forming strands. Fascicles are bundles of melanocytes that imitate the arrangement of muscle or nerve fascicles.

Strands of melanocytes in a horizontal fashion lying between collagen fibers of a sclerosed dermis can lead to a difficult differential diagnosis of sclerosing or traumatized nevus versus nevoid melanoma. Nests disposed in parallel arrays at the base of the tumor according to Idriss et al. [62] are a common feature of nevoid melanomas. This arrangement has been termed "parallel theque pattern."

4.2.2.5 Periadnexal Strands/Nests (Fig. 4.7c–g)

In the reticular dermis, melanocytes tend to form proliferations along adnexal structures, especially hair follicles (Fig. 4.7c). This is often referred to as "adnexocentricity" or "adnexotropism." It may involve the adventitial dermis only, or also the surrounding reticular dermis. Melanocytes may be present in the form of nests or as interstitial strands around a central adnexal structure. Melanocytes may also be found around nonepithelial adnexal structures, i.e., vessels (Fig. 4.7d), nerves (Fig. 4.7e, f), and muscle (Fig. 4.7g).

4.2.2.6 Plexiform Fascicles (Fig. 4.7h)

Aggregations of melanocytes form fascicles that are arranged in a way that gives the appearance of a web- or net-like structure.

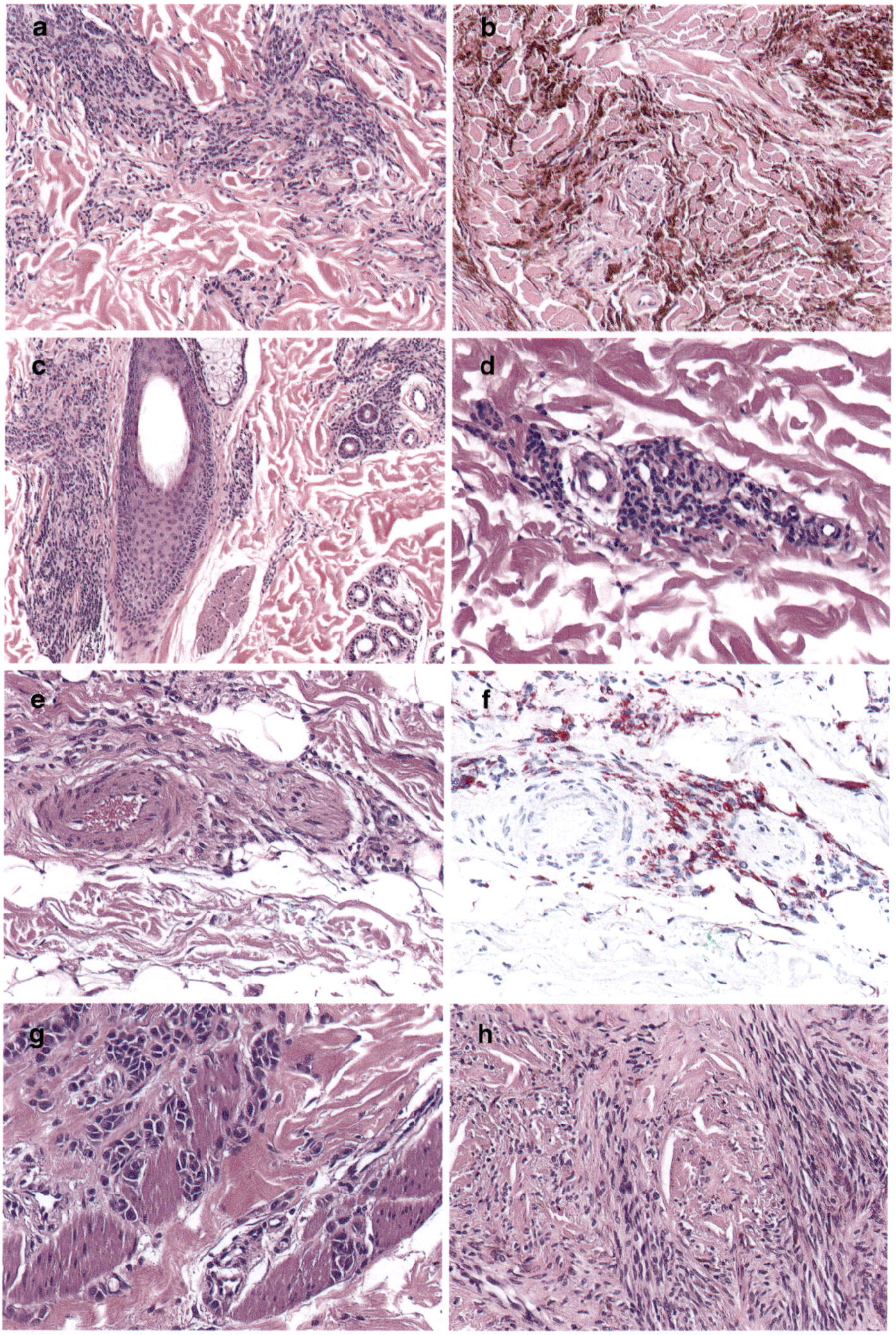

Fig. 4.7 (**a**–**h**) Dermal patterns: interstitial, periadnexal, plexiform. (**a**) Interstitial strands of melanocytes in the reticular dermis in a congenital nevus. (**b**) Interstitial strands, cords, and columns of elongated pigmented melanocytes in the reticular dermis in a common blue nevus. (**c**) Periadnexal arrangement of melanocytes: perifollicular and perieccrine melanocytes in a congenital nevus. (**d**) Perivascular melanocytes in a congenital nevus. (**e**) Perineural growth (neurotropism) of melanocytes in a melanoma. (**f**) MelanA staining of the lesion shown in (**e**) highlights the perineural distribution of the melanocytes. (**g**) Melanocytes in an arrector pili muscle (myotropism) in a Spitz nevus. (**h**) Plexiform arrangement of fascicles of melanocytes in a blue nevus. (Courtesy of the Dermatologikum Hamburg)

4.2.2.7 **Maturation** (Fig. 4.8a–d)

While the term "maturation" implies a process, it is in fact a description for a morphological phenomenon seen typically in benign melanocytic proliferations. When melanocytes in the upper part of the dermis are larger than those present in the lower part of the dermis, it is called maturation. Mostly, the increased size relates to a bigger amount of cytoplasm, but nuclei also can be larger. In contrast, melanocytes in the deeper dermis have less cytoplasm, smaller nuclei and overall a smaller diameter (Fig. 4.8a). As a consequence of these cytological characteristics, nests in the upper dermis are also larger than those in the lower dermis or no nests are present in the lower dermis and melanocytes are present only in the form of interstitial strands (see also [63], p. 16). In some lesions, maturation progresses to spindled melanocytes (Fig. 4.8b). This gradient of size and shape of melanocytes in the dermis ranging from epithelioid to lymphoid and spindled has been designated "Type A, type B, and type C nevus cells," which is a problematic terminology, because some maturation can also be seen in melanomas. Cytology of melanocytes is presented in more detail in Sect. 4.3. Maturation also is often associated with a decrease in melanin seen in melanocytes in deeper parts of the dermis (Fig. 4.8c). Pigment seen only in the upper part of a dermal melanocytic proliferation is also referred to as "Umbrella of pigment" (Fig. 4.8d).

Maturation is categorized in present (as described above), incomplete (meaning that there is smaller size of melanocytes in lower parts, but not striking), absent (melanocytes at all levels of the dermis have similar sizes), or inverse (melanocytes in the lower part of a lesion are bigger than those in the upper part).

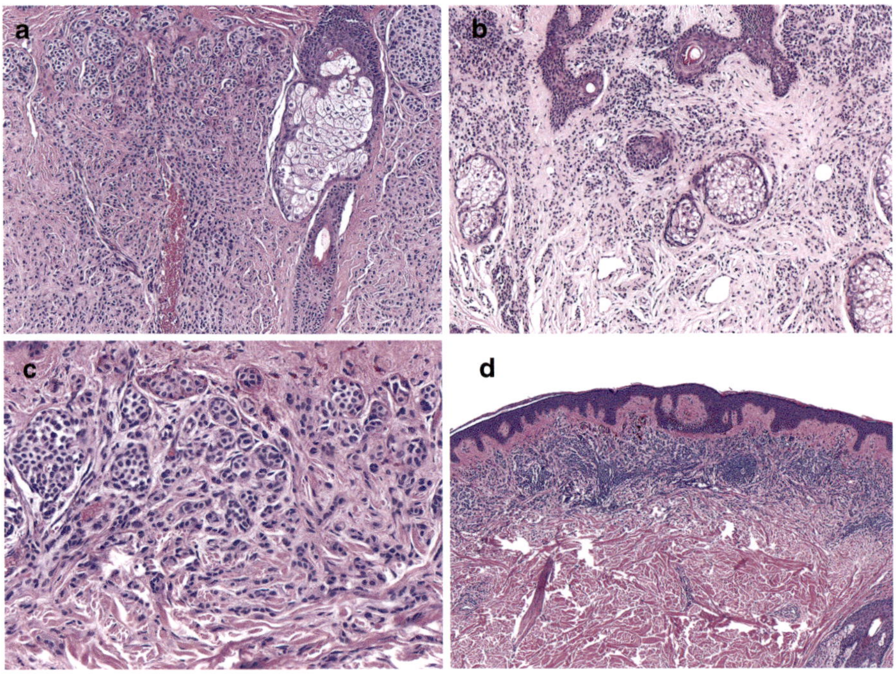

Fig. 4.8 (**a–d**) Dermal patterns: maturation. (**a**) Large nests in the upper dermis and small nests in the deep dermis in a dermal melanocytic nevus on the face. (**b**) Larger nests in the upper dermis, smaller nests and strands in the middle, and spindled thin melanocytes interstitially in the deep dermis in a congenital nevus. (**c**) Larger nests of pigmented melanocytes in the upper dermis, strands of smaller, nonpigmented melanocytes in interstitial arrangement in the deeper dermis in a congenital nevus. (**d**) Umbrella of pigment in a congenital melanocytic nevus. (Courtesy of the Dermatologikum Hamburg)

4.2.3 Subcutaneous Pattern (Fig. 4.9a–d)

4.2.3.1 Periadnexal Strands/Fascicles

Adnexal structures, especially terminal hair follicles and eccrine glandular structures may be situated partly in the subcutis, enveloped by adventitial collagen. Melanocytic proliferations involving the subcutis may form interstitial strands/fascicles along those structures, just as they do in the dermis ("adnexocentricity" or "adnexotropism").

4.2.3.2 Septal Involvement

Strands, fascicles, nests, nodules, or sheets of melanocytes are situated in the subcutaneous septa (Fig. 4.9a, b).

4.2.3.3 Lobular Involvement

Strands, fascicles, nests, nodules (Fig. 4.9c, d), or sheets of melanocytes are situated within the subcutaneous lobules.

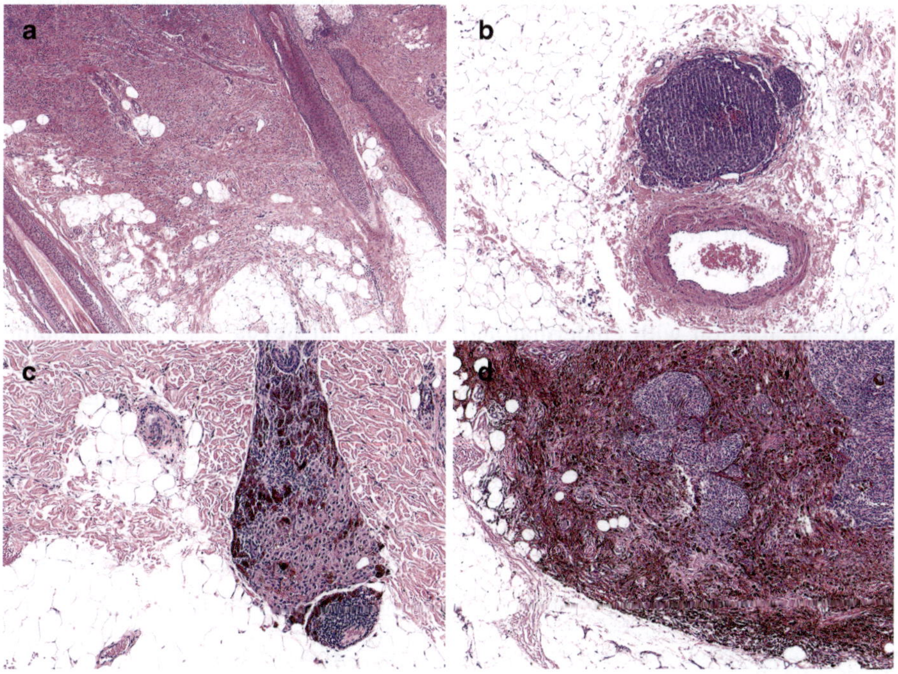

Fig. 4.9 (**a–d**) Subcutaneous patterns. (**a**) Extension of interstitial strands of melanocytes into superficial subcutaneous septa in a deep congenital nevus. Extension of periadnexal arrangement into the subcutis is seen, too. (**b**) Nodule of melanocytes in a subcutaneous septum next to a large vein in metastatic melanoma. (**c**) Nests and fascicles in superficial parts of subcutaneous lobules in a deep penetrating nevus. (**d**) Large nodules and fascicles of melanocytes in the subcutis in a blue nevus. (Courtesy of the Dermatologikum Hamburg)

4.2.4 Combination of Patterns

In some melanocytic proliferations, just one of the patterns defined above is present. One example is simple lentigo, in which single melanocytes are increased in the epidermal basal layer in regular distribution (see Fig. 4.2c). Another example is a common blue nevus in which interstitial strands and cords of elongated, bipolar melanocytes are present in the dermis (see Fig. 4.7b).

However, in most melanocytic proliferations a combination of patterns is observed and attention must be given to the arrangement of patterns to each other, especially to symmetry and to the predominance of patterns. When a melanocytic lesion in the epidermis consists of both, nests and single melanocytes, the symmetric or asymmetric arrangement of both patterns becomes very important: If arranged symmetrically, a junctional nevus[1] is the most likely diagnosis, if asymmetric, melanoma in situ needs to be considered. In a lesion with epidermal and dermal involvement, the arrangement of patterns in the epidermis needs to be compared with that seen in the dermis. If a dermal proliferation of melanocytes with a nested arrangement, adnexocentrism and maturation is associated with an epidermal proliferation of single cells that is in symmetry with the dermal part and regularly distributed, it is a congenital nevus. But, when it is asymmetrical to the dermal part with irregular distribution of melanocytes, a melanoma in situ arising in a congenital nevus is the best interpretation.

Some patterns are often associated with each other and strongly indicate a specific diagnosis, e.g., dermal nested, adnexocentric, with maturation is typical of a congenital melanocytic nevus. But it is important to understand that a lesion—even a benign one—is not homogeneously expressing these patterns. In a congenital nevus when cut in the center, an adnexocentric pattern often predominates, but when the lesion is cut off to the center, melanocytes will present in an interstitial pattern. When the lesion is sampled with a superficial technique, nesting of melanocytes will predominate, but when an excision is performed, interstitial patterns and maturation will be prominent. The epidermal part of a congenital nevus may show prominent nests when cut at the periphery, and single melanocytes when cut in the center and the nevus may seem to be a superficial congenital nevus when cut at the periphery but when studied in the center will have a deep dermal involvement. Nevertheless, at each of these different levels of cutting, the lesion will present patterns indicative of the diagnosis of a congenital nevus.

In order to apply diagnosis by pattern in melanocytic proliferations in a useful way, patterns and combinations of patterns must be linked to their most common or most likely diagnosis and differential diagnoses. In sequential steps of the diagnostic process, the patterns and combina-

[1]Here we use the term "junctional nevus" without any attribute to indicate that we refer to the class of junctional nevi but not to a specific type of nevus. Various nevi can be purely junctional, i.e., acquired nevi, Reed nevi, acral nevi, naevus spilus. This is confusing because the terms junctional, compound, and dermal nevi are also used in another way, not as generic terms, but for "common" nevi that are not otherwise specified. Whenever possible, we will try to avoid confusion and indicate which meaning we have in mind.

tions of patterns will be reevaluated taking into account cytologic features (see Sect. 4.3) and changes in epidermis and connective tissue (see Sect. 4.4). The entire diagnostic process is presented in examples in Chap. 5.

4.3 Cytology of Melanocytes

Normal melanocytes are dendritic cells situated in regular distribution in the basal layer of the epidermis and adnexal structures [64]. They have round or oval small, monomorphic, monochromatic nuclei with no obvious nucleoli. Because melanocytes have no desmosomes, they cannot connect tightly with surrounding keratinocytes but hold on to them just by their dendritic processes, which serve to transport melanin-laden melanosomes to them. Due to that, a small but characteristic cleft artifact often develops between melanocytes and surrounding keratinocytes during processing of specimens. This cleft is seen even at scanning magnification as a white sickle-shaped space surrounding the cytoplasm of the melanocyte. This should not be mixed up with a sickle-shaped artifact that may develop between the nucleus of keratinocytes and the surrounding cytoplasm.

In melanocytic proliferations, melanocytes assume a broad variety of cytologies which are all very different from the normal melanocyte in the epithelial basal layer [64]. Most of these cytologies cannot be categorized clearly in the benign or malignant category meaning that cytology alone is usually not sufficient to identify the biological nature of a melanocytic proliferation.

4.3.1 **Shape** (Fig. 4.10a–g)

4.3.1.1 Small Round

Small round melanocytes have little cytoplasm and a dark round to oval nucleus. They are typically found in the dermal part of congenital melanocytic nevi (Fig. 4.10a) but may also be seen in melanomas, especially nevoid melanomas (Fig. 4.10b) or variants of lentiginous melanoma on sun-damaged skin (so-called lentigo maligna melanoma).

4.3.1.2 Epithelioid

Epithelioid melanocytes have abundant eosinophilic or amphophilic cytoplasm and large oval or bizarre-shaped nuclei which may show one or more nucleoli. The designation is derived from their resemblance to epithelioid histiocytes (macrophages), which also have abundant eosinophilic cytoplasm. Epithelioid melanocytes are typically seen in Spitz nevi (Fig. 4.10c) and this is why in many textbooks and pathology reports they are referred to as "spitzoid cytology." However, they appear also in some examples of blue nevi, congenital nevi, BAP1-deficient nevi, in melanomas (Fig. 4.10d) and in melanocytic hyperplasia on sun-damaged skin. Epithelioid melanocytes often appear just eosinophilic or amphophilic with very little if any pigmentation, but they can have variable amounts of pigment, as it is seen in pigmented variants of Spitz nevi and quite commonly in melanomas. Still an eosinophilic or amphophilic hue of the cytoplasm should be present to apply the term epithelioid melanocyte.

4.3.1.3 Pagetoid

Pagetoid melanocytes have abundant, finely granular, blue-gray cytoplasm and are somewhat reminiscent of the cells of mammary/extramammary Paget's disease. The nuclei are large and may show prominent nucleoli. The blue-gray color derives from finely granular melanin pigment within the cells. While the size of the cells and the nuclear abnormalities are similar to those seen in epithelioid melanocytes, the cytoplasm is always blue-gray (not eosinophilic or amphophilic) in pagetoid melanocytes. Pagetoid melanocytes are almost only seen in melanomas (Fig. 4.10e), though congenital nevi in infants may show similar cells rarely.

4.3.1.4 Spindled

Spindle-shaped melanocytes are similar to spindled muscle cells and have a flat oval nucleus. They are characteristic for the pigmented spindle cell nevus Reed (Fig. 4.10f), where they appear heavily pigmented but they also may be seen in Spitz nevi, common acquired nevi, deeper dermal parts of congenital nevi (as part of the pattern of maturation), in some variants of blue nevi, and in melanomas.

4.3.1.5 Bipolar

Bipolar melanocytes represent an exaggeration of spindled melanocytes with two opposed elongated dendrites and a flat spindled nucleus. Bipolar melanocytes are reminiscent of neural cells and are typical for blue nevi of all kinds (Fig. 4.10g) including dermal melanocytoses (Fig. 4.10h, Nevus of Ota/Ito). They also may be found in deep dermal parts of congenital nevi (as part of the pattern of maturation or in so-called neurotized nevi), but they are not seen in melanomas with the rare exception of a melanoma arising in a blue nevus.

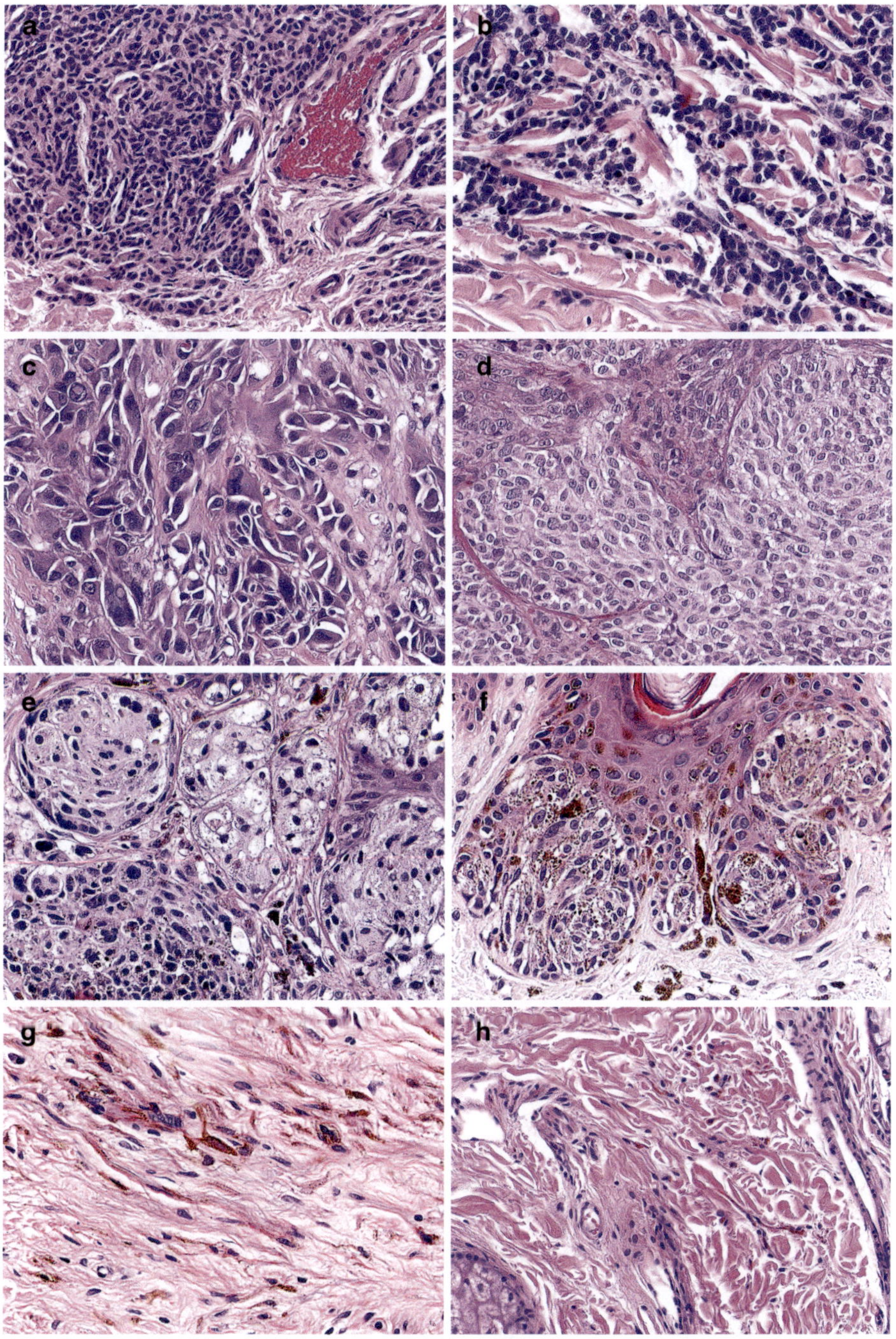

Fig. 4.10 (**a**–**h**) Cytology. (**a**) Small round melanocytes in interstitial arrangement in a congenital nevus. (**b**) Small round melanocytes in interstitial arrangement in a nevoid melanoma. (**c**) Epithelioid melanocytes in nests and single melanocytes in a Spitz nevus. (**d**) Epithelioid melanocytes in nests in a spitzoid melanoma. (**e**) Pagetoid, large pigmented melanocytes in epidermal and dermal nests of a melanoma. (**f**) Spindled pigmented melanocytes in intraepidermal nests of a pigmented spindle cell nevus (Reed nevus). (**g**) Bipolar pigmented melanocytes in a common blue nevus. (**h**) Few scattered bipolar pigmented melanocytes in a Nevus of Ota. (Courtesy of the Dermatologikum Hamburg)

4.3.1.6 Variants (Fig. 4.11a–f)

Ancient Change

Dermal nevi may show some epithelioid to spitzoid melanocytes with enlarged nuclei (Fig. 4.11a) but with homogeneous dense chromatin [65]. It is interpreted as a degenerative change in longer standing lesions and named after a similar phenomenon seen in Schwannomas.

Multinucleation

Melanocytes may exhibit multiple nuclei in benign melanocytic proliferations. In the epidermis, they take a shape similar to a Touton giant cell with ring-like arrangement of nuclei (Fig. 4.11b). In the dermis, multinucleate melanocytes often show densely aggregated nuclei forming the shape of a mulberry. The aggregations may simulate nuclear atypia at first blush, but the chromatin of the nuclei is homogenous and inconspicuous. Multinucleate melanocytes with irregularly shaped and heterochromatic nuclei occur in some melanomas and melanoma metastases but also in benign Spitz nevi.

Balloon Cell

An enlarged cell with vacuolated cytoplasm and a central nucleus simulating a sebocyte (Fig. 4.11c). Nevi with a large proportion of balloon cells are called balloon cell nevi, but balloon cells may also be seen in melanomas.

Neurotization

When bipolar melanocytes make up a large proportion of a melanocytic nevus, this is called neurotization. In that setting, structures simulating Meissner corpuscles, so-called nevic corpuscles (Fig. 4.11e) or fascicles simulating nerves can be seen (Fig. 4.11f). Such differentiation can be very similar to neurofibroma so that in some cases only the presence of a few nests of melanocytes in the upper part of the lesion enables differentiation.

Others

Plasmacytoid is used to designate melanocytes with an eccentric nucleus and eosinophilic cytoplasm (Fig. 4.11d), which mostly occur in melanomas but also in Spitz nevi. Oncocytic is a designation for melanocytes with abundant, sharply circumscribed, eosinophilic cytoplasm similar to a large, granular cell found in salivary and certain endocrine glands and making up a benign glandular neoplasm called oncocytoma (syn. oxyphilic adenoma). Signet ring cell melanocytes are melanocytes with one large vacuole pressing the nucleus to one side and forming the shape of a signet ring.

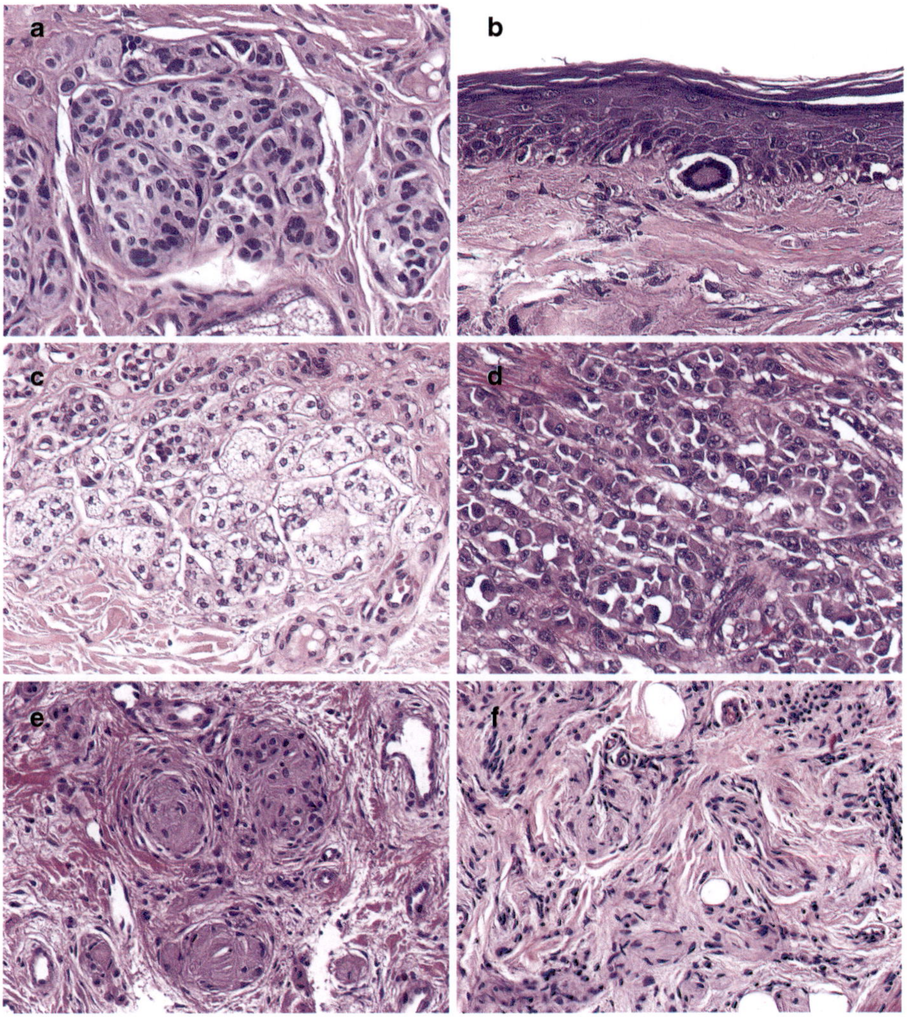

Fig. 4.11 (**a–f**) Cytology variants. (**a**) Ancient change. Enlarged melanocytes with multiple nuclei in a dermal nevus. (**b**) Multinucleate melanocyte in a melanoma in situ (**c**) Balloon cells. Vacuolated melanocytes with central scalloped nuclei simulating sebocytes in a combined congenital nevus. (**d**) Plasmacytoid melanocytes in a melanoma. (**e**) Neurotization: Nevic corpuscles. Formation of structures simulating Meissner corpuscles in a dermal nevus. (**f**) Neurotization: Fibers. Formation of fascicles simulating nerve fibers in a dermal nevus. (Courtesy of the Dermatologikum Hamburg)

4.3.2 Pleomorphism of Melanocytes (Fig. 4.12a–f)

If all melanocytes in a proliferation are more or less similar (not considering the pattern of maturation), this is called a monomorphic melanocytic lesion (Fig. 4.12a). In contrast, pleomorphism is present when melanocytes within a melanocytic proliferation show marked variation in size and shape, in nuclear characteristics, and/or in nucleus-cytoplasm ratio (Fig. 4.12d, e). In nevi usually nuclei are equidistant, monomorphic, and monochromatic (Fig. 4.12a). In melanoma (Fig. 4.12e), nuclei are often not equidistant because of their variable size and shape and because of the variable amount of cytoplasm between them. However, some nevi may also show pleomorphism of melanocytes. Typically in Spitz nevi (Fig. 4.12d) but also in some variants of blue nevi melanocytes display variation in size and shape. Nuclear characteristics of malignancy include large size, heterochromasia (difference in coloration of nuclei), and hyperchromasia (increased intensity of staining of nuclei) (Fig. 4.12d, e; page 15 in [63]). Nuclei with multiple nucleoli or with one large nucleolus (half the diameter of the nucleus) are more commonly seen in malignant proliferations. Also nucleoli in melanomas sometimes appear eosinophilic, a feature usually not seen in melanocytic nevi. Pleomorphism of nuclei should not be mixed up with multinucleation, because congenital melanocytic nevi, especially those that are largely situated in the dermis, quite often have some multinucleated melanocytes (see Fig. 4.11a). It also needs to be considered that oval nuclei of melanocytes in melanocytic nevi are cut in a section at different directions giving the appearance of some variation in size and shape of nuclei. Moreover, nuclei in melanocytic nevi may show pseudoinclusions by invagination of cytoplasmic material into the nucleus (Fig. 4.12b). Pleomorphism also needs to be differentiated from polymorphism: In combined melanocytic nevi, more than one population of melanocytes may be present together, but each of the populations is in itself monomorphic (Fig. 4.12c).

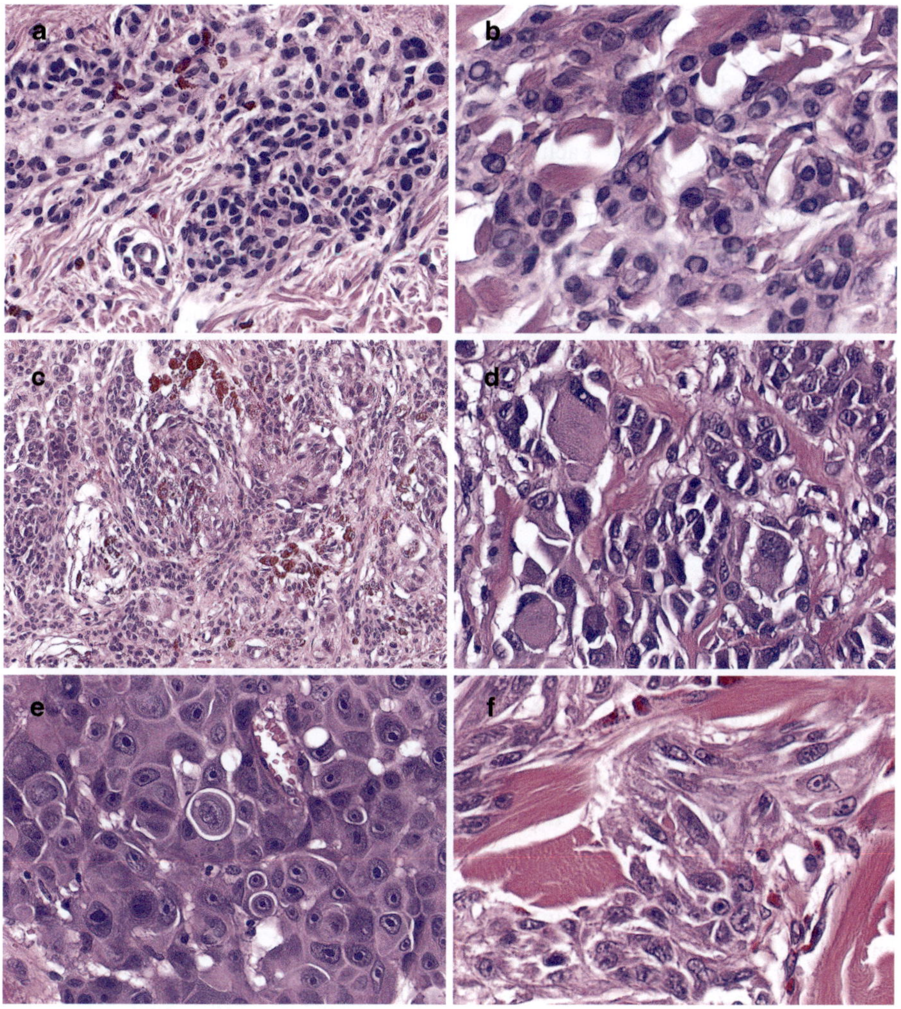

Fig. 4.12 (**a–f**) Pleomorphism. (**a**) Monomorphic melanocytes. Nuclei are equidistant and monochromatic. (**b**) Pseudoinclusions in nuclei of a melanocytic nevus. Invagination of cytoplasmic material into the nucleus. (**c**) Polymorphism. Two populations of melanocytes, each in itself monomorphic, in a combined congenital nevus. (**d**) Pleomorphism in a Spitz nevus. Nuclei are not equidistant, cells and nuclei vary in size, shape, and color. (**e**) Pleomorphism in a melanoma. Nuclei are not equidistant, cells and nuclei vary in size, shape, and color. Some nuclei have multiple nucleoli or one large nucleolus (half the diameter of the nucleus). (**f**) Color variation of nucleoli. While nucleoli usually are hyperchromatic, they may show color variation in melanomas, sometimes with an eosinophilic hue. (Courtesy of the Dermatologikum Hamburg)

4.3.3 **Crowding** (Fig. 4.13a)

Crowding refers to a distinct cytological and nuclear appearance in which nuclei of neighboring cells touch and/or overlap each other (Fig. 4.13a). It is often accompanied with, and perhaps a result of, an increased nuclear-cytoplasm ratio, i.e., reduced cytoplasm and enlarged nuclei will demonstrate nuclei in a closer arrangement. Crowding of nuclei is usually a sign of malignancy, but some rapidly proliferating normal tissues such as matrical epithelium of the hair follicle may also exhibit some crowding. In the realm of melanocytic proliferations, crowding is seen in melanomas. It should not be mixed up with multinucleation (see Fig. 4.11a). In colloquial style, some colleagues refer to this pattern as "too many cells," especially when inspecting at scanning magnification.

4.3.4 **Mitotic Figures** (Fig. 4.13b, c)

Mitotic figures are seen in cells that undergo the process of cell division. During that process, chromosomes are visible by light microscopy. In histopathology, a difference is made between normal (typical) mitotic figures and atypical mitotic figures. Normal mitotic figures are those seen during metaphase (when the chromosomes are aligned in the equatorial plane of the cell) and those seen in anaphase (when the daughter chromosomes are drawn to opposite poles of the cells). In contrast, abnormal (atypical) mitotic figures show chromosomes forming other shapes, e.g., ring-, x- or y-shape (Fig. 4.13b, c). In melanocytic proliferations, mitotic figures may be observed in the epidermal and/or dermal part of a lesion. While melanocytes in mitosis in the epidermal part are not of diagnostic importance, dermal mitotic figures may be relevant, depending on where in the dermis they are located, how many of them are present (Fig. 4.13b), and/or whether they form typical or atypical shapes [66]. In general, more than two mitosis visible within one section of a lesion are interpreted as favoring malignancy and even one mitosis when located at the base of a melanocytic proliferation, deep in the dermis, is suspicious for malignancy. However, mitoses can also be seen in melanocytic nevi, e.g., in children, after outside irritation, in growing lesions, or in proliferative nodules of congenital nevi. Abnormal mitoses can be seen in melanomas and, very rarely, in Spitz nevi (Fig. 4.13c). In contrast, even well-advanced melanomas may not show any mitotic figure or just very few typical ones. In metastatic melanoma, however, mitoses are a common finding.

When studying mitotic figures, it is important to note that it can be very difficult to decide whether a mitotic figure is truly located in a melanocyte. Mitoses may also occur in keratinocytes, in endothelial cells, or in inflammatory cells within the melanocytic lesion.

4.3.5 **Necrosis** (Fig. 4.13d–f)

Necrosis refers to the spectrum of morphologic changes that follow cell death in living tissue. Signs of necrosis are shrinkage and increased eosinophilia of the cytoplasm, pyknosis (nuclear shrinkage with increased basophilia), karyorrhexis (fragmentation of the nucleus), and karyolysis (loss of nucleus due to enzymatic degradation of DNA). Necrosis appears as single cell necrosis (Fig. 4.13d), as small clusters of necrotic cells (Fig. 4.13e), or as necrosis "*en masse*" (necrosis of large collections of cells, Fig. 4.13f).

In benign melanocytic lesions, necrosis is usually absent, exceptions being heavily traumatized lesions and Spitz nevi (which may show individual necrotic cells in the epidermis or even in the dermis). In melanomas, necrotic melanocytes can be seen especially in advanced lesions. Necrosis *en masse* can be observed in primary melanomas with considerable thickness and in metastases.

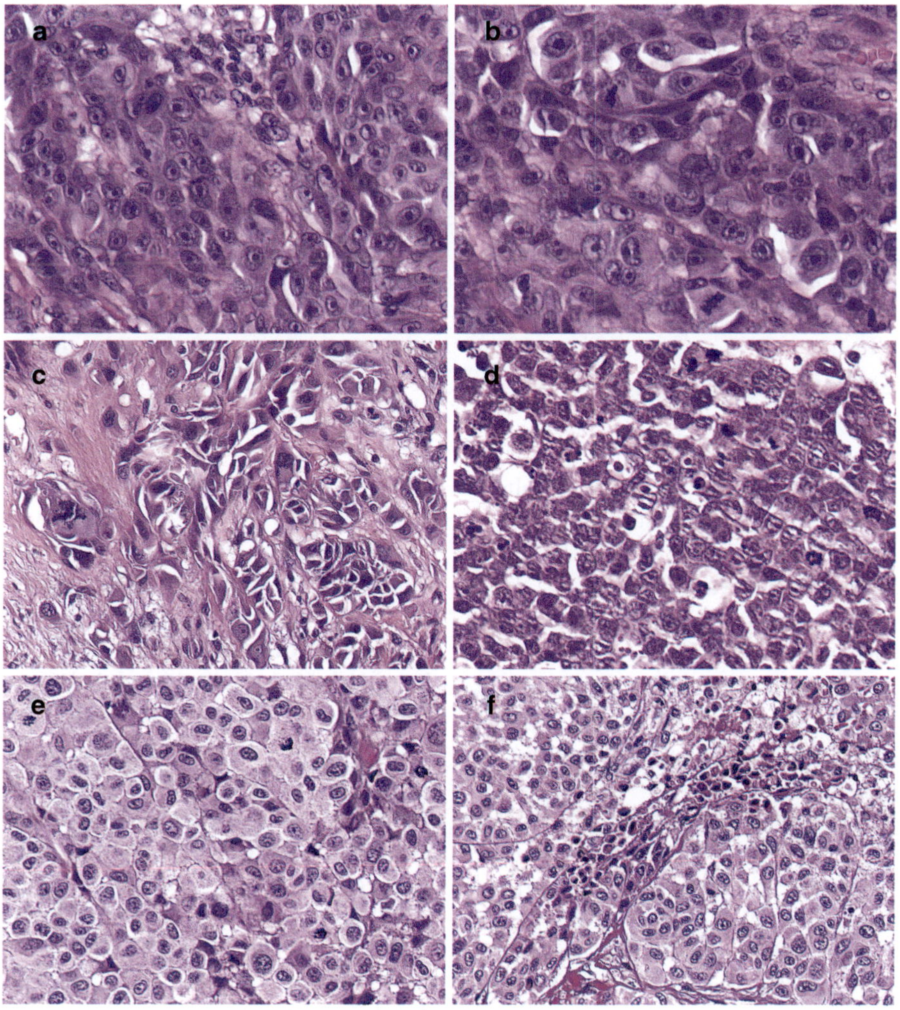

Fig. 4.13 (a–f) Crowding, mitoses, and necrosis. (**a**) Crowding. Nuclei of neighboring cells touch and/or overlap each other in the dermal part of a melanoma. (**b**) Mitoses and prominent nucleoli in the dermal part of a melanoma. (**c**) Rare atypical mitosis in a Spitz nevus. (**d**) Mitoses, including atypical forms, and single cell necrosis in a nodular melanoma. (**e**) Small collections of more eosinophilic, incipiently necrotic cells in a melanoma metastasis. (**f**) Necrosis *en masse* in a melanoma metastasis. (Courtesy of the Dermatologikum Hamburg)

4.4 Other Changes

In most melanocytic lesions, changes do not consist of a proliferation of melanocytes alone. Usually, alterations in the associated epithelial structures and in the surrounding connective tissue can be seen, too. Some of these changes are so distinctive that they are very helpful in the diagnostic process.

4.4.1 Epidermis (Fig. 4.14a–f)

When melanocytes proliferate in the epidermis, the epithelium often reacts with distinctive alterations, which are listed in the following:

4.4.1.1 Elongated Rete Ridges

Rete ridges are elongated in comparison with the surrounding uninvolved epidermis (Fig. 4.14a). Often, nests of melanocytes are positioned at the base of elongated rete ridges. This is typically seen in benign nevi, junctional or compound.

4.4.1.2 Epidermal Hyperplasia

Thickening of the epidermis by varying amounts of acanthosis and hypergranulosis. Acanthosis is a thickening of the spinous zone in comparison with the surrounding uninvolved epidermis, which may be regular or irregular. Regular acanthosis is a common finding in Spitz nevi (Fig. 4.14b) and in melanocytic lesions that have been irritated mechanically over a longer time, whereas irregular (asymmetric) acanthosis can be found in melanomas but also in traumatized nevi. Hypergranulosis is a thickened granular layer that is often accompanied by acanthosis and may be regular or irregular. Regular hypergranulosis is a common finding in Spitz nevi but it also may develop after chronic mechanical irritation. In congenital nevi, epidermal hyperplasia may imitate the architecture of a seborrheic keratosis with formation of orthokeratotic pseudohorn cysts (Fig. 4.14c). In general, regular epidermal hyperplasia is often seen in benign lesions while irregular epidermal hyperplasia and epidermal atrophy are more often seen in melanomas.

4.4.1.3 Intracorneal Pigmentation

Intracorneal pigmentation reflects epidermal pigmentation that developed 2–3 weeks before. Especially in acral lesions, intracorneal pigmentation can be informative since the cornified layer is consistently thickened. Intracorneal pigmentation in regular columnar arrangement is a feature of acral melanocytic nevi, while in acral melanomas intracorneal pigmentation is often broad and not arranged in columnar fashion. On sites other than acral, broad intracorneal pigmentation may also be seen in common junctional and compound nevi especially after exposure to sunlight or irritation.

4.4.1.4 Kamino Bodies

Kamino bodies (dull pink globules) are eosinophilic round structures seen at variable levels of the epidermis in about 50% of Spitz nevi (Fig. 4.14d), sometimes in Reed nevi, but very rarely in other nevi or melanomas [63]. The globules are made up of basement membrane, stain pink in PAS and can be highlighted with immunohistochemical antibodies against laminin or type IV collagen.

4.4.1.5 Atrophy

Flattening of the rete ridges and thinning of the epidermis are signs of epidermal atrophy which often appear in melanoma (Fig. 4.14e), but they may also be seen as a result of prior trauma in recurrent nevi. Remarkably thin epidermis is also not uncommon in fibroepitheliomatous dermal nevi, in which the finding does not indicate a malignant process. Melanocytic proliferations replacing much of the epidermis such that only a few layers persist have been described under the term "Consumption of the epidermis" (Fig. 4.14f). It often can be seen adjacent to ulceration and can be conceived of as a preliminary stage of the process of ulceration by a malignant melanocytic proliferation.

4.4.1.6 Ulceration

A defect of the epidermis within a melanocytic lesion. It may develop as a result of external trauma or caused by the biology of the melanocytic lesion. A well-demarcated, bowl shaped defect occurs after outside trauma, while irregularly shaped defects with adjacent epidermal atrophy are more likely the result of rapid proliferation of a melanocytic tumor, most likely a melanoma. It has to be taken into account, however, that melanomas also may show ulceration secondary to outside trauma.

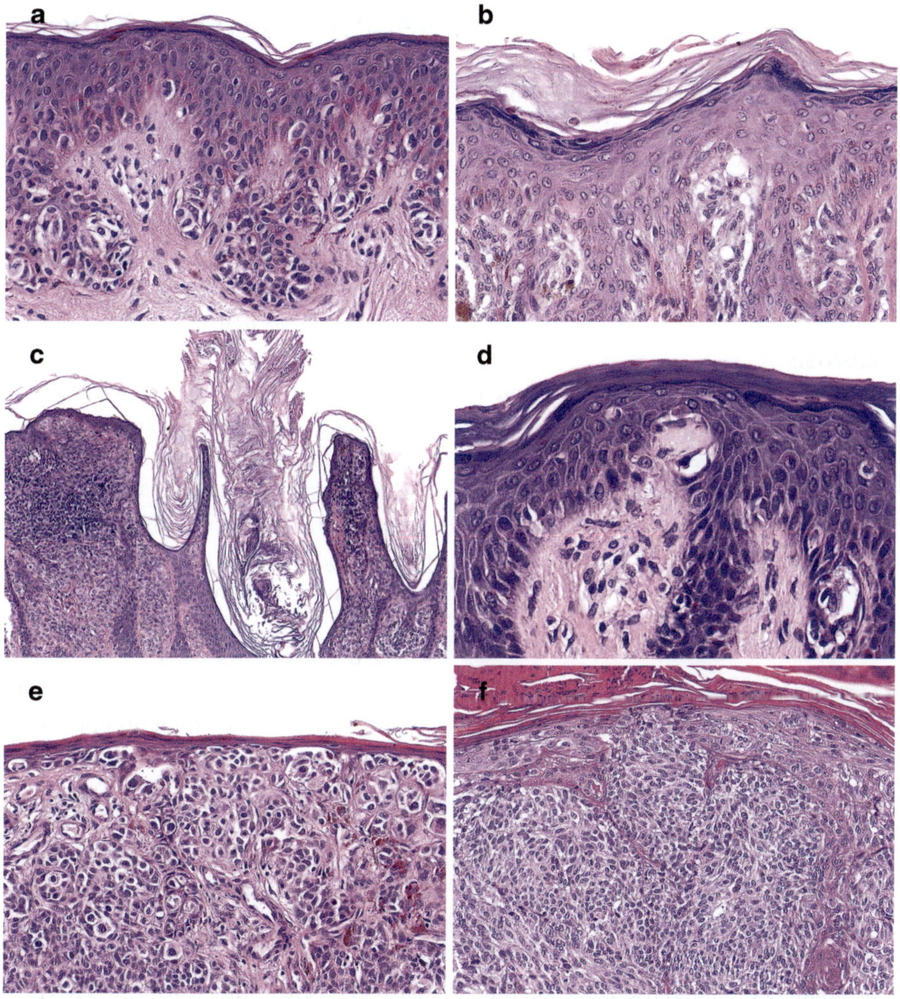

Fig. 4.14 (**a**–**f**) Epidermal changes. (**a**) Elongated rete ridges in a common acquired nevus. (**b**) Acanthosis, hypergranulosis, and hyperkeratosis in a Spitz nevus. (**c**) Seborrheic keratosis-like epidermal hyperplasia in a congenital nevus. Note the thin epidermis between dilated infundibular channels, which is of no concern in the situation of an entirely dermal melanocytic proliferation. (**d**) Kamino body (dull pink globule). Pale pink round structure within the epidermis in a Spitz nevus. (**e**) Thin epidermis with flattened rete ridges in a melanoma. (**f**) Melanocytes replacing the epidermis almost entirely in a melanoma (so-called consumption of the epidermis). (Courtesy of the Dermatologikum Hamburg)

4.4.2 Collagen (Fig. 4.15a–f)

A variety of connective tissue changes can be seen in association with melanocytic proliferations. Among them are types of fibrosis, in which collagen changes are accompanied by an increase in number of fibroblasts, and forms of sclerosis, in which collagen bundles are thickened but fibroblasts are not increased in number.

4.4.2.1 Fibroplasia

The term fibroplasia has been introduced to designate thickened, wiry collagen bundles in the papillary dermis which envelop rete ridges and which are seen in microscopic sections as vertical or horizontal bundles (Fig. 4.15a). It is a type of sclerosis often seen in junctional or compound melanocytic nevi, but also sometimes in melanoma.

4.4.2.2 Sclerosis

In some types of blue nevi (Fig. 4.15b) and in some Spitz nevi (Fig. 4.15c), thickened collagen bundles are present between proliferations of melanocytes in the dermis. Confusingly, the same type of connective tissue is referred to as sclerosis in the term "sclerosing blue nevus," and as desmoplasia in the term "desmoplastic Spitz nevus."

4.4.2.3 Desmoplasia

Desmoplasia is defined as a connective tissue change induced by a neoplastic proliferation. In the designation of melanocytic lesions, it appears in the terms desmoplastic Spitz nevus and desmoplastic melanoma. However, the type of connective tissue induced by each of these two lesions is very different. In desmoplastic melanoma, it is characterized by an increased number of larger stromal cells, increased extracellular fibers, and varying amounts of mucin, but in desmoplastic Spitz nevus it is sclerosis with thickened collagen bundles (Fig. 4.15c) similar to those seen in sclerosing blue nevi. Therefore, desmoplasia is not referring to one specific type of connective tissue change.

4.4.2.4 Scar

As a result of previous trauma, the dermal connective tissue shows collagen bundles arranged horizontally (Fig. 4.15d), with interspersed vertically oriented vessels. The number of fibroblasts is higher in fresh scars compared with longstanding scarring. Adnexal structures and elastic fibers are reduced in scars and the overlying epidermis often shows flattened rete ridges.

4.4.2.5 Collagen Changes in Regression

Inflammatory infiltrates in response to neoplasms (see Sect. 4.4.4.3) are often followed by alterations of the connective tissue [67]. Typically, the connective tissue is loose with delicate collagen fibers and mucin deposition (Fig. 4.15e). Vessels are oriented vertically and rete ridges are flattened. Regressed areas in seborrheic keratosis, in basal cell carcinoma, and in melanoma can look very similar, so that in a fully regressed lesion a robust specific diagnosis may not be possible. However, zones of regression in melanoma often show band-like melanophages in the upper dermis, and melanocytes missing or residual single melanocytes in irregular distribution may be found in the epidermis. In advanced melanoma, partial regression is a relatively common finding while complete regression is quite rare.

4.4.2.6 Solar Elastosis

Replacement of regular collagen in the dermis by blue-gray fibers which do not show a net-like arrangement but rather appear haphazardly arranged and may form large masses filling the entire dermis (Fig. 4.15f). The morphological feature is mostly seen on chronically sun-exposed skin, but it can also appear to a lesser degree in areas devoid of sun exposure as a result of biological aging. In melanocytic lesions, solar elastosis below the lesion is interpreted as an indirect sign of a lesion developing later in life, and therefore more likely to be a melanoma (assuming that a longstanding melanocytic lesion protects the dermis underneath from sun damage and would result in preserved collagen below the lesion).

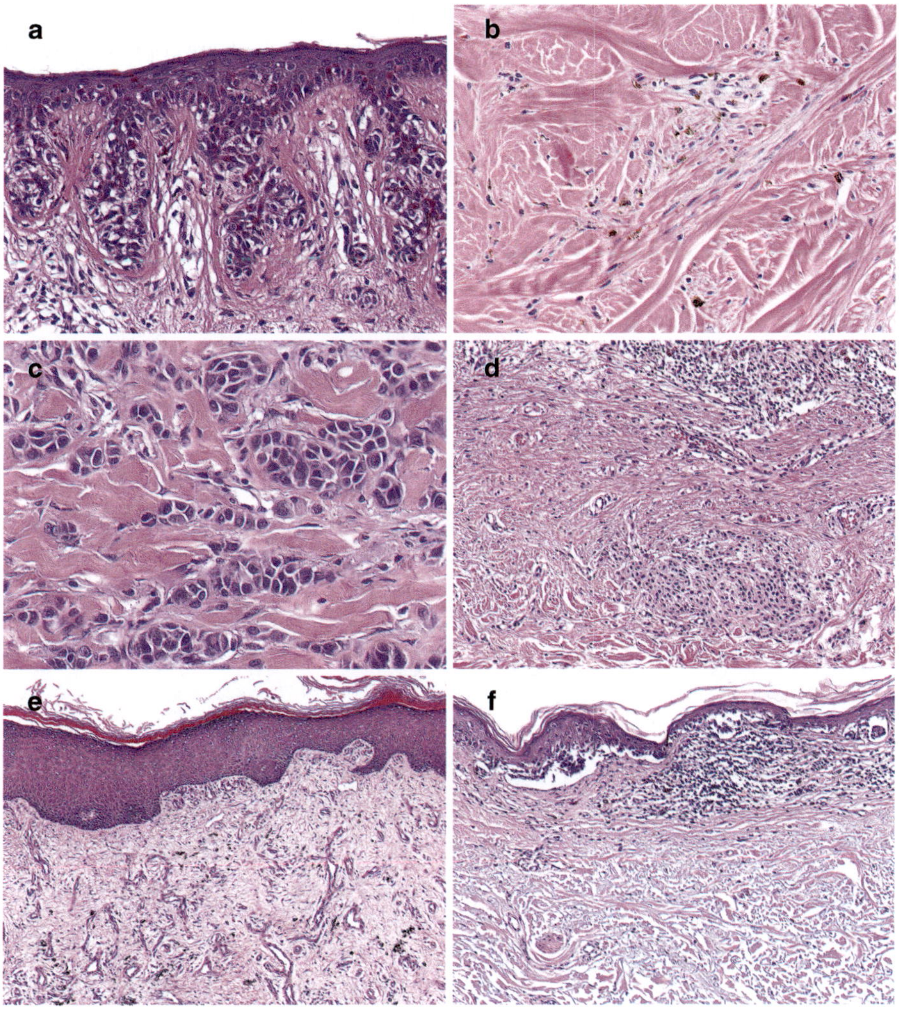

Fig. 4.15 (**a**–**f**) Connective tissue changes. (**a**) Fibroplasia. Wiry collagen bundles enveloping elongated rete ridges in a compound nevus. (**b**) Sclerosis. Thickened collagen bundles in a sclerosing blue nevus. (**c**) Sclerosis. Thickened collagen bundles in a sclerosing (desmoplastic) Spitz nevus. (**d**) Scar. Horizontally arranged collagen bundles and increased fibroblasts and vessels in the dermis after incomplete removal of a congenital melanocytic nevus (remnants of the nevus are seen in small nest below the scar in the residual reticular dermis). (**e**) Regression. Altered connective tissue with fine collagen bundles, vertically oriented vessels, melanophages, and scattered lymphocytic infiltrates. (**f**) Solar elastosis underneath a melanoma in situ. Blue-gray fibers replacing collagen in the dermis indicate chronically sun-damaged skin. (Courtesy of the Dermatologikum Hamburg)

4.4.3 Vessels (Fig. 4.16a–d)

The shape and distribution of vessels in a lesion can help in differentiation between benign and malignant proliferations.

4.4.3.1 Vascularization

Regular distribution of vessels favors a benign process while irregular distribution is more common in malignant proliferations. In dermal nevi, especially in those with a fibroepitheliomatous shape, large dilated vessels in regular distribution are often seen (Fig. 4.16a). In melanomas, vertically oriented vessels are present in zones of regression.

Vascularization should not be mixed up with so-called pseudovascular spaces which are artificial spaces lined by melanocytes, not by endothelial cells, and which are commonly seen in dermal nevi (Fig. 4.16b).

4.4.3.2 Vascular Invasion

The presence of melanoma cells in a vessel (Fig. 4.16c, d), which can be either a blood vessel or a lymphatic. Biologically it is a sign of metastatic spread and hence interpreted as a morphologic finding indicating a bad prognosis. Therefore, it is important to be certain about this observation and the presence of melanoma cells in a vascular space should be confirmed using immunohistochemical markers for melanocytes, lymphatics, and blood vessels. Nests of melanocytes impinging in a vessel from the outside may sometimes imitate vascular invasion.

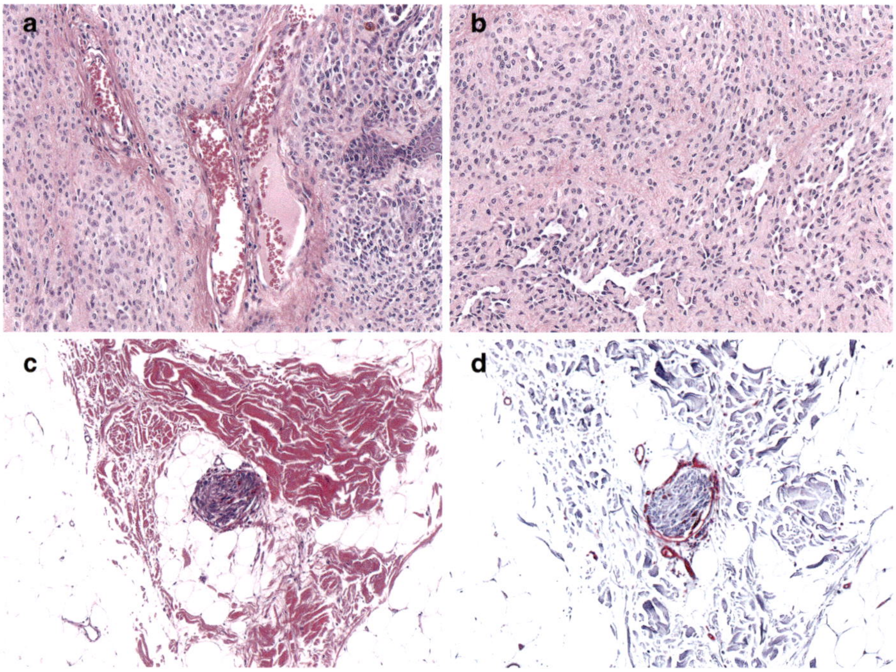

Fig. 4.16 (**a–d**) Vascular changes. (**a**) Dilated vessels increased in number in a fibroepitheliomatous dermal nevus (Unna nevus). Vessels are lined by thin endothelial cells and filled with erythrocytes and serum. (**b**) Pseudovascular spaces in a dermal nevus. The cells lining the artificial space are melanocytes. They appear plump and they often form papillary protrusions. No serum or erythrocytes are seen within the space. (**c**) Vascular invasion. Pigmented pleomorphic melanoma cells in a vessel in the subcutis; (**d**) CD31-staining of lining endothelial cells. (Courtesy of the Dermatologikum Hamburg)

4.4.4 Inflammatory Infiltrates (Fig. 4.17a–f)

Some amount of inflammatory infiltrate is often seen in melanocytic lesions, both benign and malignant, and does not help much in the diagnostic process. However, some lesions have a distinctive pattern of inflammation that can be diagnostically helpful.

4.4.4.1 Halo Phenomenon

A dense band-like infiltrate that obscures a melanocytic lesion is referred to as "Halo phenomenon" (Fig. 4.17a). The designation derives from the infiltrate seen in Halo nevus, which is usually dense, band-like and obscures the dermal part of the proliferation, sometimes also the dermoepidermal junction. When the infiltrate is present but no Halo seen clinically, this is called the Halo phenomenon. It is important to know that granulomatous infiltrates can be present in a halo phenomenon, thereby giving the wrong impression of pleomorphism and loss of maturation. In such cases, immunohistochemistry is necessary to properly identify the dermal cell types.

4.4.4.2 Meyerson Phenomenon

Melanocytic lesions may be overlayed by a spongiotic dermatitis with a mixed infiltrate housing lymphocytes and eosinophils (Fig. 4.17b). Clinically, the lesion is surrounded by erythema and may be covered by crust or scale.

4.4.4.3 Patchy Lymphocytes/Plasma Cells

Inflammatory infiltrates are designated as patchy when collections of inflammatory cells are present in various areas of a largely dermal melanocytic neoplasm. Whereas patchy lymphocytes are a common finding in sclerosing Spitz nevi, a patchy distribution of lymphocytes together with plasma cells is often seen in desmoplastic melanoma. In desmoplastic melanomas, the melanocytic nature of the lesion can be hard to identify morphologically, especially when no intraepidermal melanoma in situ is associated. In the setting of an ill-defined spindle cell neoplasm in the dermis and extending into the subcutis, patchy infiltrates of lymphocytes and plasma cells are a hint to desmoplastic melanoma (Fig. 4.17c).

4.4.4.4 Melanophages

Melanophages are macrophages that have ingested melanin. They are a common finding in melanocytic neoplasms but also in pigmented keratinocytic neoplasms and in inflammatory diseases, especially in diseases with interface dermatitis such as lichen planus or fixed drug eruption. Depending on the depth of melanophages in the dermis and the degree of pigmentation they can account for the clinical impression of a brown, black, gray, or blue color of a lesion. Histologically melanophages may be mistaken for melanocytes because not uncommonly they are more pigmented than melanocytes. If no immunohistochemical stains are used, the dendritic morphology and the size of melanin granules help to identify melanophages. In melanophages, the granules of melanin are typically larger (Fig. 4.17d) while melanocytes show fine granules. Melanophages also need to be differentiated from hemosiderophages. Pigment in hemosiderophages has a green hue when the condenser is removed and they stain positive in iron staining.

4.4.4.5 Lymphocytic Infiltrates in Regression

Subepidermal band-like infiltrates of lymphocytes are one morphologic expression of regression in a melanoma (Fig. 4.17e). The infiltrate is often accompanied by band-like deposition of melanophages (Fig. 4.17f) and by connective tissue changes (see Fig. 4.15e).

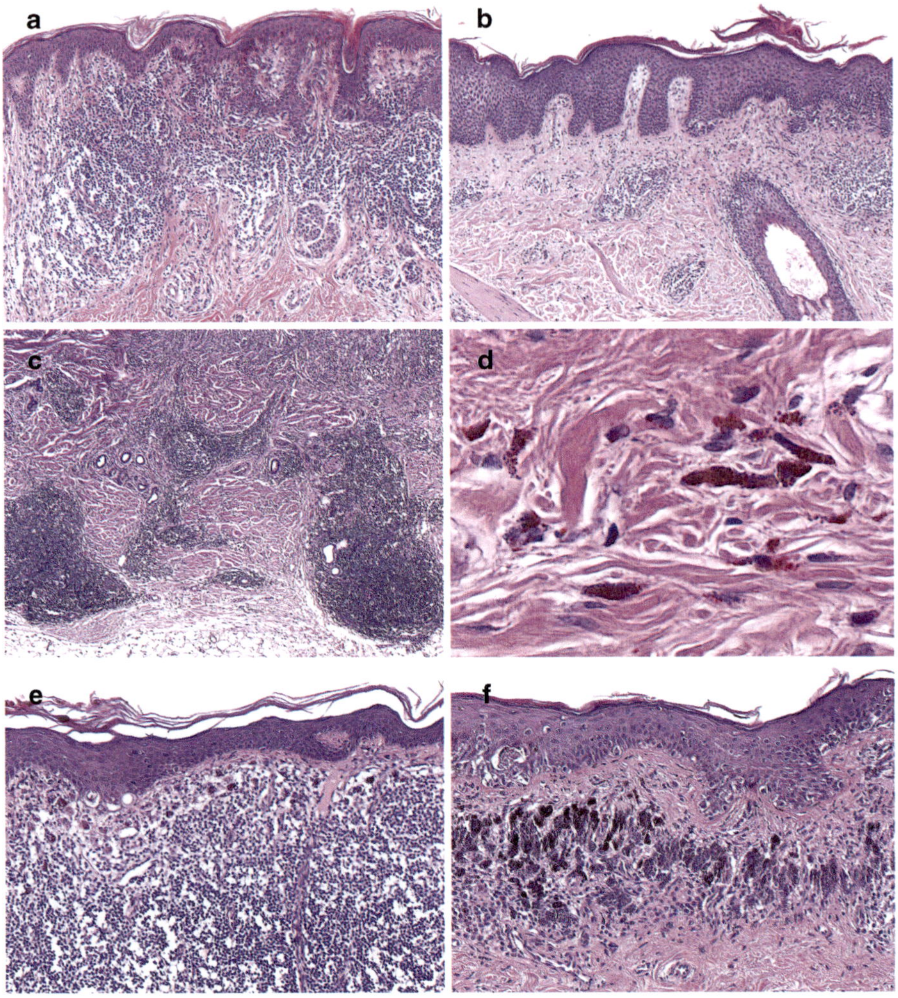

Fig. 4.17 (**a**–**f**) Inflammatory infiltrates. (**a**) Band-like lymphocytic infiltrate in a Halo nevus. (**b**) Spongiotic dermatitis overlying and extending beyond the melanocytic lesion in a Meyerson nevus. The infiltrate may have numerous eosinophils. (**c**) Patchy lymphocytic infiltrate in a desmoplastic melanoma. (**d**) Large pigment granules in melanophages. (**e**) Band-like lymphocytic infiltrate in an area of regression of a melanoma. (**f**) Band-like melanophages in an area of regression of a melanoma. (Courtesy of the Dermatologikum Hamburg)

Integration of Patterns 5

Integration of patterns requires profound knowledge about the occurrence of patterns in specific melanocytic lesions. While some patterns are exclusively seen in one type of lesion (e.g., bipolar melanocytes in blue nevi), many of the patterns described above may appear in both benign and malignant proliferations of melanocytes. Some patterns are associated with site (e.g., suprabasal melanocytes in acral lesions) or to previous trauma (e.g., irregular epidermal proliferations in recurrent nevi, so-called pseudomelanoma).

In many cases, a simple combination of patterns is already very suggestive of a benign diagnosis. This is exemplified in the sentence "small and mostly nested: it's a nevus," which has been taught at many dermatopathology training centers over the last 50 years as a very helpful basic rule. Another example is prominent maturation together with adnexocentric distribution of melanocytes which indicates a congenital nevus. However, in the latter case, the addition of two more epidermal patterns, i.e., an asymmetric epidermal component with predominance of single melanocytes and melanocytes above the basal layer will change the diagnosis into "melanoma in situ arising in association with a congenital nevus." Therefore, all patterns seen in a lesion should first be observed correctly and then be integrated stepwise without jumping to a conclusion too early in the process.

5.1 Combination of Patterns and Differential Diagnosis

In most cases, it is the combination of patterns together with silhouette and cytology that enables a specific diagnosis. Clinical presentation and dermatoscopy, if available, will help to confirm the conclusion. In some cases, however, the features observed remain conflicting and a sure diagnosis cannot be made based on morphology alone. This is especially true for samples that do not show the entire lesion so that symmetry and circumscription cannot be assessed.

Tables 5.1, 5.2, and 5.3 summarize patterns of melanocytes and combinations of patterns together with diagnoses in which they occur often. While these lists do not attempt to be all-encompassing, they should provide a rough categorization of common differential diagnoses and diagnostic challenges. Suggestions on how to approach problems in differential diagnosis are given in the last column. Ideally these tables should be used as models which can be expanded by a dermatopathologist/pathologist by adding their own experience.

A. Böer-Auer et al., *Pattern Analysis for Histopathologic Diagnosis of Melanocytic Lesions*,
https://doi.org/10.1007/978-3-031-07666-4_5

Table 5.1 Epidermal patterns of melanocytes and differential diagnoses

Patterns	Combination	Diagnoses	Solving differential diagnoses
Single melanocytes increased, regular	None	Simple lentigo	Small lesion, slight elongation of rete ridges
		Melanocytic hyperplasia in sun-damaged skin	Flattened rete ridges, solar elastosis, epithelioid cytology may be present, compare with contralateral biopsy of normal skin
		Surface of a dermal nevus	No sun damage, nests in the dermis
		Surface of a fibrous papule	No sun damage, thick collagen bundles, plump fibroblasts, vessels increased
		Nevus spilus	Large lesion, slight elongation of rete ridges, no sun damage, clinical picture!
Single melanocytes increased, regular	None	Seborrheic keratosis with melanocytes ("Melanoacanthoma")	Acanthosis and hyperkeratosis with pseudocysts (classic for seborrheic keratosis), melanocytes also in upper epidermal layers
		Epidermal nevus with melanocytic hyperplasia	Verrucous acanthosis and lamellar hyperkeratosis
Single melanocytes increased, regular	None	Large cell acanthoma	Enlarged keratinocytes with enlarged nuclei, no crowding of nuclei
Single melanocytes increased, irregular	None	Melanoma in situ	Focal nesting or back-to-back melanocytes, large lesion
		Recurrent nevus/traumatized nevus	Subepidermal fibrosis with horizontal arrangement of collagen, search for dermal monomorphic nests/strands below the scar as remnants of incomplete removal. Irregular epidermal melanocytes are confined to the area of fibrosis
Single melanocytes increased, irregular	Melanocytes above the basal layer	Melanoma in situ	Focal nesting or back-to-back melanocytes, large lesion
		Recurrent nevus/ traumatized nevus	Subepidermal fibrosis with horizontal arrangement of collagen, search for dermal monomorphic nests/strands below the scar as remnants of incomplete removal. Irregular epidermal melanocytes are confined to the area of fibrosis
		Melanocytic hyperplasia in melanoma re-excision	Melanocytes small, no nesting, in juxtaposition to scar or suture entry
Nests, even in size, at base of rete ridges	None	Junctional nevus	Elongated rete ridges, symmetric, well circumscribed
		Epidermal part of a congenital nevus	A sample cut, or taken from the periphery of a congenital nevus, can look just like a junctional nevus, check deeper sections for involvement of reticular dermis, especially perivascular and periadnexal
Nests, uneven in size	None	Junctional nevus, irritated, traumatized, or inflamed	Signs of trauma: parakeratosis, crust, erosion, ulceration, subepidermal fibrin, superficial fibrosis
		Epidermal part of a congenital nevus	Check deeper sections for involvement of reticular dermis by melanocytes
		Melanoma in situ, early/ nested	Focal single cells and/or scattered melanocytes

Table 5.1 (continued)

Patterns	Combination	Diagnoses	Solving differential diagnoses
Nests and single melanocytes, regular	Nests predominate over single melanocytes	Junctional nevus	Elongated rete ridges, symmetric
		Spitz nevus, junctional	Epithelioid cytology, amphophilic cytoplasm, Kamino bodies, melanocytes above the junction
		Reed nevus, junctional	Pigmented spindled cytology, hyperpigmented keratinocytes, band-like melanophages in upper dermis
		Congenital melanocytic nevus, surface	Check deeper sections for involvement of reticular dermis by melanocytes
Nests and single melanocytes, regular	Single melanocytes predominate over nests	Early junctional nevus	Lesion evolving from simple lentigo. Small, symmetric, no sun damage, slight elongation of rete ridges
		Naevus spilus	Large lesion, slight elongation of rete ridges, focal accentuation of nests in regular arrangement, no sun damage, clinical picture!
Nests and single melanocytes, irregular	Nests predominate over single melanocytes	Nested melanoma of the elderly	Asymmetry of the lesion, sun damage in the dermis, pleomorphism, age!
Nests and single melanocytes, irregular	Single melanocytes predominate over nests	Melanoma in situ	Asymmetry, poor circumscription

Table 5.2 Dermal patterns and differential diagnoses

Patterns	Combination	Diagnoses	Solving differential diagnoses
Nests	Maturation	Congenital nevus	Epidermal hyperplasia, terminal hair follicles, intraepidermal proliferation of melanocytes regularly distributed and symmetric over the dermal part, adnexocentrism, no crowding, monomorphic
		Spitz nevus, dermal	Variable epidermal part, if present should be mostly nested, symmetric, well circumscribed, epithelioid cytology, pleomorphism, no crowding, rare mitoses, sclerosis
		Melanoma	Intraepidermal irregular proliferation of melanocytes present the vast majority of melanomas; in some melanomas, maturation is seen, but it is much less prominent than in nevi. Check for pleomorphism, HMB45 expression, mitoses, asymmetric silhouette
Nests	No maturation	Melanoma	Intraepidermal irregular proliferation of melanocytes are present in the vast majority of melanomas
		Melanoma metastasis	Pleomorphism, mitoses, necrosis, crowding
		Blue nevus, cellular type	Second population of bipolar melanocytes, no epidermal involvement, no necrosis, no crowding, no mitoses
Interstitial strands	Maturation	Congenital nevus	Often adnexocentric distribution in deeper section, symmetric epidermal involvement can be present in the form of regular single cells and/or nests, papillomatous surface, terminal hair follicles within the lesion
		Sclerosing (Desmoplastic) Spitz nevus	Epithelioid cytology, pleomorphism, sclerosis, symmetric, well-circumscribed epidermal involvement can be present, nests should predominate

(continued)

Table 5.2 (continued)

Patterns	Combination	Diagnoses	Solving differential diagnoses
Interstitial strands	No maturation	Blue nevus, common type	Bipolar melanocytes, no epidermal involvement
		Blue nevus, cellular type	Bipolar melanocytes and a second epithelioid melanocytic proliferation, no epidermal involvement, no crowding, no mitoses
		Melanoma, primary	Asymmetry; epidermal part with predominance of single cells, suprabasal melanocytes, poor circumscription, crowding; mitoses not always present
		Melanoma metastasis	Crowding, mitoses, necrosis, usually no epidermal involvement
Nodules	No maturation	Blue nevus, cellular type	Second population of melanocyte with bipolar cytology must be present
		Melanoma, primary	Asymmetry, in the vast majority of cases epidermal part with predominance of single cells, suprabasal melanocytes, poor circumscription, crowding. Mitoses not always present
		Melanoma metastasis	Crowding, mitoses, necrosis, usually no epidermal involvement (except in rare epidermotropic metastasis over the dermal nodule)
		Proliferative nodule in congenital nevus	Age, surrounding monomorphic nests and/or strands of a congenital nevus. Mitoses common, typical forms
Plexiform fascicles	No maturation	Blue nevus	Bipolar melanocytes, no epidermal involvement, sclerotic collagen, no mitoses
		Deep penetrating nevus	Enlarged pigmented melanocytes, no mitoses, often combined with a conventional congenital nevus
		Pigmented epithelioid melanocytoma	Epithelioid and dendritic cells, heavily pigmented
Single cells, interstitial	No maturation	Dermal Spitz nevus	Epithelioid, amphophilic morphology, sclerosis
		BAP1-deficient nevi	Epithelioid with amphophilic cytoplasm, prominent nucleoli, often combined with "common" dermal nevi
		Desmoplastic melanoma	Spindled melanocytes; MelanA often not expressed, pleomorphism highly variable, mitosis may be lacking, sometimes irregular intraepidermal melanocytic proliferation
		Blue nevus	Bipolar melanocytes, melanophages
		Dermal melanocytosis (Ito/Ota, Mongolian Spot[a])	Bipolar melanocytes, clinical presentation!

[a] We discourage the use of the term "Mongolian" spot because we believe it is inappropriate to name diseases after ethnic groups

Table 5.3 Subcutaneous patterns and differential diagnoses

Patterns	Combination	Diagnoses	Solving differential diagnoses
Nests/interstitial strands	Maturation	Deep congenital nevus	In continuity with a congenital nevus in the dermis
Nests/interstitial strands	No maturation	Melanoma	Mitoses, necrosis, pleomorphism
		Deep penetrating nevus	Enlarged pigmented melanocytes, no mitoses, often combined with a conventional congenital nevus
Nodules	No maturation	Deep penetrating nevus	Enlarged pigmented melanocytes, no mitoses, often combined with a conventional congenital nevus
		Blue nevus Masson, "Neuronevus Masson"	Involvement of dermis and subcutis, second population of bipolar melanocytes must be present
		Melanoma metastasis/nodular melanoma	Crowding, mitoses, necrosis, usually no epidermal involvement

5.2 The Full Histologic Examination Procedure on the Basis of Examples

The following six examples of melanocytic lesions are presented each with a list of patterns observed in them followed by an integration weighting the observations and concluding a diagnosis. For educational purposes, this exercise is restricted to histomorphology on routine H/E slides. It intends to demonstrate how integration can be accomplished purely from morphological observation of well-defined patterns. Of course, in real life, clinical information, clinical appearance, and evolution of a lesion would be taken into account and, in difficult cases, ancillary methods such as immunohistochemistry and sometimes molecular techniques would need to be added. These aspects are addressed in the subsequent chapter on "Integration of Context."

The examination procedure always starts at scanning magnification assessing silhouette, circumscription, and symmetry. Then the epidermis is studied at intermediate magnifications over the entire front of the lesion followed by the same procedure in dermis and subcutis. Last, the cytology is assessed at high magnification. In a real slide, all sections seen on the slide should be assessed with the same procedure. After a close-up assessment it is very important to go back to scanning magnification and rethink the previous assessment of silhouette and circumscription.

5.2.1 Example 1

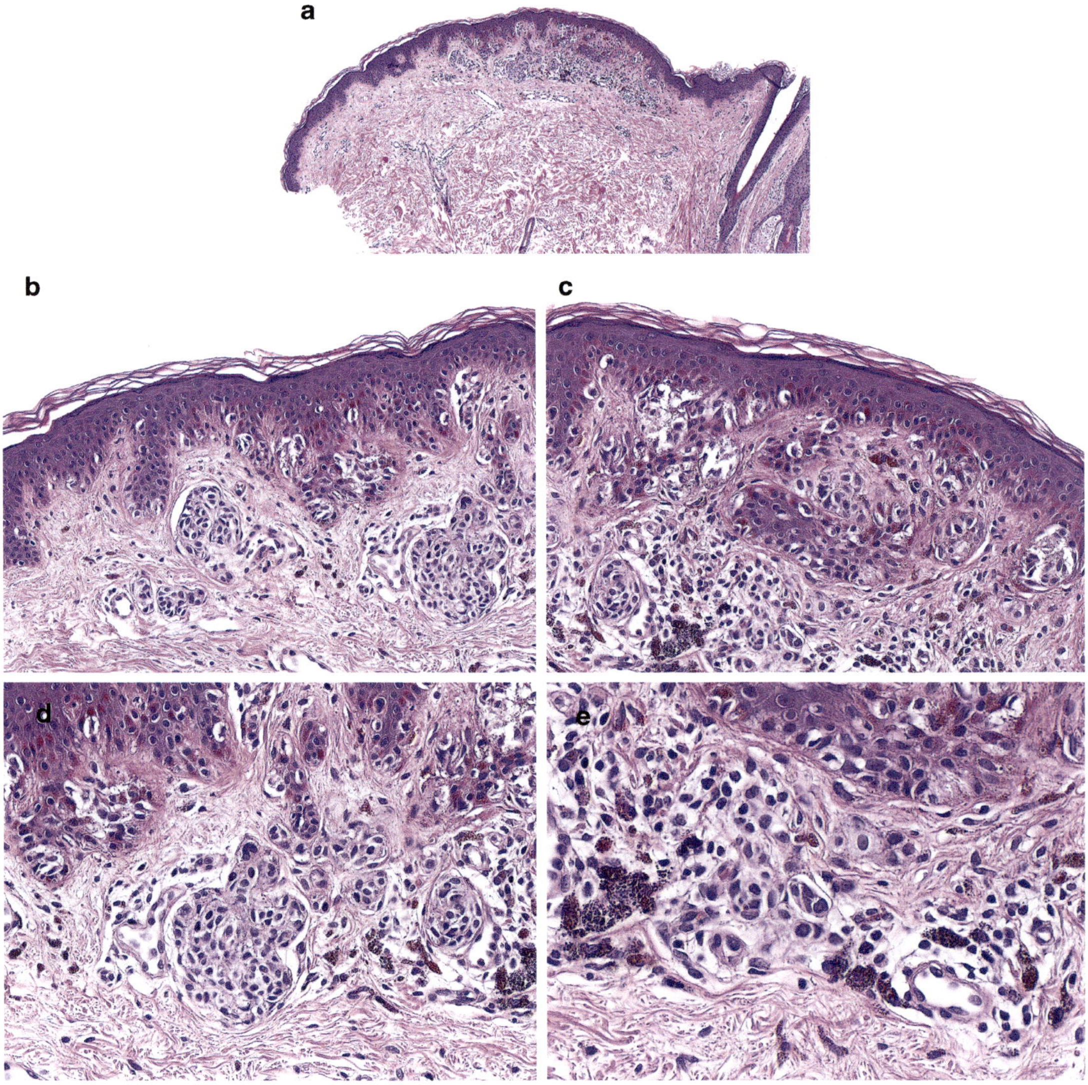

Fig. 5.1 (**a–e**) Example 1: compound nevus. (Courtesy of the Dermatologikum Hamburg)

Overall Pattern: Epidermal and Dermal, Nested, Small, Symmetric

Detailed Description

Silhouette

- Largely symmetrical
- Well circumscribed
- Small

Patterns

Epidermis

- Small nests at the base of rete ridges
- Some single cells between the nests, situated in the basal layer, regularly distributed
- Nests predominate over single cells
- No suprabasal melanocytes

Dermis

- Nests of melanocytes restricted to the papillary dermis
- Nests small, round, moderate variation in size

Cytology

- Monomorphic
- No crowding
- No nucleoli

Other Changes

- Elongated rete ridges
- Hyperpigmentation of basal keratinocytes

Integration

Within the epidermis, the lesion ends with a nest on both sides and is therefore well circumscribed (Fig. 5.1a–c). The epidermal part of the lesions is regularly arranged over the dermal part. A slight asymmetry is caused by melanophages and inflammatory infiltrate in the dermis (Fig. 5.1d, e), which may also account for an asymmetric clinical appearance. Large granules identify the asymmetric pigmented cells in the dermis as melanophages (Fig. 5.1e). In the lesion, a nested pattern is predominant. Epidermal melanocytes are positioned in the basal layer (Fig. 5.1b, c); dermal nests are restricted to the papillary dermis (Fig. 5.1a).

Diagnosis: Compound nevus.

5.2.2 Example 2

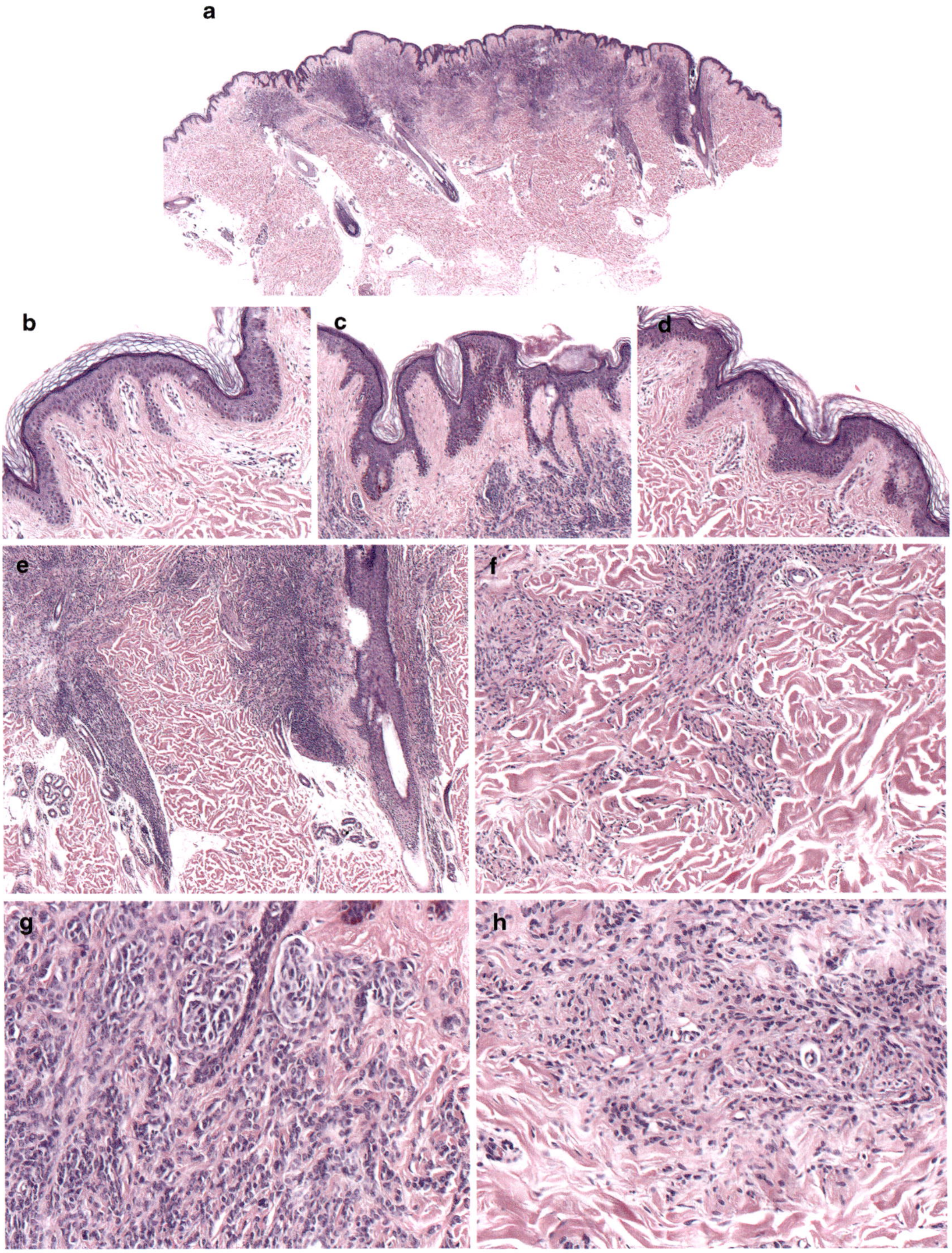

Fig. 5.2 (**a–h**) Example 2: Congenital melanocytic nevus. (Courtesy of the Dermatologikum Hamburg)

Overall Pattern: Dermal, Periadnexal, and Interstitial

Detailed Description

Silhouette

- Well circumscribed
- Largely dermal

Patterns

Epidermis

- Single cells situated in the basal layer increased in number, regularly distributed
- No suprabasal melanocytes

Dermis

- Nests of melanocytes in the upper dermis
- Periadnexal and interstitial melanocytes in strands
- Maturation

Cytology

- Monomorphic
- No crowding
- No nucleoli

Other Changes

- Elongated rete ridges
- Seborrheic keratosis-like epidermal hyperplasia with a papillated surface
- Hyperpigmentation of basal keratinocytes

Integration

Within the epidermis, the lesion shows only single melanocytes in the basal layer, regularly distributed (Fig. 5.2c). The epidermal part of the lesion is regularly arranged over the dermal part (Fig. 5.2a). The epidermis is markedly hyperplastic in a seborrheic keratosis-like fashion (Fig. 5.2b–d), which is seen often in congenital melanocytic nevi. The dermal proliferation is nested in the upper part and extends along adnexal structures and interstitially into the deeper dermis (Fig. 5.2c, e). The size of melanocytes in the deep dermis is smaller than those in the upper dermis as a sign of maturation (Fig. 5.2g, h). Some dermatopathologists refer to the type of dermal melanocytes seen here as type A (epithelioid) or type B (lymphoid) cells, but we do not use those terms in clinical or scientific practice.

Diagnosis: congenital melanocytic nevus.

5.2.3 Example 3

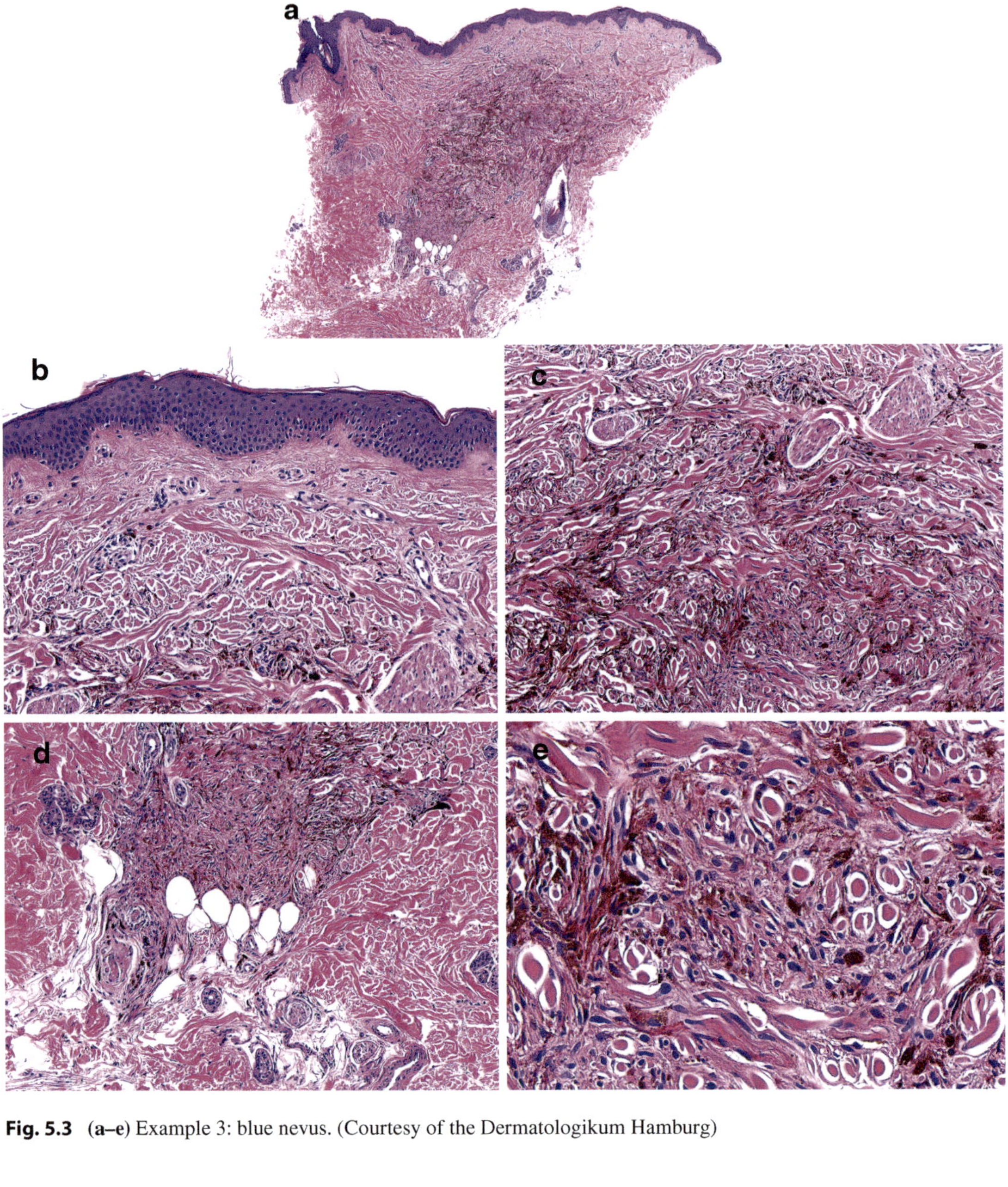

Fig. 5.3 (**a–e**) Example 3: blue nevus. (Courtesy of the Dermatologikum Hamburg)

Overall Pattern: Dermal, Interstitial

Detailed Description

Silhouette

- Well circumscribed, but somewhat asymmetrical
- Dermal, extending focally into superficial subcutis

Patterns

Epidermis

- None

Dermis

- Interstitial strands and fascicles

Cytology

- Spindled and bipolar, with fine melanin granules
- Monomorphic
- No crowding
- No nucleoli, no mitoses
- No prominent maturation

Other Changes

- Thickened collagen bundles at the periphery of the proliferation
- Numerous melanophages with large melanin granules

Integration

Within the epidermis, there are only a few regularly distributed single melanocytes in the basal layer (Fig. 5.3b). The proliferation of melanocytes is situated only in the dermis with focal extension into the superficial subcutis (Fig. 5.3a, c, d). Dermal melanocytes are arranged in an interstitial pattern in which circumscription and symmetry are not obvious. The arrangement, however, is uniform throughout the lesion. Irregularity is only present in the degree of pigmentation, which varies throughout the lesion both, in regard to pigmentation of melanocytes and to accompanying melanophages. Large granules identify the heavily pigmented cells in the dermis as melanophages. The melanocytes have a spindled and bipolar cytology, some with wavy nuclei similar to that seen in neural cells (Fig. 5.3.e). Pleomorphism, mitoses, and necroses are absent. This cytology, the regular arrangement and the lack of epidermal involvement are typical of a blue nevus. Sclerotic collagen bundles in blue nevi can be similar to those seen at the periphery of dermatofibromas, as it is seen here. Extension into the subcutis is not uncommon in blue nevi.

Diagnosis: blue nevus (so-called common blue nevus).

5.2.4 Example 4

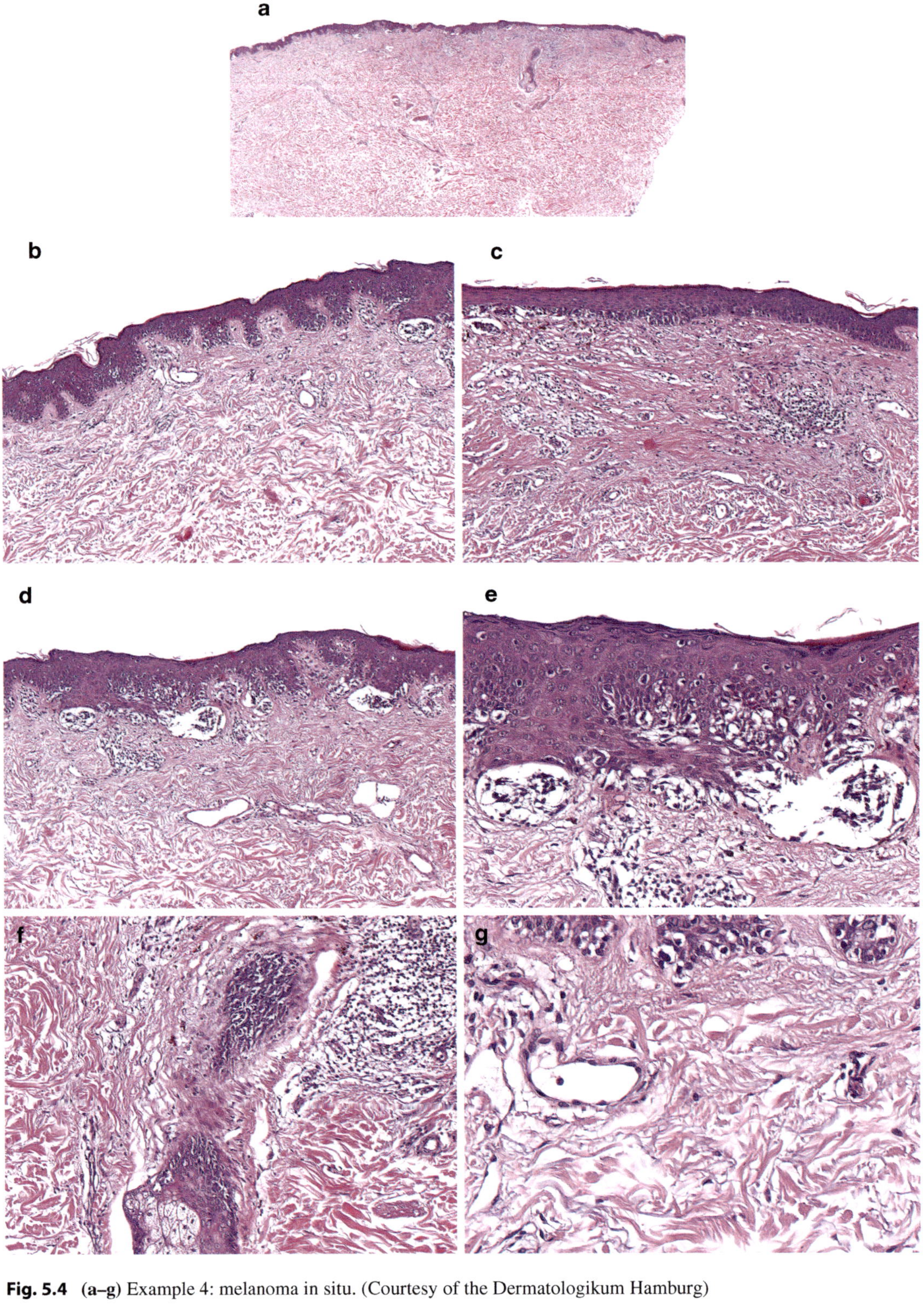

Fig. 5.4 (a–g) Example 4: melanoma in situ. (Courtesy of the Dermatologikum Hamburg)

Overall Pattern: Epidermal, Poorly Circumscribed, Single Melanocytes Predominate

Detailed Description

Silhouette

- Broad lesion
- Asymmetric
- Poorly circumscribed at both sides

Patterns

Epidermis

- Nests and single melanocytes, irregularly distributed
- Single cells predominate, especially at the periphery
- Confluence of nests
- Single melanocytes in suprabasal layers including the granular layer
- Prominent proliferations of single melanocytes in follicular epithelium

Dermis

- None

Cytology

- Relatively scant cytoplasm
- Slightly enlarged and irregular hyperchromatic nuclei
- No crowding, no nucleoli, no mitoses

Other Changes

- Flattened rete ridges and epidermal atrophy on one side of the lesion
- Prominent clefting around nests of melanocytes, also towards the dermis
- Area of fibrosis with horizontal collagen fibers
- Patchy lymphocytic infiltrates
- Patchy melanophages
- Solar elastosis below the lesion

Integration

At scanning magnification, this lesion is asymmetric, which is most obvious in the shape of the epidermis with focal flattening of rete ridges and epidermal atrophy (Fig. 5.4a–c). It seems relatively well circumscribed at first blush; however, intermediate and high magnifications show that single melanocytes extend far beyond the last nest on both sides (Fig. 5.4b, c), making this a large and poorly circumscribed proliferation. At high magnification the cytology is relatively bland, but scattered suprabasal melanocytes can be identified over the entire front of the lesion (Fig. 5.4e). The zone of fibrosis on the right is difficult to interpret. It has similarities to a superficial scar but in the context of patchy lymphocytic infiltrates and melanophages it is more likely a zone of regression (Fig. 5.4c). The localization of this lesion on sun-damaged skin (Fig. 5.4g) together with asymmetry, poor circumscription, and single cell predominance enable a diagnosis of melanoma in situ and the prominent clefting is another feature supporting the interpretation. In a lesion like this it is mandatory to do deeper cuts and immunostainings, e.g., with MelanA staining to check for a dermal component, especially in the context of an area of regression.

Diagnosis: Melanoma in situ.

5.2.5 Example 5

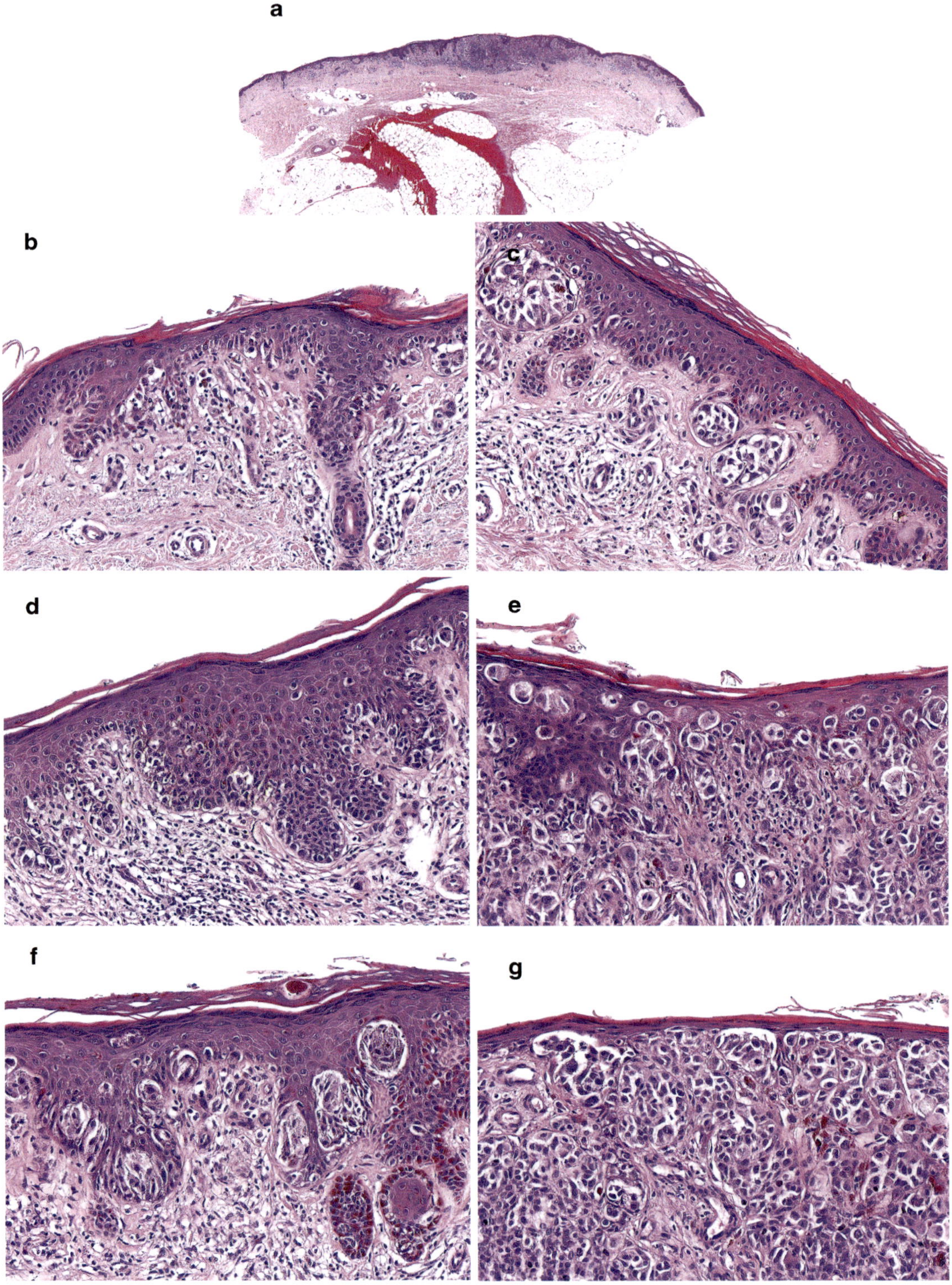

Fig. 5.5 (**a–i**) Example 5: invasive melanoma. (Courtesy of the Dermatologikum Hamburg)

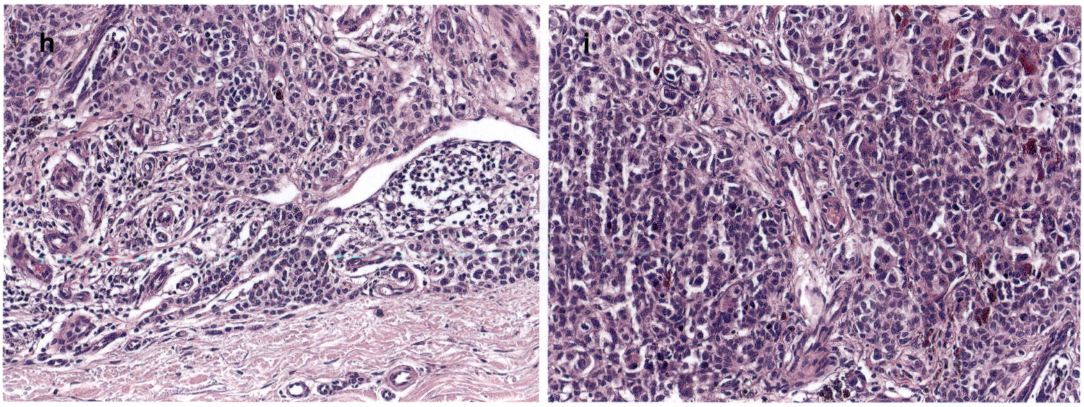

Fig. 5.5 (Continued)

Overall Pattern: Asymmetric, Broad, Epidermal and Dermal

Detailed Description

Silhouette

- Broad lesion
- Asymmetric
- Relatively well circumscribed at both sides

Patterns

Epidermis

- Nests and single melanocytes, irregularly distributed
- Nests vary in size and shape
- In some areas single cells predominate over nests
- Single melanocytes and nests are present in suprabasal layers including the granular and cornified layer, and suprapapillary epidermis

Dermis

- Nests of variable size
- Confluence of nests to larger aggregations
- Maturation in some areas lacking

Cytology

- Epithelioid and pagetoid
- Pleomorphic
- Crowding

Other Changes

- Epidermal atrophy ("consumption")
- Solar elastosis below the lesion

Integration

The lesion is strikingly asymmetric, even though it ends with nests on both sides in this section (Fig. 5.5a–c). The epidermal proliferation is positioned asymmetrically over the dermal part (Fig. 5.5a). The epidermis is focally thinned to only a few layers (Fig. 5.5g). The intraepidermal proliferation has zones with predominance of single cells and numerous melanocytes are present in suprabasal layers (Fig. 5.5 c–e). In the dermal part, some areas show maturation (Fig. 5.5.h) but in other zones, large epithelioid cells are present in the deep dermis (Fig. 5.5i).

Diagnosis: invasive melanoma.

5.2.6 Example 6

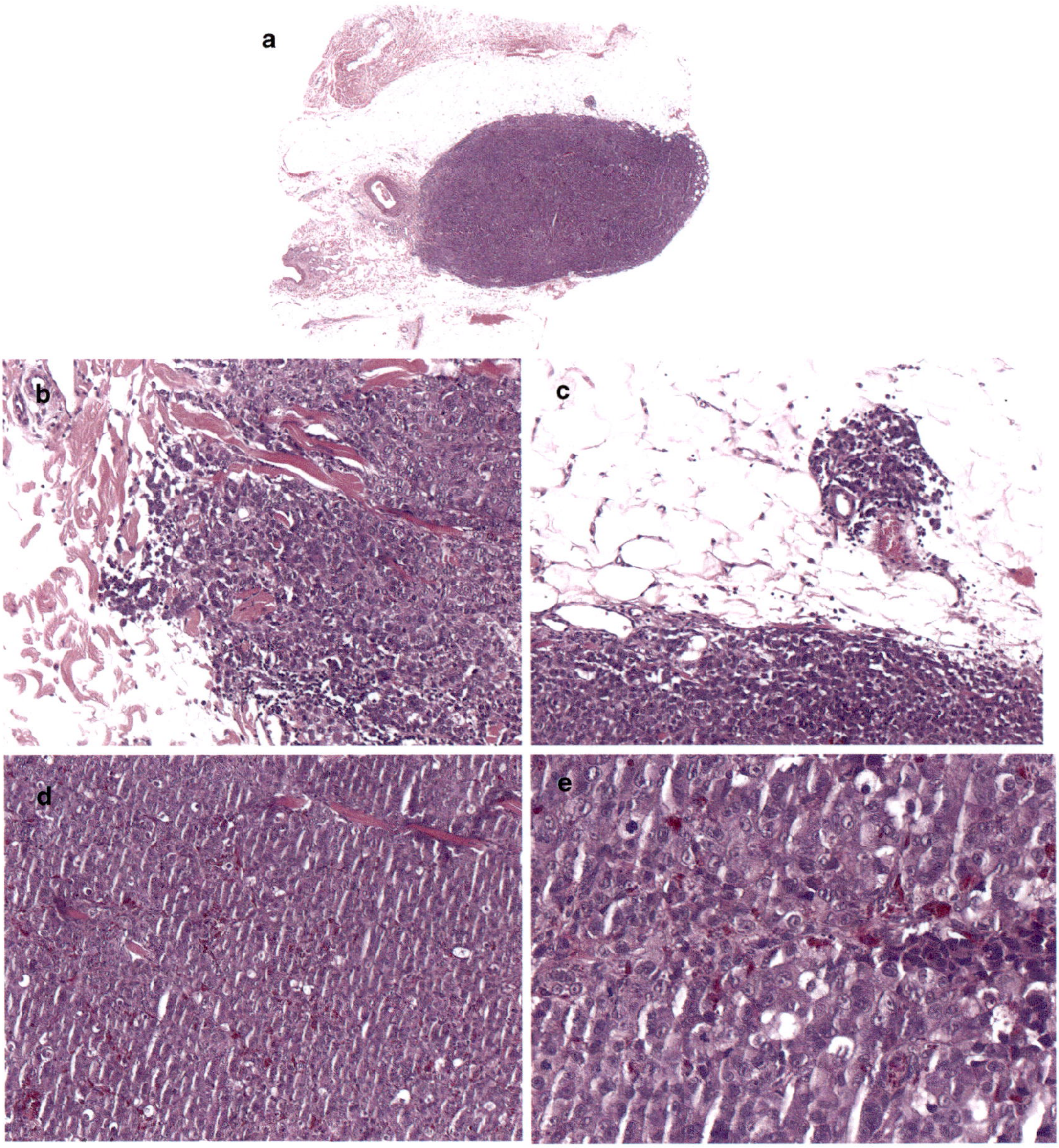

Fig. 5.6 (**a–e**) Example 6: melanoma metastasis. (Courtesy of the Dermatologikum Hamburg)

Overall Pattern: Subcutaneous, Nodular

Detailed Description

Silhouette

- Large nodule in the subcutis
- Mostly well circumscribed

Patterns

Subcutis

- Septal and lobular
- Large nodule and small nodule
- Sheets of cells replacing pre-existing tissue
- In some areas strands of cells in interstitial arrangement

Cytology

- Epithelioid melanocytes with fine melanin granules
- Crowding of nuclei
- Pleomorphism
- Prominent nucleoli
- Mitotic figures
- Necrosis *en masse*

Other Changes

- Melanophages

Integration

The close and crowded arrangement of pleomorphic melanocytes indicates malignancy (Fig. 5.6a, e). The architecture of a nodular lesion in the subcutis without epidermal and dermal parts is best interpreted as metastatic melanoma, which is further supported by the cytology, the number of mitoses, and the areas of necrosis (Fig. 5.6d, e). While the lesion seems well circumscribed as scanning magnification, there is an area of interstitial arrangement of cells (Fig. 5.6.b), which means that the lesion is actually not so well circumscribed in that focus. The smaller nodule at the side of the large aggregation (Fig. 5.6c) is not attracting much attention, but it demonstrates a striking variation in size and shape of aggregations, which also points towards a diagnosis of a malignant proliferation. In this case, the pleomorphic cells can be assumed to be melanocytes, because they have some fine intracellular pigment granules and they are accompanied by numerous melanophages (Fig. 5.6e). In other cases with similar architecture, this feature may be lacking and immunohistochemistry is required to confirm that the cells are truly melanocytes.

Diagnosis: melanoma metastasis.

5.3 Limitations of Pattern Analysis

In Tables 5.1, 5.2, and 5.3 we summarize common combinations of patterns of melanocytes and try to match the differential diagnoses considered in a specific combination of patterns with diagnoses given in the current WHO classification of melanocytic tumors [30]. It becomes apparent that some diagnoses, e.g., junctional nevus, appear repeatedly in the table because the condition may manifest itself with variable combinations of patterns, very few lesions appear just once, e.g., dermal melanocytosis, because they always look the same. This is akin to the situation of patterns of inflammatory skin diseases where, as an example, lupus erythematosus is found in the pattern "perivascular dermatitis" when it is a biopsy from a butterfly rash or in the pattern "panniculitis" when it involves the subcutis in the form of lupus profundus. Moreover, melanocytic lesions, just like inflammatory skin conditions, have a "life of lesion" meaning that they may change their appearance throughout the course of development from early to late. During that process, patterns of melanocytes seen under the microscope may change. Moreover, they may present with different combinations of patterns depending on how the lesion was grossed. If sections come from the periphery of the lesion, the combination of patterns likely will differ from that seen in a section cut in the center of the lesion.

In contrast, some disease entities given in the WHO classification of melanocytic tumors are not mentioned in Tables 5.1, 5.2, and 5.3 because they are not primarily defined by a specific pattern of melanocytes but rather by a secondary change or a specific feature such as accompanying inflammatory infiltrates or anatomic site. An example is Meyerson nevus which is typified by spongiosis and inflammatory infiltrate housing eosinophils. The Meyerson changes can be found in a junctional nevus, in a compound nevus, or in a dermal nevus. Another example is an acral nevus, which typically will show melanocytes above the basal layer, but that site-specific pattern occurs in junctional nevi, in compound nevi, in acquired and in congenital nevi, meaning that "acral nevus" includes in fact various types of nevi in acral localization.

Some entities of the WHO classification of melanocytic tumors are difficult to match with combinations of patterns given in Tables 5.1, 5.2, and 5.3 because the terms are used with variable definition and therefore likely refer to more than one disease entity. Examples would be "common nevus" or "dysplastic nevus." The term "common nevus" is frequently used by clinicians, albeit it has never been defined consistently. Sometimes it is contrasted with "atypical" or "dysplastic" nevus. Most commonly, however, "common nevus" stands for dermal nevus. Historically, dermal nevi have also been named eponymously either Unna nevus (a papillomatous dermal nevus on the trunk) or Miescher nevus (a dome-shaped dermal nevus on the face). From the point of view of pattern analysis both, Unna and Miescher nevi, are typified by a dermal pattern with periadnexal arrangement of small and monomorphous melanocytes in nests and strands (Figs. 5.7 and 5.8) indicative of a congenital nevus.

For reasons of completeness and because some of our readers surely will search for such terms we decided to include them here in Table 5.4. Together with each diagnosis we provide a description of associated changes and possible combinations of patterns of melanocytes and, where necessary, a comment or critique of the term.

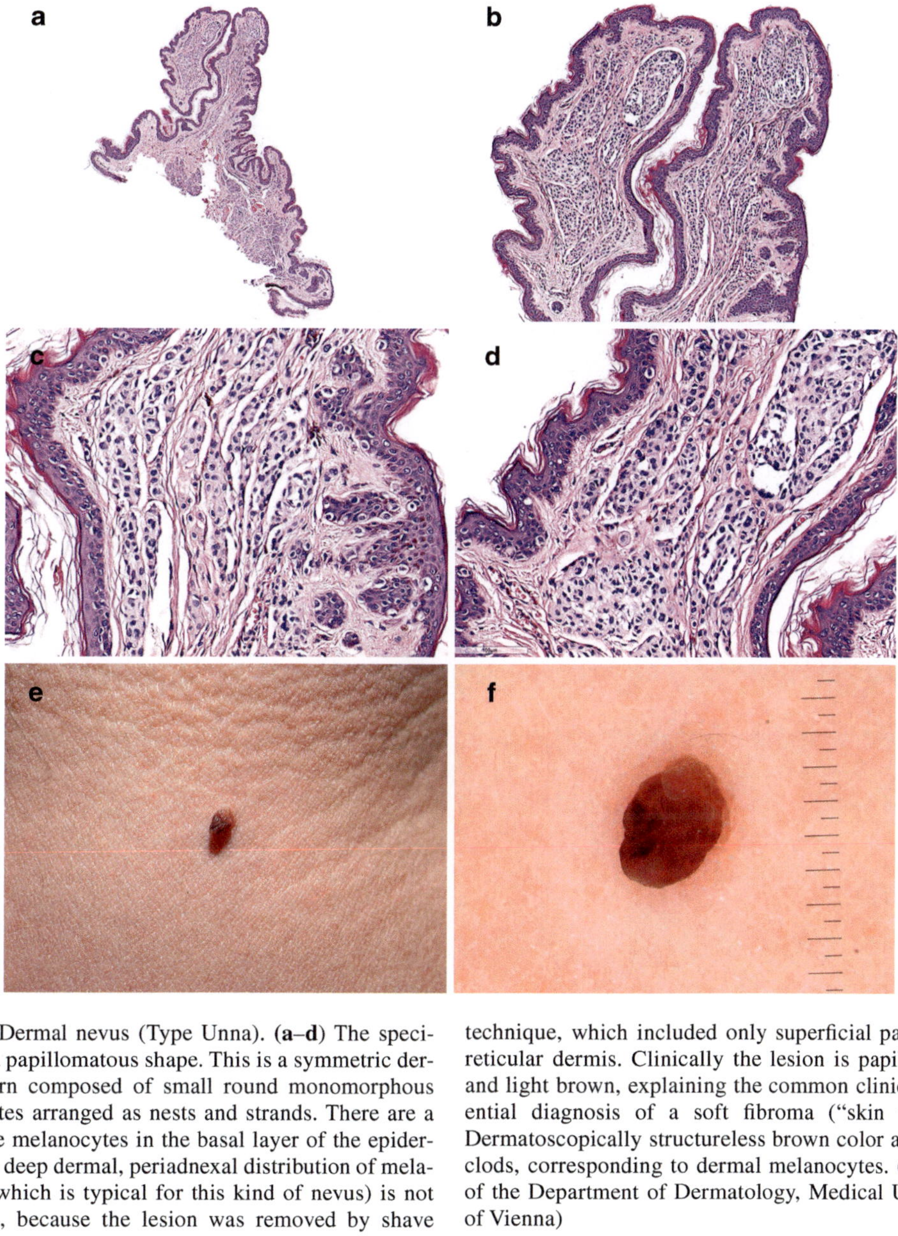

Fig. 5.7 Dermal nevus (Type Unna). (**a–d**) The specimen has a papillomatous shape. This is a symmetric dermal pattern composed of small round monomorphous melanocytes arranged as nests and strands. There are a few single melanocytes in the basal layer of the epidermis. (**e**) A deep dermal, periadnexal distribution of melanocytes (which is typical for this kind of nevus) is not seen here, because the lesion was removed by shave technique, which included only superficial parts of the reticular dermis. Clinically the lesion is papillomatous and light brown, explaining the common clinical differential diagnosis of a soft fibroma ("skin tag"). (**f**) Dermatoscopically structureless brown color and brown clods, corresponding to dermal melanocytes. (Courtesy of the Department of Dermatology, Medical University of Vienna)

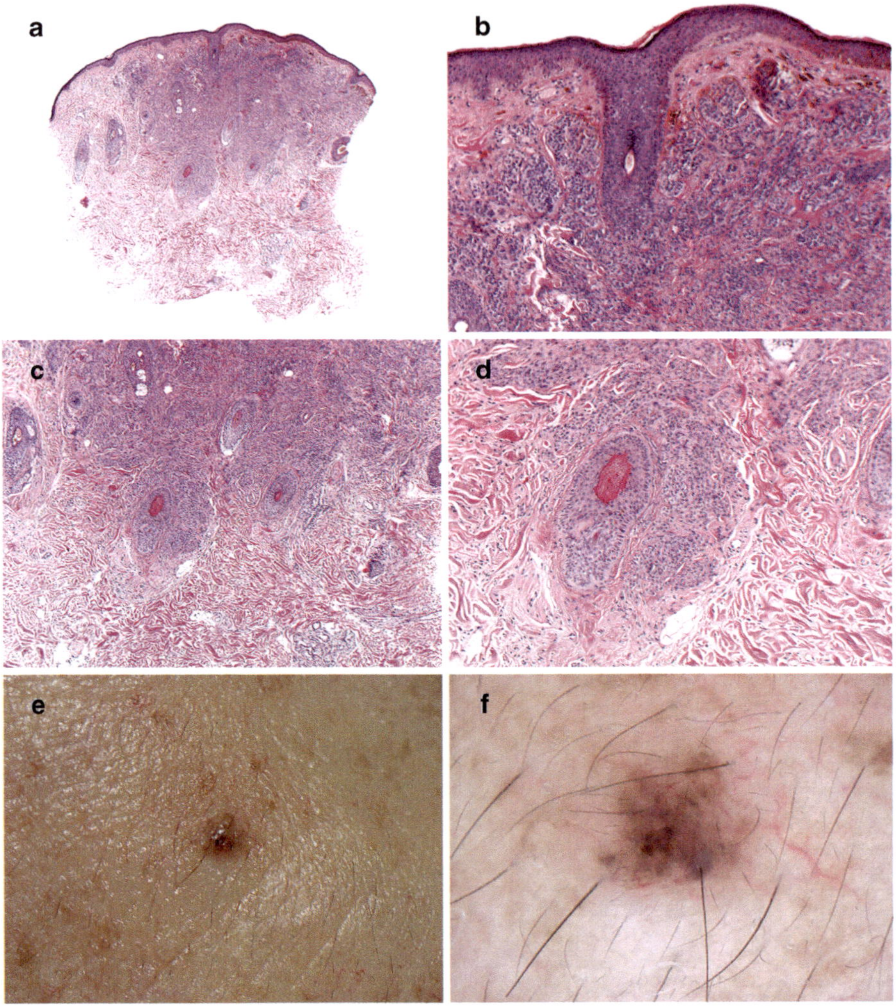

Fig. 5.8 Dermal nevus (Type Miescher). (**a–d**) The specimen has a dome-shaped surface. This is a symmetric dermal pattern composed of small round monomorphous melanocytes arranged diffusely and as nests in perifollicular arrangement typical of congenital nevi. Superficial melanocytes harbor increased melanin pigment, with surrounding melanophages. (**e**) Clinically the lesion is dome shaped with light-brown to dark-brown color. (**f**) Dermatoscopically there is structureless brown, corresponding to dermal melanophages. Central dark-brown to gray clods correspond to melanophages and melanocytes with increased pigment in the superficial dermis, and may lead to the clinical differential diagnosis of basal cell carcinoma. (Courtesy of the Department of Dermatology, Medical University of Vienna)

Table 5.4 Diagnoses defined by secondary changes, body site, or conceptual framework

Associated changes	Patterns of melanocytes	Diagnosis	Comment
Spongiosis and an infiltrate of lymphocytes and eosinophils	Epidermal only or epidermal and dermal Single melanocytes and nests at the base of rete ridges	Meyerson nevus	Meyerson nevus is defined by the presence of spongiosis and inflammatory infiltrate containing eosinophils The epidermal changes may obscure the melanocytic lesion; immunohistochemistry helps to identify the patterns of melanocytes
Band-like infiltrate of lymphocytes and histiocytes, sometimes granulomas	Epidermal, epidermal and dermal, or dermal only Often periadnexal pattern in the dermis	Halo nevus	In most instances, Halo nevus is a small congenital nevus, but since it represents a process of regression, epidermal and/or dermal parts of the lesion may be missing Due to the effects of the infiltrate cytologic features of Halo nevi can appear somewhat pleomorphic
Anatomic site: palms and soles, nail apparatus, ear, mamilla, scalp, umbilicus, genital, milkline	Irregular distribution of single melanocytes in the epidermis Single melanocytes in suprabasal layers	Special site nevus, acral nevus	These sites of the body are grouped under the heading "special" because nevi may show irregularly distributed and/or suprabasal melanocytes On mamilla and umbilicus features of trauma may be superimposed
Dermal nevus with congenital features	Dermal with periadnexal pattern	Common nevus	Depending on location this type of nevus has also been named Miescher nevus (face) or Unna nevus (trunk)
Combination of two or more cellular components	Dermal and epidermal and dermal, often with congenital features	Combined nevus	The most common combinations are "common" nevus with blue nevus, "common" nevus with Spitz nevus, and "common" nevus with deep penetrating nevus. BAP-1 inactivated nevi may also appear in combination with a "common" nevus
Inconsistent, features, depending on school of training	Architectural disorder, junctional shoulders, bridging of nests, cytological atypia	Dysplastic nevus, Clark nevus, atypical nevus; large atypical nevus; B-K mole; atypical mole; melanocytic dysplasia; nevus with architectural disorder and melanocytic atypia	Architectural disorder and cytologic atypia, the necessary and sufficient features of "dysplastic" nevi, are not clearly defined and are subject to a high degree of subjectivity, resulting in low interobserver agreement in the diagnosis of "dysplastic" nevi [68]

6 Integration of Context

Histomorphology is at the heart of pattern analysis, but is sometimes insufficient for a definitive diagnosis. Inclusion of information beyond histomorphology, such as patient age, anatomic location, medical history, and clinical and dermatoscopic images (if available), is essential in difficult cases. Immunohistochemical or molecular studies may be useful to solve some diagnostic dilemmas but we do not recommend using these tools uncritically. Information beyond histomorphology can sometimes be misleading and confusing, especially when it relates to fields outside one's area of expertise. Pathologists who do not have training in clinical dermatology tend to distrust clinical information even when it could be useful, or they tend to put too much weight on molecular findings with dubious significance. In contrast, dermatologists who specialize in dermatopathology tend to place too much weight on clinical information or dermatoscopic images.

It would, however, be a big mistake to disregard the clinical context entirely. This type of error is called "base rate neglect." The same constellation of findings may have different significance depending on whether it is observed in a high- or low-prevalence population. Unfortunately, there is a common misconception that pathologists should not be influenced by findings outside of pathology. This is certainly true when it comes to describing histomorphology, which should be as independent and objective as possible, but it is certainly false when it comes to integrating all findings into a final diagnosis. In many situations, and the pathology of melanocytic skin lesions is no exception, the final diagnosis is expected from pathology. This means that the role of the pathologist is not just to provide a piece of the puzzle, but to solve the puzzle. This can sometimes only be accomplished by incorporating information outside of pathology. If the pathologist's expertise does not allow for the integration of all the information, or if this information is withheld from the pathologist, then pathology is not the gold standard, but merely one piece of the puzzle, and it is up to someone else, preferably the clinician responsible for the patient, to put all the pieces together.

The best approach to integrating additional information is to first look at the slide without knowledge of the context. In most cases, this is sufficient and the unbiased and independent evaluation of the slide alone will lead to a single, definitive diagnosis. Additional information is not required, but can be used for confirmation if desired. In typical cases, ancillary tests, such as immunohistochemistry, will not be needed. We are aware that in some laboratories immunohistochemistry is routinely performed for all melanomas and there are even some local standards that mandate it. Furthermore, some pathologists prefer to assess the symmetry and circumscription of a melanocytic lesion by immunohistochemical stainings with melanocyte markers. In general, however, ancillary tests should be ordered when

A. Böer-Auer et al., *Pattern Analysis for Histopathologic Diagnosis of Melanocytic Lesions*,
https://doi.org/10.1007/978-3-031-07666-4_6

the diagnosis is uncertain and when the test is likely to answer a specific question critical to the diagnosis. If, for example, a definitive diagnosis cannot be made by histomorphology alone, contextual information and additional testing should be obtained to increase or decrease the likelihood of differential diagnoses. The part of the biopsy of an acral lesion shown in Fig. 6.1 looks like a nevus but one quick look at the clinical image may save you from making a big mistake (Fig. 6.2). This is the rare case of a melanoma that developed in association with an acral nevus and a partial biopsy can be misleading due to sampling error.

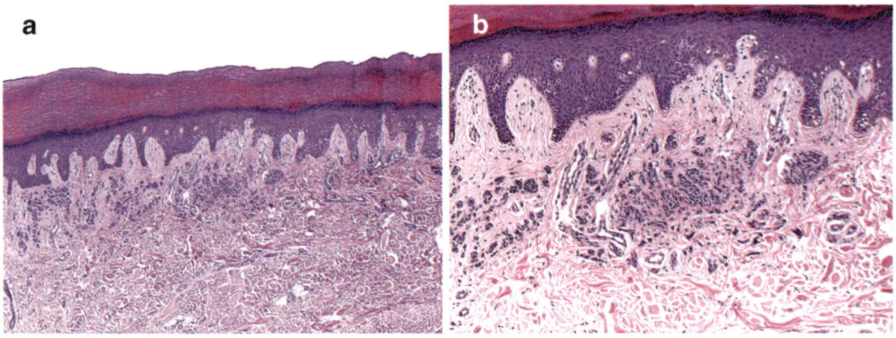

Fig. 6.1 (**a**, **b**) The melanoma that is associated with this acral nevus is hardly visible in this part of the specimen and can be easily missed if it is not correlated with the clinical image shown in Fig. 6.2. (Courtesy of the Department of Dermatology, Medical University of Vienna)

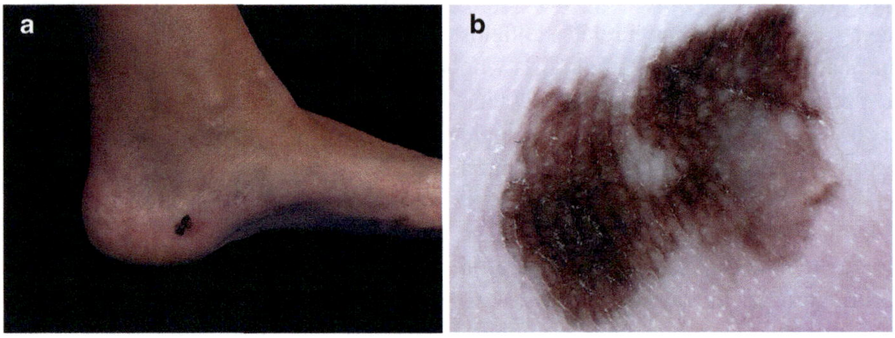

Fig. 6.2 (**a**, **b**) Clinical (**a**) and dermatoscopic (**b**) image that correspond to the specimen shown in Fig. 6.1. These images are not consistent with the diagnosis of nevus. This is a melanoma that developed in association with an acral nevus and a partial biopsy can be misleading. (Courtesy of the Department of Dermatology, Medical University of Vienna)

We recognize that there are situations that are uncertain by default, such as ruling out melanoma in situ in the nail matrix, and in these situations immunohistochemical studies are truly essential. We will provide examples of these situations later in this chapter. Before that, we will discuss the three main pillars of contextual information and ancillary tests that are most commonly needed in routine clinical practice: clinical context, in vivo imaging including dermatoscopy, and immunohistochemistry. The first two pillars will be discussed in more detail, and the audience we have in mind is pathologists with little or no knowledge of clinical dermatology. At the end of the chapter we will discuss ancillary molecular tests and their usefulness.

6.1 Clinical Context

Ideally, the referral slip will contain all essential information, such as the patient's age, sex, skin type, anatomic site, lesion size, history, clinical differential diagnoses, and other relevant information such as known genetic predispositions to melanoma, and ideally, the referral slip will not overload the pathologist with irrelevant information. We all know that in reality this is not always the case but we should at least convince our referrers that this information is important because it can steer the final diagnosis one way or the other. Most, but not all, melanomas are pigmented and the usual differential diagnoses clinically are nevi, pigmented seborrheic keratoses and pigmented basal cell carcinoma. Amelanotic melanomas are usually biopsied or excised under a different differential diagnosis such as wart, angioma, or basal cell carcinoma.

The incidence of melanoma, like that of most malignant neoplasms, increases with age. The peak incidence of melanoma is at age 55. Melanoma is extremely rare in prepubertal children. Melanomas in prepubertal children occur either in congenital nevi, or when they occur de novo, they often have Spitz-like features. De novo melanomas in children are often removed by the referring physician under another diagnosis such as wart or nevus. The risk of melanoma developing in a congenital nevus increases with the size of the nevus, but is generally low even in giant congenital nevi. In the past, the risk has been overestimated because of reporting bias. Most melanomas in adults occur de novo and only 20–25% of all melanomas occur in association with a nevus [44, 69]. Most nevi appear and grow in childhood and during adolescence. This means that a changing lesion in an adult has other significance than a changing lesion in a child.

Melanoma may occur at any site but shows some anatomic preferences. The back is the most common anatomic site for melanomas in males, while in females, melanomas occur more frequently on the lower leg. Some melanoma subtypes such as desmoplastic melanoma and lentigo maligna melanoma occur preferentially on chronic sun-damaged skin. Mucosal melanoma is rare and usually occurs later in life, although this finding may be influenced by later detection.

Some nevus subtypes prefer some anatomic sites and others such as Spitz and Reed nevi are more common in children than in adults. Spitz and Reed nevi often grow rapidly and cause concern to parents. For unknown reasons, Spitz nevi are relatively common on the face in children, but they can occur in any location. There is no preferred site for Reed nevi. Lesions with patterns of Spitz or Reed nevi in adults should be viewed with greater caution. The risk that a proliferation with a Spitz-like pattern is actually a melanoma rather than a nevus increases with age. However, there is no generally accepted age threshold, and Spitz and Reed nevi have also been diagnosed in individuals older than 60 years, although this is an exception. In the authors' opinion, the diagnosis of Spitz or Reed nevus should be made with caution in persons older than 50 years. For reasons that are probably related to the external factors such as hair epilation, nevi with Spitz-like features are relatively common on the legs in young to middle-aged females. This is a typical example of how gender, anatomic site, and age may influence histopathology in a complex way. An expert dermatopathologist will take this into account when making a final diagnosis.

Nevi on special sites such as the mucosa, milkline, scalp, genito-anal region, and nevi of the nail matrix are often congenital even if invisible at birth. Small congenital nevi are usually not present or not visible at birth and are therefore sometimes called "tardive" congenital nevi by clinicians, but most often their congenital nature is not comprehended and they are referred to as "acquired nevi," "atypical," "dysplastic" nevi, "common" nevi, or "Clark nevi." Histopathologically, they often share "congenital" features such as the dermal pattern and adnexocentricity. Congenital nevi may clinically mimic melanoma and may fulfill the ABCD criteria. They may be asymmetric and multicolored with irregular borders and the diameter may be larger than 1 cm. Congenital nevi of the nail matrix are of special concern because they may be indistinguishable from melanomas clinically. Good clinicians will know that and will usually be very reluctant to biopsy melanocytic proliferations of the nail matrix in prepubertal children. If monitored over time, congenital nevi of the nail matrix often decrease in size and become lighter or even vanish completely.

In facial lesions, the diagnosis of a "junctional," "dysplastic," "atypical," or "Clark nevus" should be made with great caution. Purely junctional nevi do not usually occur on the face, especially in older patients with evidence of chronic sun damage. In these cases, the diagnosis of melanoma in situ should always be considered even if the typical criteria of melanoma are not pronounced or largely absent. To a lesser extent this is also true for non-facial purely junctional lesions on chronically sun-damaged skin, especially if they are broad and poorly circumscribed. Severe chronic sun damage increases the likelihood of melanoma and the threshold for the diagnosis of melanoma should be lowered.

Melanoma is common in individuals with lighter skin type (Fitzpatrick skin type I and II) and rare in individuals with darker skin, especially in Fitzpatrick skin type V and VI. Some melanoma subtypes, such as acral and mucosal melanomas, can be found with a similar frequency across all skin types. About 10% of melanomas occur in melanoma prone families. Melanoma susceptibility is associated with specific phenotypes and genotypes and this information may be of interest to pathologists because it will increase the likelihood of melanoma. There are high- and low-penetrance melanoma susceptibility genes and usually only the high-penetrance genes will have practical value. The most commonly found germline mutations occur in the CDKN2A gene, which is found in 20–40% of melanoma prone families. Less commonly, mutations are found in other susceptibility genes such as CDK4, BAP1, TERT, POT1, ACD, TERF2IP, and MITF, which together account for only 10% of germline mutations in melanoma families. It is important to note that the penetrance of germline mutations, especially of germline mutations in the CDKN2A gene, varies and may be modulated by other factors. Germline mutations in high-penetrance melanoma susceptibility genes are often linked to the phenotype of multiple moles. If this phenotype occurs in the background of a family history of melanoma, it has been called "familial multiple mole melanoma syndrome" (FAMMM) or "dysplastic nevus syndrome". The definitions of FAMMM and the "dysplastic nevus syndrome" vary and have been modified over time [69, 70]. As a result, these terms have been used inconsistently by clinicians. We prefer to use the term FAMMM instead of "dysplastic nevus syndrome" because the term "dysplastic" and the controversies that arose from it did a lot of damage to our field and did certainly not improve the understanding of the biology of melanocytic proliferations.

It is important to know that FAMMM increases the likelihood of melanoma irrespective of the underlying germline mutations and this should be taken into account when dealing with a particular lesion. In many families with FAMMM, no germline mutation can be detected. On the other hand, the risk of melanoma may also be significantly increased due to germline mutations that do not increase nevus counts. The prototypic example is Xeroderma pigmentosum, a hereditary condition that is typified by high UV-sensitivity and high risk of skin cancer, including keratinocyte cancer and melanoma (see also Fig. 1.1 of Chap. 1)

6.2 In Vivo Imaging

"A picture is worth a thousand words." This phrase is overused, but nevertheless true. To put it more directly, we believe that in vivo images of melanocytic proliferations are an integral part of gross pathology. In vivo images are an essential component of clinical decision making and may provide useful information to the pathologist. The most common types of in vivo imaging techniques relevant to the topic of this book are conventional photographs, either as overview or close-up images, dermoscopy (dermatoscopy), and in vivo confocal microscopy. The latter examination achieves a resolution close to that of conventional light microscopy. Ex vivo dermatoscopy and ex vivo confocal microscopy are increasingly being used by pathologists and are blurring the traditional boundaries between dermatology and dermatopathology.

Total body or overview photographs are commonly used in practice for documentation and follow-up of patients with multiple nevi [71]. They are of limited importance to the pathologist because they are not usually included with the referral. In addition, because of their sensitive nature with respect to privacy, total body images are not easily accessible, even through electronic health records. Even when available, the information is of limited value in diagnosing a particular lesion. However, it is good to know that sequential whole-body imaging is used by clinicians to select either new or changing lesions for biopsy or excision to rule out melanoma (Fig. 6.3).

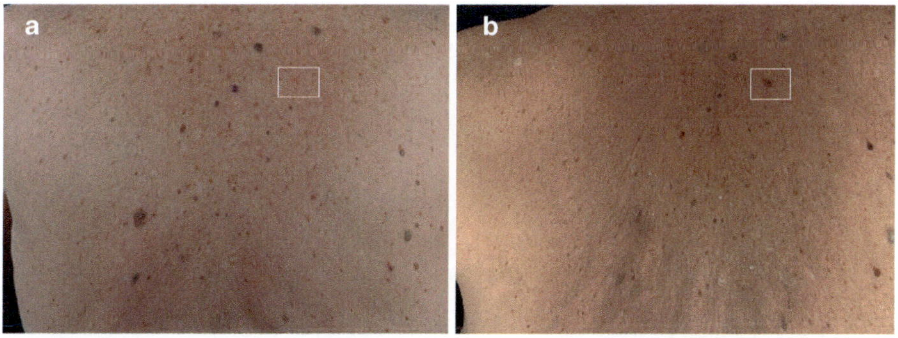

Fig. 6.3 (**a**, **b**) A new lesion appearing on the back of a patient with multiple moles documented by total body photography. The left photograph (**a**) was taken 6 years before the right photograph (**b**). The new lesion was a melanoma. (Courtesy of the Department of Dermatology, Medical University of Vienna)

This objective information about the biologic behavior of melanocytic lesions may be important in making a definitive diagnosis in cases of doubt. Total body photography is also a great tool to understand the concept of the "ugly duckling" approach, which attempts to find the one outlier among multiple similar looking lesions [72, 73]. It is a comparative approach that takes the variability of nevi in a particular patient into account. It assumes that "individuals have a nevus archetype and that deviations from this archetype may indicate malignancy" [2] (Fig. 6.4).

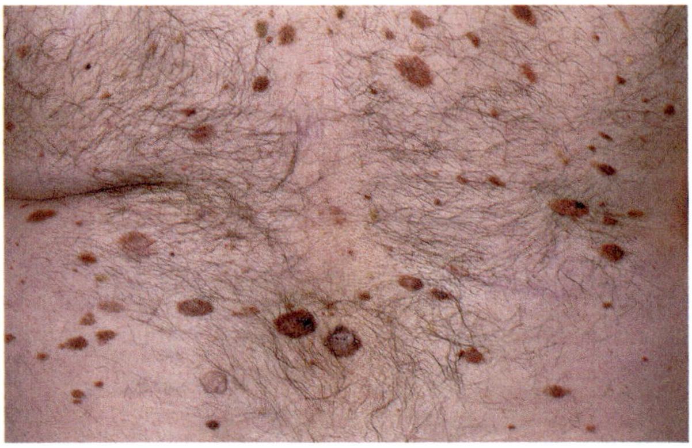

Fig. 6.4 In patients with multiple nevi or the FAMMM syndrome, clinicians often select lesions according to the "ugly duckling" principle. This patient has many large moles. If removed, most of them would show histopathologic patterns and features of congenital nevi. The lesion on the lower back with multiple shades of brown and eccentric hyperpigmentation is different from the others and would be selected for excision by most clinicians. It was not a melanoma, though, it was a compound nevus with congenital features. Congenital nevi may mimic melanoma. (Courtesy of the Department of Dermatology, Medical University of Vienna)

Clinical close-up and dermatoscopy photos are probably the most common types of visual documentation used by clinicians. In many cases, clinical close-ups will be sufficient to make a diagnosis. Dermatoscopy usually adds information but it needs some expertise. As in dermatopathology, the interpretation of clinical close-ups and dermatoscopy images follows the principles of pattern analysis. The only difference to pathology is that the basic elements that form the patterns in the macroscopic world are not melanocytes, because the resolutions reached with the unaided eye and dermatoscopy are not high enough. Symmetry and asymmetry, however, are basic principles of pattern analysis in all visual worlds, irrespective of resolution. While the pathologist only observes the arrangement of melanocytes in vertical sections that are a few micrometers thick, the clinician is able to observe the distribution of pigment in the entire lesion. The clinician's view is the horizontal plane but he also receives information about the vertical distribution of melanin, because melanin appears black and brown if located in the epidermis and gray and blue if situated in the dermis. Examination with dermatoscopy reveals more structural details than examination with the unaided eye (Fig. 6.5). With the unaided eye, symmetry and asymmetry is based merely on the distribution of color, while with dermatoscopy it is based on color and structure. Dermatoscopic structures are lines, dots and clods, and circles; these three elements form all patterns in dermatoscopy. Dermatoscopy is very simple if taught the right way and the basic principles can be understood in less than 1 h. Pathologists, who usually have a certain visual talent and are good in discerning patterns, will have no difficulty learning it quickly.

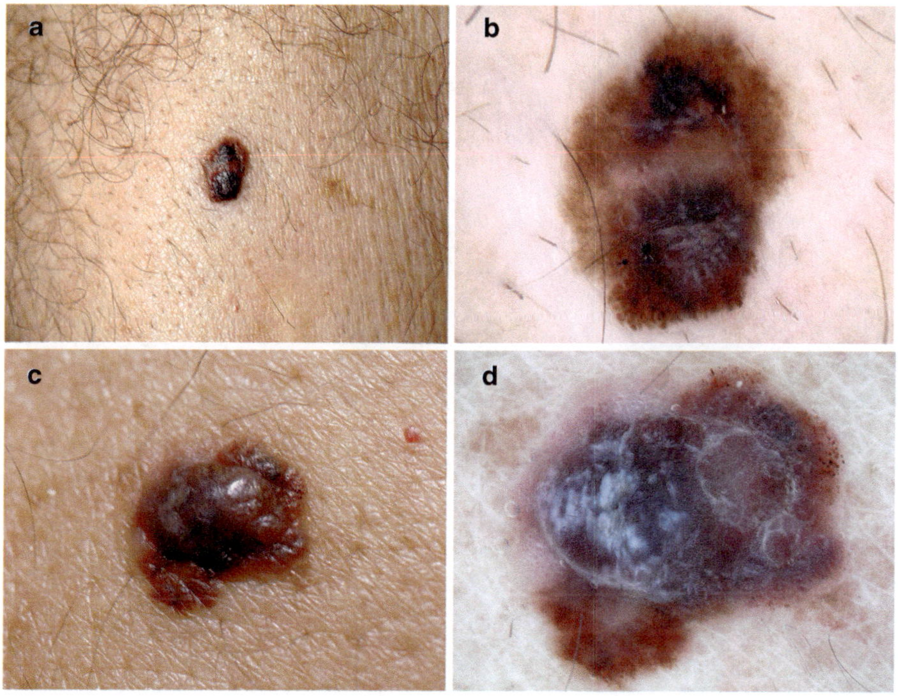

Fig. 6.5 (**a–d**) Two melanomas viewed with the unaided eye (**a**, **c**) and with dermatoscopy (**b**, **d**). Dermatoscopy shows more details. Both melanomas are chaotic with regard to the arrangement of colors and structures. In both melanomas, multiple patterns (dots, clods, lines, and structureless areas) are present. The dermatoscopy of the melanoma in the second row shows blue color and white lines, which indicate a thick tumor, most probably thicker than 1 mm. (Courtesy of the Department of Dermatology, Medical University of Vienna)

In vivo reflectance confocal microscopy is currently not as broadly available as dermatoscopy. While most clinicians who biopsy or remove melanocytic lesions will have a dermatoscope, in vivo confocal microscopes are mainly found in specialized centers. Confocal microscopy is an excellent adjunctive examination that may increase the likelihood of a suspected diagnosis to certainty or may exclude a diagnosis. Because it is time consuming and because the acquisition costs are considerable, it is usually used in specific situations. A typical situation would be whether or not to perform a biopsy or excision of a flat pigmented facial lesions (Fig. 6.6).

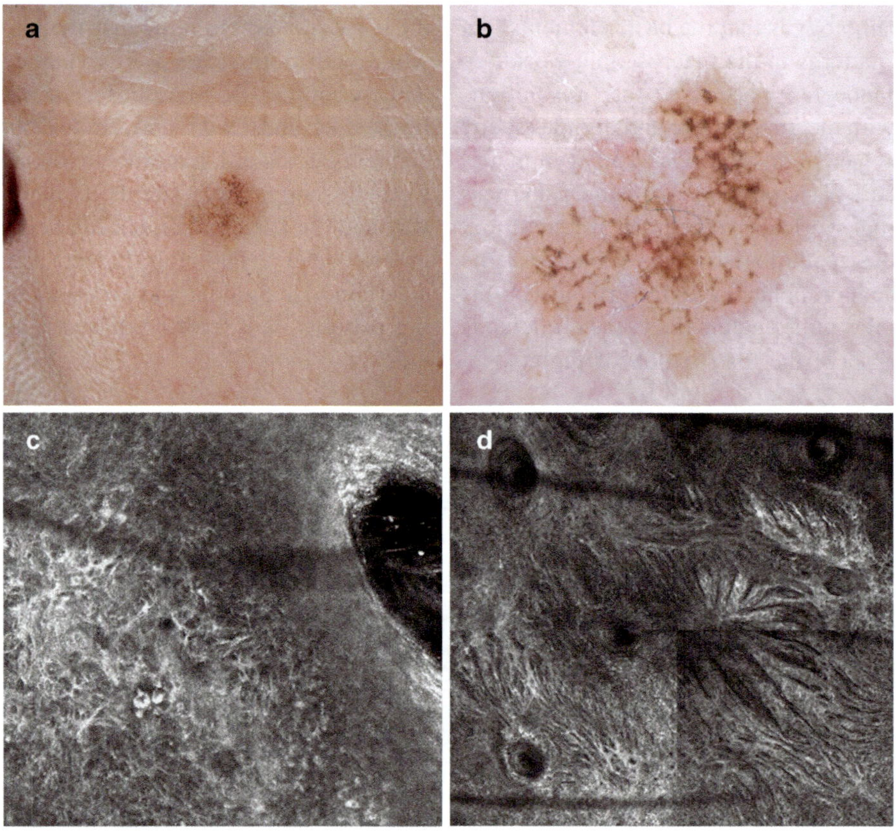

Fig. 6.6 (**a–d**) In vivo reflectance confocal microscopy of a melanoma in situ. When viewed with the unaided eye (**a**) the flat pigmented lesion on the cheek could be a melanoma in situ or a solar lentigo. By dermatoscopy (**b**), melanoma in situ becomes more likely but still not certain enough to excise the lesion without confirmation by a biopsy. With confocal microscopy (**c**, **d**) the diagnosis of melanoma in situ becomes certain. Dendritic melanocytes are present at the basal layer of the epidermis and in the follicular infundibulum. (Courtesy of the Department of Dermatology, Medical University of Vienna)

6.3 Ex Vivo Dermatoscopy

Some dermatopathologists use ex vivo dermatoscopy as part of their standard gross examination of the tissue before grossing. Dobrosavlijevic et al. demonstrated that ex vivo dermatoscopy increased specificity for all types of tumors but especially for melanoma, for which it also increased sensitivity [74]. The advantages are obvious. It may help to optimize grossing, it increases the point of view by adding another dimension (the horizontal view), and it may be useful for the diagnosis of doubtful lesions if the clinician did not care to include a photo (Fig. 6.7). Moreno-Romero and coworkers described a procedure they called "derm-dotting," which can be performed in vivo and ex vivo [75]. They used nail polish to mark small suspicious areas by dermatoscopy to guide the pathologist, which could be useful to detect melanomas that develop in association with a nevus.

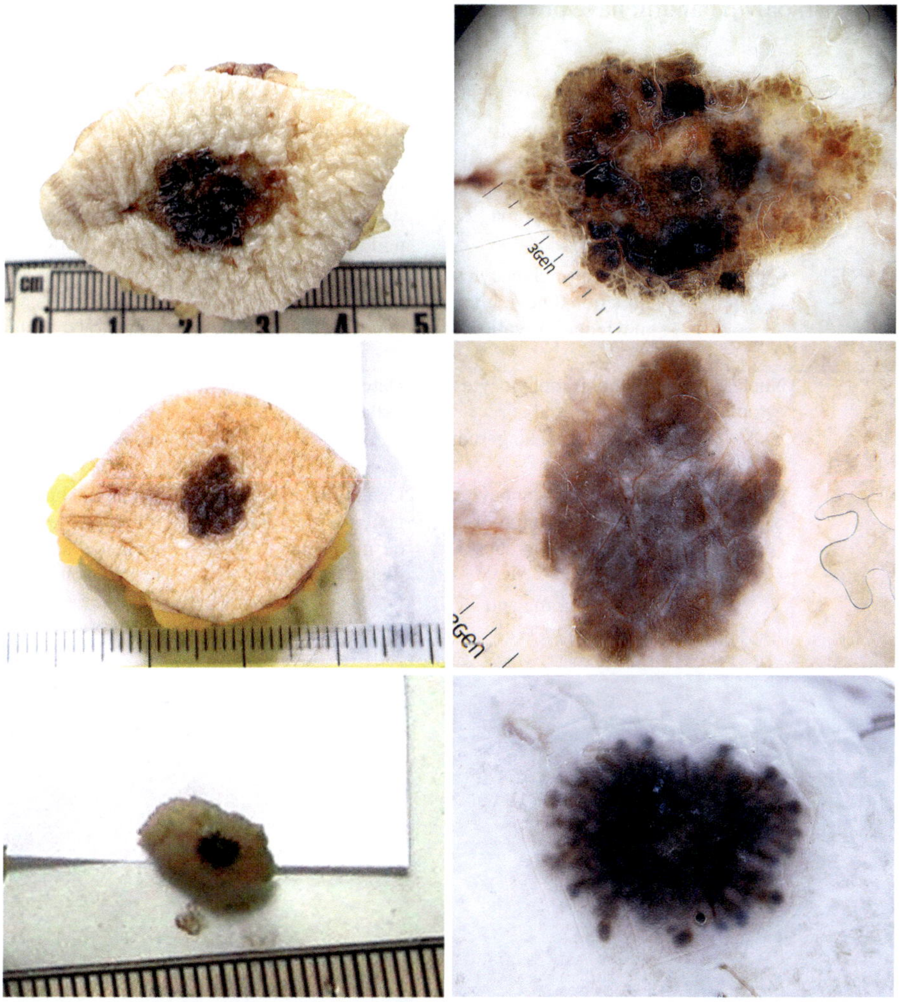

Fig. 6.7 Three cases of ex vivo dermatoscopy. **First row**: a melanoma with chaotic arrangement of colors and structure in ex vivo dermatoscopy (right). **Second row**: this was diagnosed as a "melanocytic nevus with high-grade dysplasia" by the dermatopathologist but from the ex vivo dermatoscopy it could as well be a melanoma in situ, given the irregular arrangement of colors in a flat lesion surrounded by chronic sun damage. **Third row**: a classical Reed nevus with radial lines at the periphery indicating quick growth. (Courtesy of Danijela Dobrosavljevic Vukojevic)

6.4 Immunohistochemistry

Immunohistochemistry allows for detection and visualization of protein expression, usually associated with a cell lineage or certain functional properties of a cell. In the context of melanoma, it is used to identify melanocytes through positive identification or distinction to other cell lineages, or to better reveal architecture and spread of a melanocytic proliferation. While many candidates for this task were proposed in the past, only a handful have prevailed the test of time in routine diagnostic dermatopathology, especially for the context of pattern analysis (Table 6.1). We understand this is an opinionated selection of antibodies, where other laboratories may choose different candidates from the pool of available ones [76]. As the use of a brown chromogen can lead to misinterpretations in pigmented lesions, we prefer to use a red chromogen (Fig. 6.8) as a default for any melanocytic marker, albeit you also see Diaminobenzidine (DAB) in cases contained in this book.

Table 6.1 Details of commonly used antibodies for identifying nature and architecture of melanocytic neoplasms

Antibody	Staining	Positive-controls	Exemplary use cases	Not useful for
HMB45/gp100	Cytoplasmic	PEComa, junctional nevi, blue nevi, angiomyolipoma [77]	Ascertain dermal melanocytic component	Detecting resting mature melanocytes, spindle cell melanoma, or desmoplastic melanoma
			Assess melanocytes in nail matrix	
MelanA/MART-1	Cytoplasmic	Regular melanocytes, junctional nevi, blue nevi, angiomyolipoma [77]	Distinguish neurofibroma from neurotized dermal nevi	Exact delineation of melanoma, as MelanA tends to "overstain"
S100	Nuclear and cytoplasmic	Regular melanocytes, nerve strands, adipocytes, langerhans cells	Detect desmoplastic melanoma	Distinguishing melanocytic lesion from a nerve sheath tumor
SOX10	Nuclear	Regular melanocytes, melanocytic tumors, regular sweat ducts	Detect melanocytes in general, including desmoplastic melanoma [79]	Distinguishing macrophages from melanocytes in re-excision scars [81]
		Spiradenoma and cylindroma [78]	Distinguish from fibrohistiocytic tumors [80]	

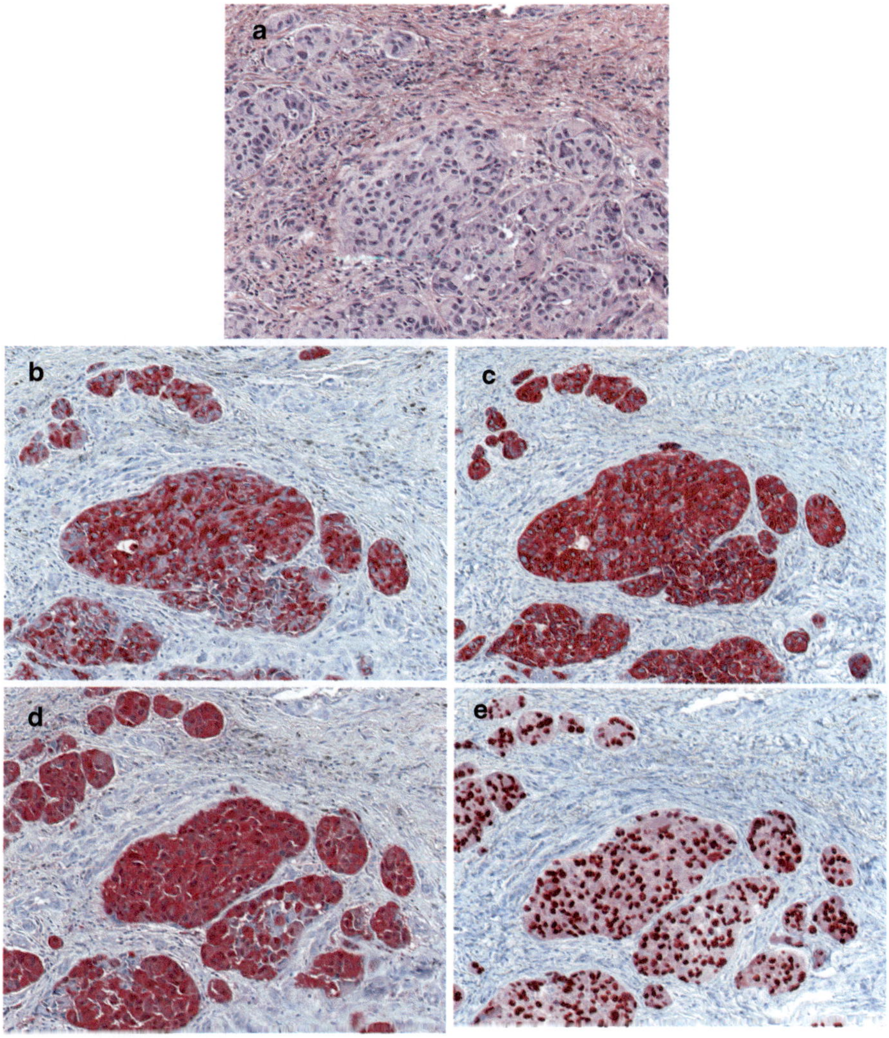

Fig. 6.8 Common immunohistochemical stainings of melanocytic lesions exemplified in a melanoma metastasis. (**a**) Conventional H/E staining showing crowded pleomorphic melanocytes, arranged in nests, with nuclei varying in size and shape. (**b**) HMB45 showing cytoplasmic staining. (**c**) MelanA with cytoplasmic staining. (**d**) S100 with nuclear and cytoplasmic staining. (**e**) SOX10 with exclusively nuclear staining. (Courtesy of the Department of Dermatology, Medical University of Vienna)

6.4.1 Use Cases

6.4.1.1 Diagnosing Melanoma Without Immunohistochemistry

Use of immunohistochemistry for melanocytic lesions in general was discussed to be associated with younger age and low confidence in diagnosis [82]. It is, in our view, not an invariable necessity to apply immunohistochemistry to diagnose morphologically clear-cut melanoma. Often, nature, extent, and invasion depth are recognizable in H/E stainings alone (Fig. 6.9). In such cases, immunohistochemistry may only increase costs and duration for a final report, but not diagnostic accuracy. Added remuneration of immunohistochemical stainings should not lead a practicing dermatopathologist to ask for additional diagnostic tests.

Contrastingly, use of immunohistochemistry may even be a root cause for adding diagnostic quandaries to a case. Aberrant expression of epitopes is seldom, but possible [83], e.g., MelanA positive dermal cells can occur even in nonmelanocytic neoplasms [84], and "pseudo"-melanocytic nests in lichenoid dermatoses can also show positive specific immunohistochemical stainings [85].

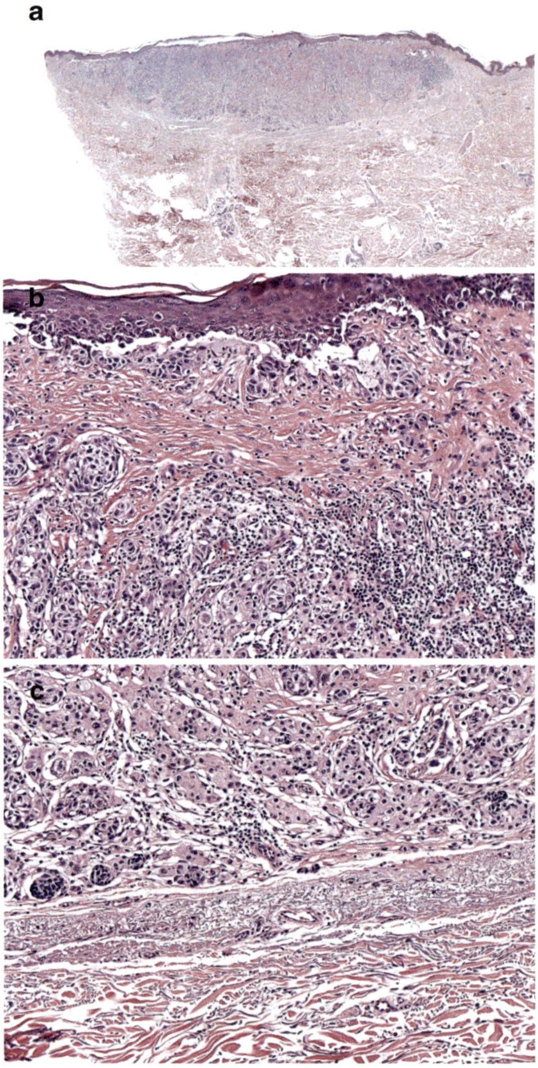

Fig. 6.9 (**a**–**c**) An invasive melanoma without the strict necessity of immunohistochemical staining. The excision shows an asymmetric proliferation of melanocytes, with clefting and single melanocytes (**a**), within the epidermis (**b**). Nests of melanocytes are also discernible within the epidermis, with a clear-cut border at the bottom (**c**) allowing for measuring invasion depth. (Courtesy of the Department of Dermatology, Medical University of Vienna)

6.4.1.2 Rule out a Melanocytic Process

There are histologic, but also clinical mimickers for melanoma, where it can be of value to rule out a melanocytic process. In such cases, we regard a combination of two sensitive markers the most sensible choice for inclusion in an immunohistochemical panel. If only one marker can be chosen, SOX10 may be more informative as it will not stain intraepidermal Langerhans cells. To distinguish against other diseases, markers for the relevant non-melanocytic differential diagnoses are necessary [86] (Fig. 6.10), if a mucosal lentigo is the main differential diagnosis only melanocytic markers suffice usually (Fig. 6.11).

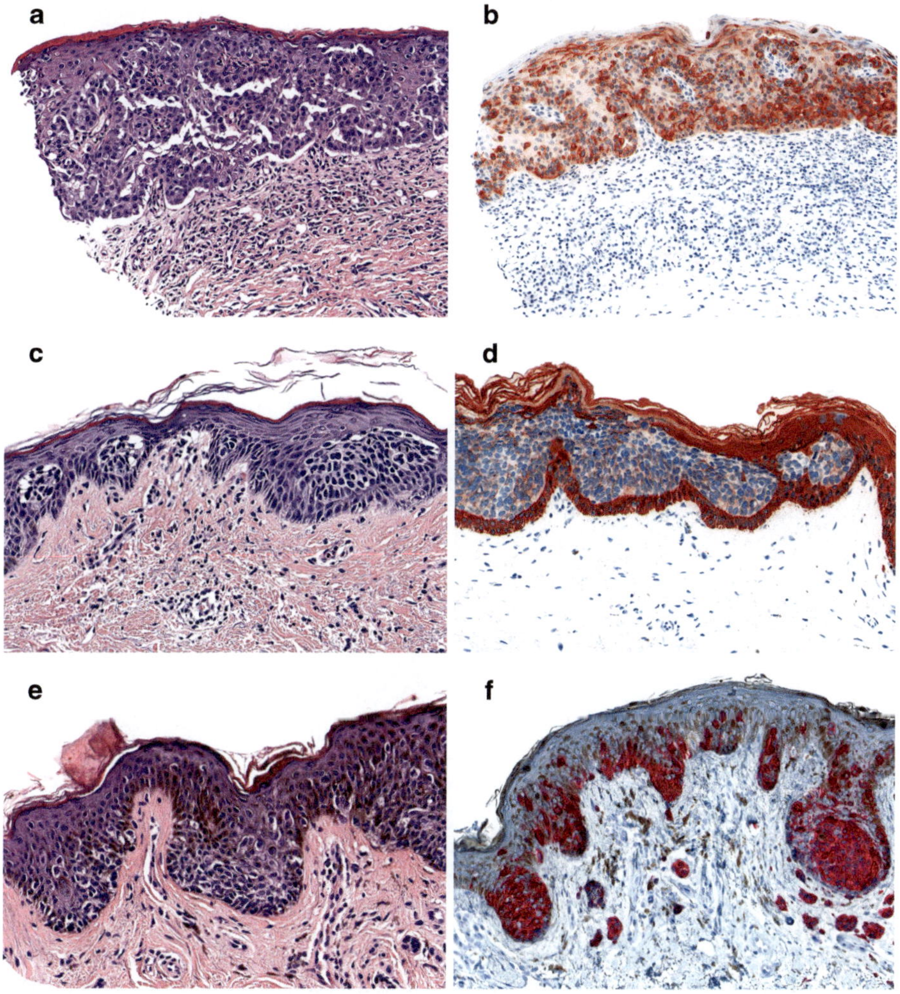

Fig. 6.10 Immunohistochemistry for distinguishing pagetoid intraepidermal proliferations. (**a**, **b**) Extramammary Paget's disease shows CEA positivity. (**c**, **d**) A Pagetoid Bowen's disease with decreased but detectable Cytokeratin AE1/3 positivity—this proliferation was CEA negative. (**e**, **f**) Melanoma with melanocytes in the epidermis and upper dermis identifiable with S100 staining. (Courtesy of the Department of Dermatology, Medical University of Vienna)

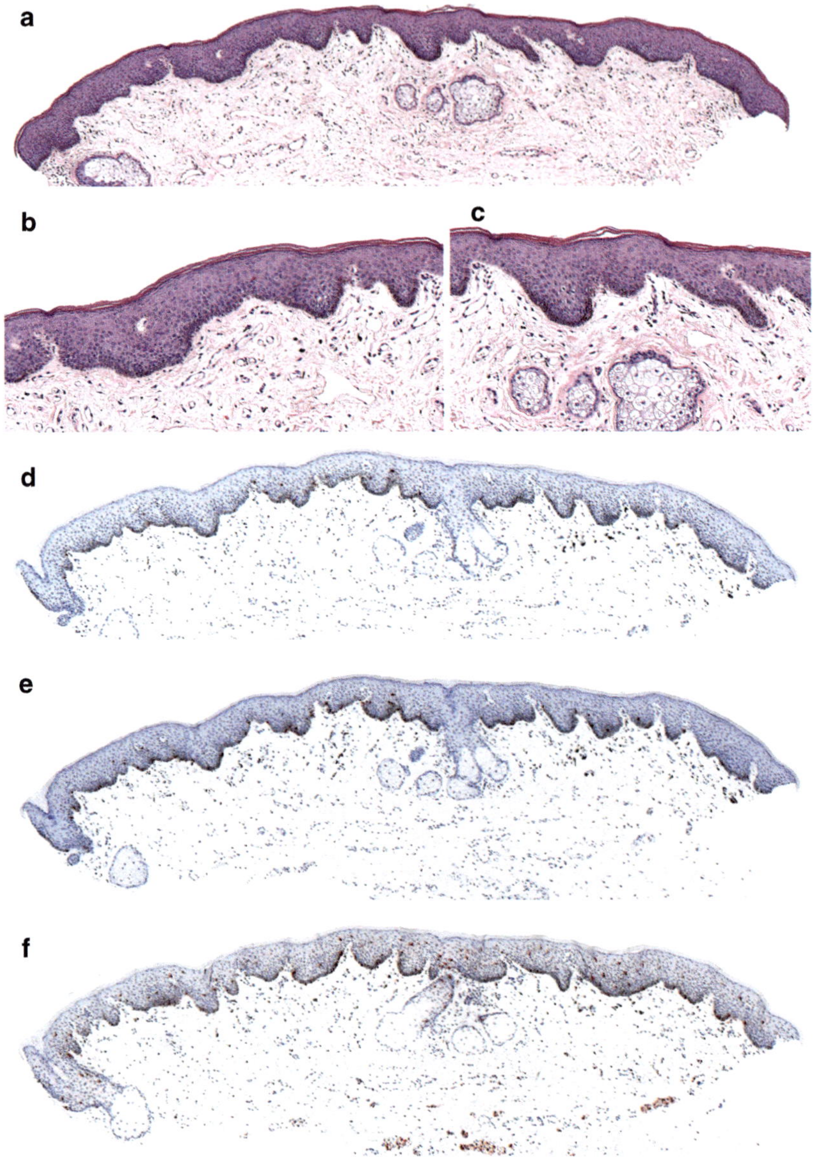

Fig. 6.11 Immunohistochemistry for ruling out a melanocytic process on a mucosal lesion. (**a–c**) H/E staining of a case, sent in to rule out melanoma, shows delicate acanthosis and basal hyperpigmentation, a proliferation of melanocytes is not identifiable with certainty. (**d–f**) Immunohistochemically there are only regularly distributed melanocytes in HMB45 (**d**), MelanA (**e**) and S100 (**f**), where the latter shows positive staining mostly due to suprabasal Langerhans cells. The case was finally signed out as a mucosal lentigo. (Courtesy of the Department of Dermatology, Medical University of Vienna)

6.4.1.3 Discovery of Histologically Invisible Melanoma

Immunohistochemistry is almost invariably necessary in the diagnosis—or exclusion—of in situ melanoma on the face (lentigo maligna; Fig. 6.12), acral sites, and nail matrix. While HMB45, S100, and MelanA are highly sensitive for the detection of lentigo maligna, one should be cautious of overinterpretation, as chronically sun-damaged skin can show increased melanocytes as well. Stainings are easiest to interpret in combination, and with the section spanning the lesion border.

Regarding interpretation of specimens of the nail matrix, visualizing thick and increased dendrites visible with HMB45 are a soft, but not undisputed, hint towards melanoma in situ of the nail matrix. Evaluation of an unequivocal melanocytic nail lesion, in our view, must always be evaluated together with the clinical picture. Melanocytic lesions in the nail matrix usually show more positivity for HMB45 than MelanA.

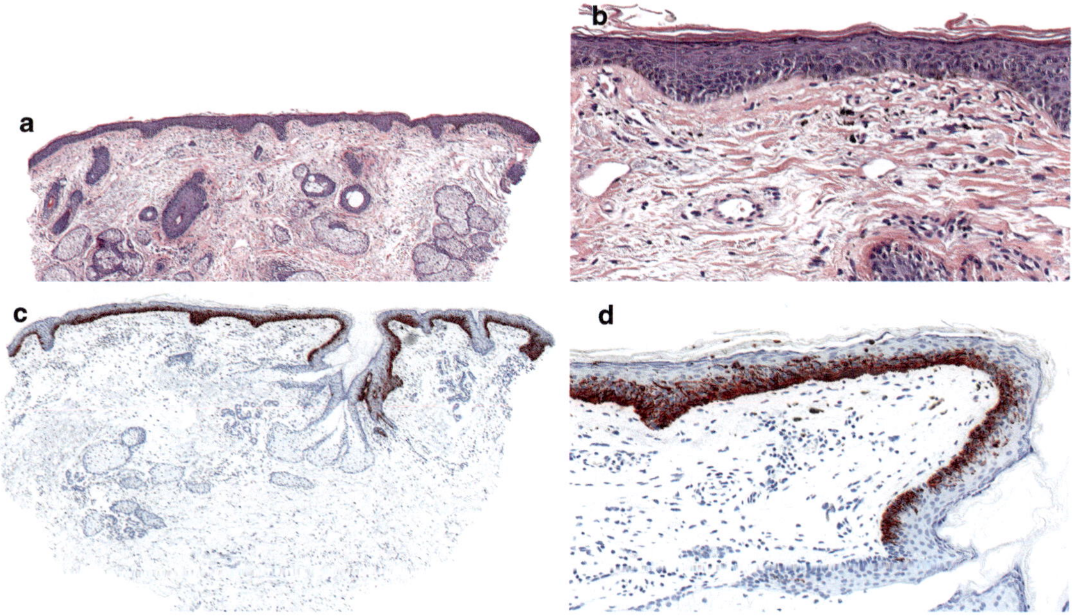

Fig. 6.12 Revealing a melanocytic proliferation with immunohistochemistry. (**a**, **b**) H/E staining of a punch biopsy with a clinical suspicion of melanoma. Melanocytes seem to be increased in number, but are not clearly identifiable. (**c**, **d**) Staining for HMB45 reveals a melanocytic proliferation covering the complete basal layer of the specimen, also traveling into the follicular epithelium. (Courtesy of the Department of Dermatology, Medical University of Vienna)

6.4.1.4 Desmoplastic and Spindle Cell Melanoma

Desmoplastic melanomas commonly show negative reactions when staining for otherwise specific markers such as HMB45, MelanA, MITF, or Tyrosinase. ***S100*** and ***SOX10*** [87] are most helpful for diagnosing this subtype in the majority of cases, and followingly to detect tumor remnants in re-excision scars (Fig. 6.13). In rare negative cases, others described NGFR [88, 89] may provide an additional possibility for detection, but the authors have not used it so far. As a caveat, both S100 and SOX-10 can show scattered stainings in malignant peripheral nerve sheath tumors [87].

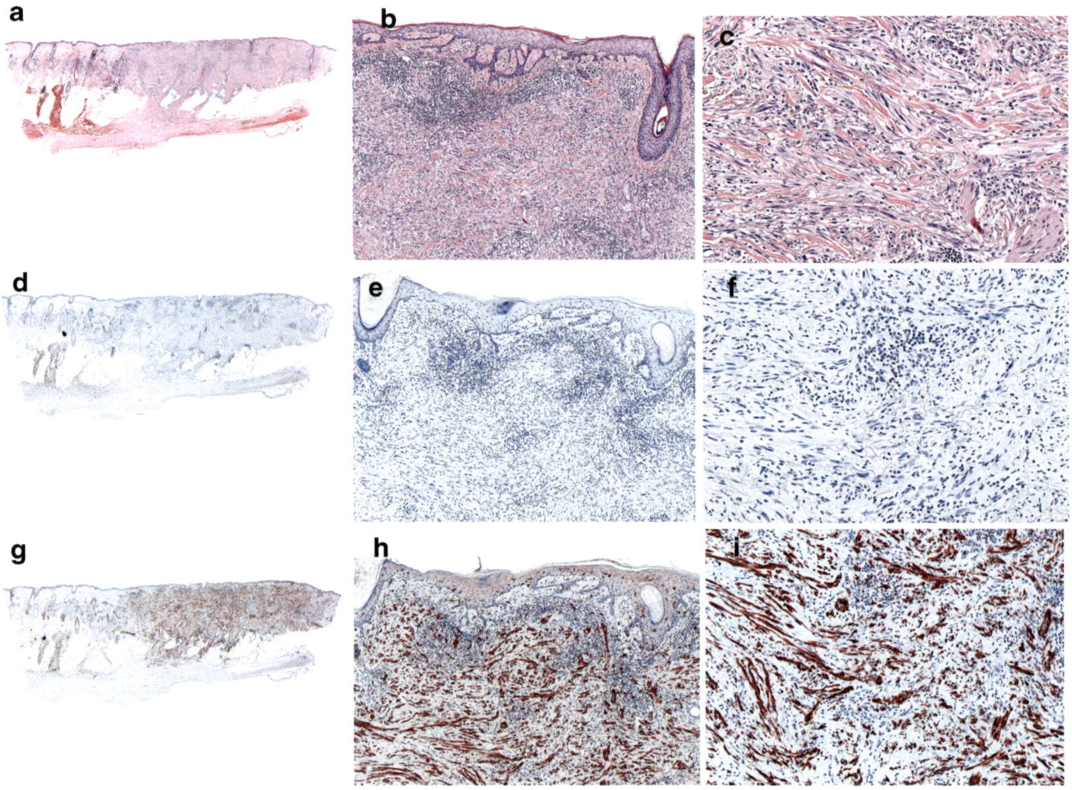

Fig. 6.13 Prototypical presentation of a desmoplastic melanoma. (**a–c**) H/E staining of a surgical resection of the previously diagnosed desmoplastic melanoma. The dermis shows circumscribed fibrosis reaching into the subcutaneous septa, populated with a spindle cell proliferation and a patchy inflammatory infiltrate. (**d–f**) Negative staining with MelanA. (**g–i**) Positive staining of the spindled cells with S100 reveals invasion into the subcutaneous tissue. (Courtesy of the Department of Dermatology, Medical University of Vienna)

6.4.1.5 Measuring Melanoma Thickness

Conventionally, melanoma thickness is assessed by measuring the vertical distance between the deepest part of the tumor and the granular layer of the epidermis. What sounds simple, and often is, can become problematic in certain situations. When dermal parts of a melanoma are found along a follicle, the question arises whether to measure from the granular layer of the surface epidermis or the follicular epithelium. In such cases, the lesion should be screened for a dermal involvement not associated with a follicle and should be measured there. If no such area can be found, we indicate the "depth" from the follicular epithelium, but explicitly state in the report that this is how we proceeded. However, we are willing to change this practice if compelling evidence emerges to support a different approach. Current standards for reporting are constantly evolving, and the reporting pathologist should be aware of the most current versions of the WHO classification and AJCC staging system [50] (see also Chap. 3).

A more common problem in our experience are nests of melanocytes in the upper dermis associated with a clear-cut melanoma within the epidermis. In such a situation, it is often difficult to distinguish with certainty invasive melanoma from an associated dermal nevus by morphology alone. Diffuse ***PRAME***-positivity can be a hint towards a dermal melanoma in comparison to an associated dermal nevus [90]. Negativity, or a decreasing positivity, of ***HMB45*** in dermal melanocytes, can be a hint towards a dermal nevus in comparison to an invasive melanoma portion.

6.4.1.6 Atypical Spitzoid Lesions

In our view, ancillary studies with immunohistochemistry seldomly clear up a previously problematic spitzoid lesion. One exception from that rule is, if we find a BRAF mutation in an otherwise spitzoid lesion we count this as a strong indicator for a melanoma as this mutation is rare in a true Spitz nevus. VE1 is one option to test for such a mutation immunohistochemically with reasonably good positive and negative predictive values [91], but sequencing is a more reliable technique in our view, when available. Ki67[1] can be helpful in identifying increased proliferation in deep parts of a spitzoid lesion—as a hint to melanoma, but relevant mitoses are usually visible within H/E stainings already.

6.4.1.7 BAP1 Deficient Nevi

Melanocytes of BAP1-deficient neoplasms have a conspicuous epithelioid morphology, potentially causing misdiagnosis and confusion with spitzoid lesions [93]. These are detectable by showing a lack of nuclear BAP1 staining in immunohistochemistry, but since staining for this antigen is not available in many laboratories, and often difficult to establish technically, it is advisable to refer such cases to a specialized laboratory in case of suspicion. Importantly, BAP1 loss is not a single marker defining malignancy, thus, integrating immunohistochemical detection of BAP1-loss into other morphologic and clinical findings is still necessary.

[1] Some prefer to use Phosphohistone H3 (PHH3) antibodies to Ki67 as a marker more specific to mitosis [92].

6.4.1.8 Malignancy Prediction Through Immunohistochemistry

The desire to offload the distinction of melanoma from melanocytic nevi to ancillary testing is decades old. Many approaches are published, such as counting Ki67 as an indicator for melanoma [94], measuring complete loss of p16 in melanomas [95], estimating missing HMB45 in dermal nevi [96], or diffuse expression of PRAME (PReferentially expressed Antigen in MElanoma) in MElanoma) in melanomas [97]. PRAME and p16 may have some value in distinguishing nodal nevi from nodal melanoma metastasis [98, 99], nodular proliferations in congenital nevi [100], or evaluating conjunctival lesions [101]. Unfortunately, a meta-analysis has shown p16 to be of rather limited use outside evaluation of lymph nodes [98]. Homogeneous PRAME expression, as a successor, was reported to be present more commonly in melanomas than nevi [97, 102], and also suggested to be of better usability for assessing acral melanocytic neoplasms in comparison to p16 [103]. Unfortunately, PRAME expression was also found in non-melanocytic neoplasms such as cellular neurothekeoma [104], and especially in atypical junctional nevi and Spitz nevi [97, 105, 106].

In sum, albeit initial study results often looking promising, in practice we have not found relying on single immunohistochemical stainings to be of unequivocal and robust usefulness for a dependable distinction "melanoma or nevus" in primary diagnostics. This is especially true for the common diagnostic dilemmas of *atypical lentiginous junctional lesions* or *atypical spitzoid lesions,* where there is currently no highly dependable value in single additional immunohistochemical stainings.

This should not lead to the conclusion above that stainings should not be used at all for aiding one's diagnosis, but the final interpretation should always keep in mind imperfect diagnostic accuracy, where a combination of multiple stainings [96] and synthesis with other information [107] is most helpful. Also, special use-cases like estimating lymphatic spread [108] or tumor-infiltrating lymphocytes and PD-L1 expression, can certainly be of added value but are outside the scope of this work.

6.5 Molecular Findings

Multiple methodologies, ranging from focused conventional sequencing, FISH and mass spectrometry, to aCGH, qRT-PCR, methylation profiles [109, 110], and next generation sequencing (NGS) [111] are available as ancillary tests for melanocytic lesions. A major part of the current literature for solving diagnostic quandaries is based on FISH and CGH. In *fluorescence in situ hybridization (FISH),* probes specific either for a (small) genomic region or centromeres allow visualization of those segments. It can thus also detect changes in different regions of a lesion, but is limited to single probed loci or crude chromosomal copy number aberrations. In *array comparative genomic hybridization (aCGH)* tumor DNA is labeled, and hybridized to an array, where fluorescence can be compared to reference DNA. Gains and losses of chromosomal areas can be measured spanning the entire genomic DNA. About a third of the tumor should show a specific aberration for it to be reliably detected. This is almost a traditional technique by now, as classic CGH as a diagnostic tool for melanocytic lesions was suggested by Bastian et al. as early as 2003 [112]. A more current technique is *next generation sequencing (NGS),* which in comparison to traditional sequencing techniques allows for a much higher throughput. With NGS potentially a whole human genome can be sequenced in a short timeframe, but often a "targeted" NGS approach is used to cover a panel of potentially relevant genomic targets to save time, costs, and analytic workload, while obtaining a better coverage of targeted areas. Nothing more should be written about the technological background herein, as covering it in enough detail is far beyond the scope of this book.

Having now mentioned the most common techniques, in our view molecular methods are not useful to solve questions *for the most common lesions in average daily practice.* Instead they have value for constellations and questions that will only rarely occur in daily practice, and usually be forwarded to and solved by highly specialized laboratories who are familiar with current primary literature—who don't need our advice anyways. Also, we expect the vast majority of readers, like us and many others [113], not to have routine access to complex and expensive techniques, and therefore will have to rely on reference laboratories. As knowledge and techniques continuously advance, we advise reporting dermatopathologists to seek contact with such a specialist at the time of question whether additional methodologies such as the ones mentioned herein, or any future ones, can be expected to be meaningful in a specific case.

Now, looking at today's knowledge, what are specific patterns where we *do* see potential value of ancillary testing in routine practice? Those are in our view morphologically ambiguous epithelioid ("spitzoid"), "nevoid," "desmoplastic" and "blue"-like lesions that cannot be resolved by other means. Here, if an ancillary test is interpretable unequivocally as malignant or benign, one has gained information. If an ancillary test is equivocal as well though, which is a situation one should be prepared to find in practice, not much is gained for the following clinical course of action. In which situation do we currently not see relevant use explicitly? Ambiguous in situ or very thin lesions. This is because the expected added clinical value for the pathologist, treating physician, and patient is low and doesn't justify added time, costs, and complexity.

6.5.1 General Concepts

6.5.1.1 Expected-Mutation Mismatch

Certain groups of melanocytic neoplasms are associated with selected mutations, a current overview of mutation targets can be seen in tables of the WHO classification [30]. For example, blue nevi commonly show GNAQ, GNA11 or CYSLTR2 mutations, or Spitz nevi alterations in HRAS, ALK, ROS1, RED or NTRK1/2. If one now examines an atypical lesion in question trying to decide between Spitz nevus and melanoma, finding a $BRAF^{V600E}$ mutation, this may be one signal towards melanoma as such a mutation would be rather unexpected in a Spitz nevus.

6.5.1.2 Interobserver Agreement

Adding clinical information, as well as clinical and dermatoscopic images, improves interobserver agreement, and reduces the amount of "unknown" sign-outs [29]. The same was shown by Benton et al., where adding next-generation sequencing data increased agreement of an expert group in evaluating complex Spitzoid neoplasms [114]. While we see the former applicable and necessary for everyday practice, the latter will be limited to specialists and consultation-level cases.

6.5.1.3 Prognosis and Therapy

Apart from putting a lesion into a diagnostic group, which is the core task also within this book, additional prognostic information may be required after diagnosing a melanoma. Targeted search for BRAF, NRAS, or KIT mutations may be helpful, or even necessary when choosing a therapy for metastatic melanoma. Monosomy 3 is correlated with risk of metastasis in choroidal melanoma [115], DNA copy number changes with clinical behavior [28], and mutational burden with disease recurrence [116]. This field is a moving target, and in our view will continue to be, thus familiarity with recent data from primary literature will be necessary.

6.5.1.4 Bias

Many centers will not have access to molecular testing in routine practice and will thus probably be biased against the use of new technology. On the other hand, those with access to such techniques, or maybe even profiting financially and academically from them will for certain be biased for their use [117, 118]. We encourage the reader to be aware of this, and have an open but critical mind wherever genomic testing is discussed.

6.5.2 Selected Situations

6.5.2.1 TERT

TERT promoter mutation and hypermethylation, but also TERT amplifications, are proposed to be early events in melanoma, but were also found in different nevus types [119, 120]. Thus, especially with highly sensitive assays and low detected levels, TERT mutations should rather be one data point added into the integration of a case, but never demand the diagnosis of a melanoma or a "dysplastic" "precursor." It may have additional and other use cases, as TERT alterations were shown to be correlated with metastatic disease in conjunctival melanoma [121].

6.5.2.2 Spitzoid/Epithelioid Lesions

Early work using FISH described gains in 6p25 or 11p13, and especially homozygous deletions in 9p21 as significantly associated with clinically aggressive behavior in atypical spitzoid neoplasms [26]. With FISH analyses being time consuming and expensive, more recent work tried to analyze whether PRAME immunohistochemistry could serve as a surrogate, or even replacement for FISH, but found only mild-to-moderate agreement in assessment [107]. Naturally, more elaborate techniques evolved, one of them being next-generation sequencing (NGS). In a small case series, targeted NGS detected BRAF, MET, NTRK1, and ROS fusion only in benign lesions, whereas only malignant counterparts harbored EML4 fusions mutations in BRAF, MAP2K1, TERT, and NF1 [111]. Such enumerations of genes should only be regarded as illustrative and never exhaustive, as new target panels, lesion sets, and higher coverage may detect many others. What such studies do show is that NGS could in fact be a helpful technique in ambiguous lesions in the future.

Synthesis of multiple tests can be more helpful, even with modern high-resolution techniques such as NGS. Valiga et al., for example, combined assessment of NGS with PRAME immunohistochemistry to diagnose a sarcomatoid melanoma [122]. Ancillary techniques should not be regarded in isolation, because they are usually involved at a point when a lesion will be reported by a panel of pathologists. Interestingly, in such settings, NGS was experimentally shown to improve inter-rater agreement on problematic spitzoid neoplasms [114].

6.5.2.3 Blue-Like Lesions

Using FISH probes for RREB1 (6p25), MYB (6q23), CCND1 (11q13), and Cep6 (centromere 6), Pouryazdanparast et al. [123] and Gerami et al. [124] were able to distinguish epithelioid blue nevi from blue nevus-like melanoma. Maize et al. reported that with CGH, histologically malignant lesions show a distinct number and pattern of chromosomal aberrations, and that ambiguous lesions were divisible into those with and without chromosomal aberration [125]. Similar results were found by Chan et al., but importantly only 67% of melanomas arising in blue nevi showed copy number aberrations [126]. We interpret such findings that there is indeed a fair chance for resolving an ambiguous situation, but it is not guaranteed.

6.6 Adding It Up: But How?

In our opinion, diagnostic uncertainty in medicine will never completely disappear, but modern technologies are pushing the boundaries. So we need to find ways and strategies to deal with this uncertainty and discuss it openly with colleagues and patients. When an objectively correct diagnosis is not within reach, the goal shifts to optimal management. In unclear situations, as many objective criteria as possible should be collected and weighted. The best and most natural way to formally combine multiple levels of information into a final judgment is Bayesian inference. In this process, the probability for a hypothesis, in our case a diagnosis, is always updated based on new data. The starting point is a pretest probability, which in the simplest case is equal to the frequency of a diagnosis in the population of all referrals. Assume you see 1 melanoma per 100 referrals, then that should be the starting point for your considerations. Now, when you look in the microscope, the probability of a diagnosis of melanoma increases if you see a melanocytic proliferation and decreases to zero if you do not. The probability increases further if you see certain histomorphologic criteria and if the clinical diagnosis is melanoma, but it may also decrease, for example, if the patient is a prepubescent child. This is a very crude and simplified representation of inference from conditional probabilities, but it roughly corresponds to practical thinking. For those readers who are interested in the formal approach of Bayesian inference we recommend the book "*Bernoulli's Fallacy: Statistical Illogic and the Crisis of*

Modern Science" [127], which is not only a profound critique of the current scientific standards of reporting statistics but also a great introduction into Bayesian thinking. At the end of this thinking process, the probability of a particular diagnosis is usually so high that we do not hesitate to make that diagnosis. However, this is not always the case, because sometimes a residual uncertainty remains. In our opinion, residual diagnostic uncertainty should be made transparent in a histopathology report without assigning it to biological uncertainty. How this is achieved varies from laboratory to laboratory, country to country, community to community, and pathologist to pathologist.

7 Pattern Analysis in Practice

The purpose of this chapter is to spend some time together with us at a virtual multiheaded microscope. We invite you, the reader, to watch us approach easy and challenging cases and learn from it. Unlike any other textbook, we will share not only our knowledge but also our doubts and will not pretend to know it all. We will let you know how we arrived at a final diagnosis and how we balance criteria in difficult cases. In the field of dermatopathology there is something we call "objective ignorance." By this we mean that even if we had complete information, if we were able to assess the position and state of every atom of the lesion at hand, we could not know for sure how it will behave biologically. Nevertheless, we will have to make judgments and call a lesion benign or malignant. This is even more challenging in daily practice, where we always have incomplete information that increases our ignorance even further. Pattern analysis should help us to make the best possible judgements under these circumstances. In addition to pattern analysis, we also recommend applying general measures of "decision hygiene" to reduce bias, noise, and error and to think in conditional probabilities as stated in the last paragraph of Chap. 6. Decision hygiene will be explored in greater detail in Chap. 8.

Before we begin, we want to repeat here what we already stated in Chap. 5. Classifications come and go. The current WHO classification of melanocytic neoplasms, for example, will be replaced by others in the future. Pattern analysis, on the other hand, is timeless, it can be mapped to every classification, to those that exist today and to those that will exist in the future. We have not committed ourselves to a classification that may be outdated tomorrow. We, however, acknowledge the need to comply with the rules of the prevailing orthodoxy when it comes to issuing pathologic reports. For this reason, we will give the diagnosis that would apply according to the most recent WHO classification, whenever we deem this useful.

In our experience, diagnostic challenges typically occur in certain constellations, and this chapter is organized accordingly. Difficult constellations may be characterized by histomorphologic pattern, anatomic location, or type of biopsy technique. We recognize that the subheadings we use in this chapter are fuzzy, and some cases may appear under different subheadings. The subheadings are neither perfectly defined categories nor general patterns, but only roughly reflect the common features of the most critical situations encountered in practice.

A. Böer-Auer et al., *Pattern Analysis for Histopathologic Diagnosis of Melanocytic Lesions*,
https://doi.org/10.1007/978-3-031-07666-4_7

7.1 Patterns

7.1.1 Junctional

The junctional pattern is one of the most common challenges in practice. We encounter it every day. The task is to differentiate melanoma in situ from its benign simulators, which vary depending on the context. The main simulators are Reed nevi, recurrent nevi, acquired junctional nevi, nevus spilus, and, especially in older patients with chronically sun-damaged skin, UV-induced melanocytic hyperplasia. Partial biopsies can be particularly difficult without additional information. Histomorphologic evaluation of junctional melanocytic proliferations should describe whether the lesion is small or broad, whether the melanocytes are arranged primarily as single cells or as nests, and whether the nests are of equal size and equidistant from each other. If single cells predominate, they should also be evaluated for their arrangement and distribution and whether they involve the follicular infundibulum. Immunostaining may be useful to better assess whether the lesion is symmetric or asymmetric and poorly or well circumscribed. Pagetoid spread of melanocytes can also sometimes be better assessed with immunostaining. Additional findings should always be considered, for example, if chronic sun damage or fibrosis of the dermis and flattening of the epidermis are present. If regression, scarring, or inflammation is present, please also refer to the examples shown in the subchapter regression, sclerosis, recurrence, and inflammation. Sometimes deeper levels will reveal a few nests of small and monomorphous melanocytes in the papillary dermis in the center of the lesion. This usually indicates a nevus.

7.1.1.1 Example 1: Nests and Single Cells (Fig. 7.1)

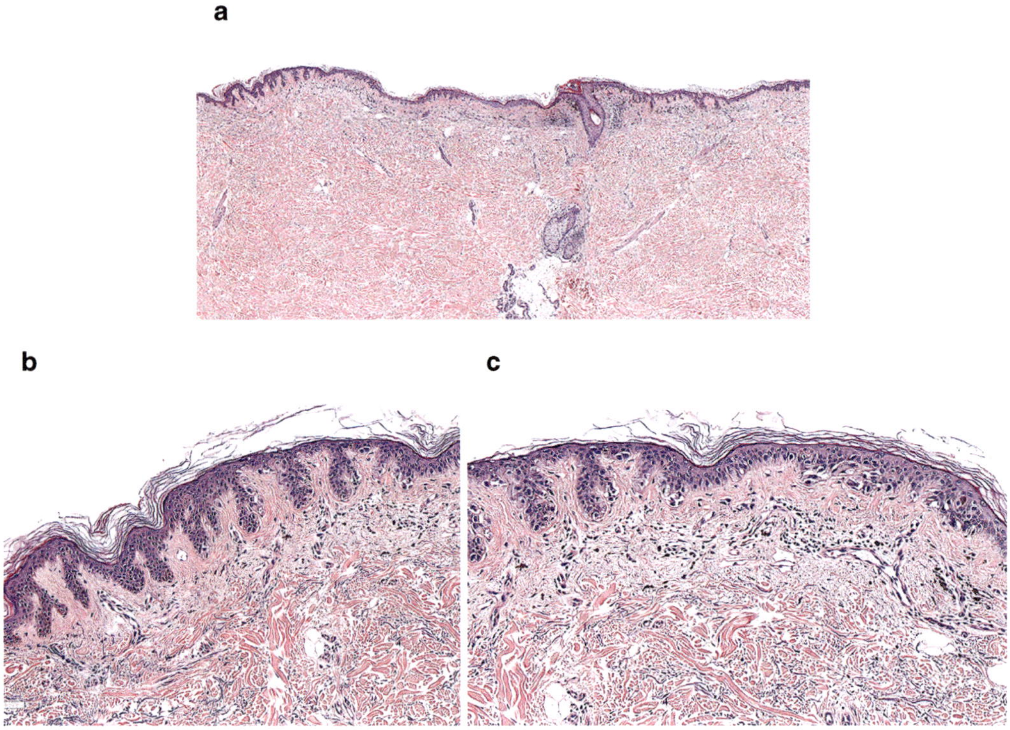

Fig. 7.1 (**a–k**) Junctional pattern, Example 1. (Courtesy of the Department of Dermatology, Medical University of Vienna)

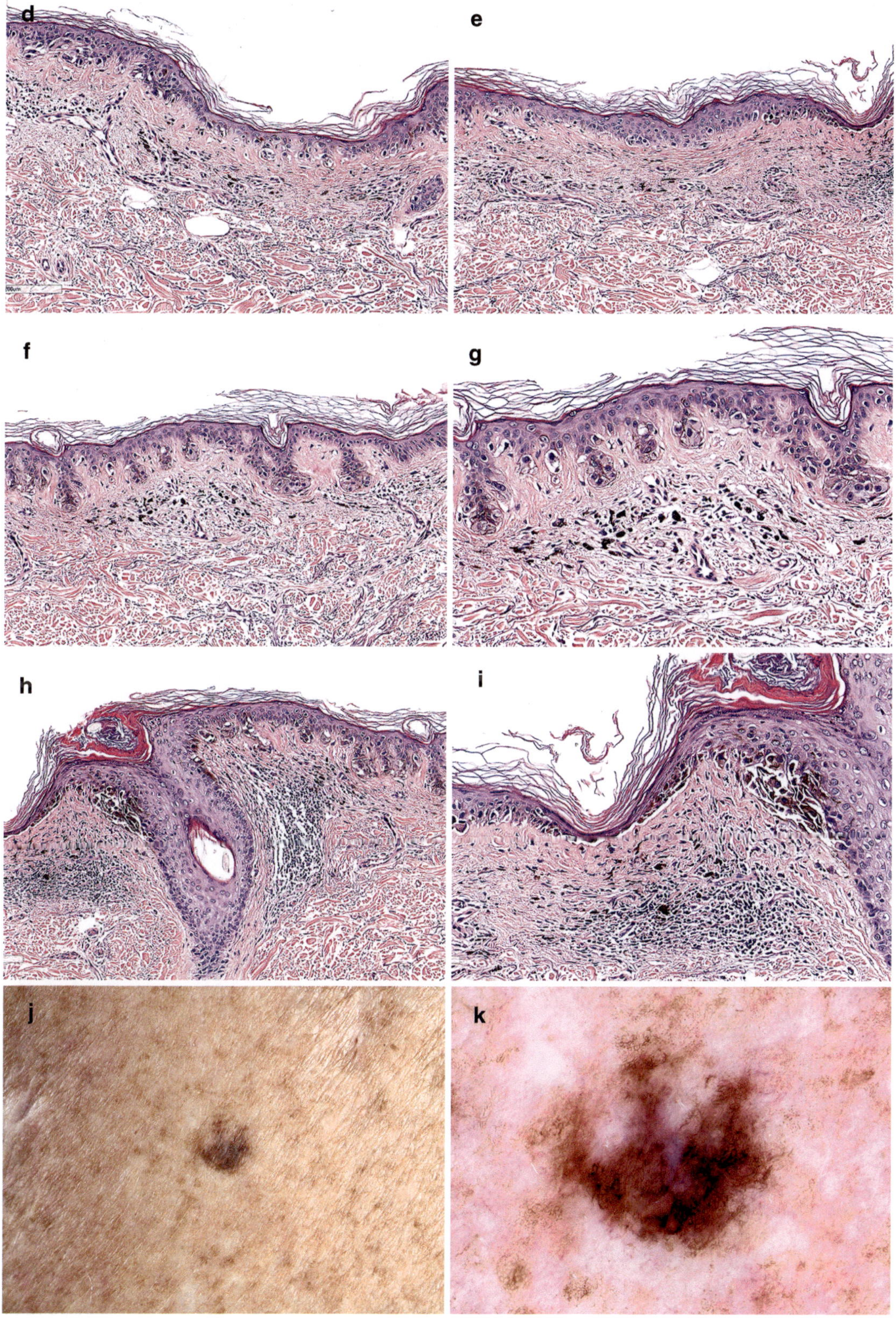

Fig. 7.1 (continued)

Overall Pattern: Nested and Single Cells, Epidermal, Asymmetric

Detailed Description

Silhouette

- Asymmetric
- Poorly circumscribed
- Epidermal

Patterns

Epidermis

- Nested at the junction.
- Nests vary in size and shape and are not equidistant. In some parts, however, nests are regularly distributed.
- Some horizontal confluence of nests.
- Single melanocytes between nests.
- Involvement of infundibular epidermis.
- Only a few melanocytes in suprabasal layers.

Cytology

- Small round, enlarged, and spindled, richly pigmented

Other Changes

- Focal fibrosis in the dermis and some solar elastosis.
- In some parts the epidermis is flattened.
- Numerous melanophages in the papillary dermis.
- Patchy infiltrate of lymphocytes in the papillary dermis.

Integration

Pathologically, the differential diagnosis is acquired junctional nevus versus melanoma in situ. Clinically, this is a changing lesion in a male adult older than 50 years on the back surrounded by chronic sun damage (Fig. 7.1j), which increases the likelihood of melanoma. The dermatoscopy shows a chaotic lesion with a reticular pattern and signs of regression in the form of white structureless areas (corresponding to the fibrosis underneath the flattened epidermis) and gray dots (corresponding to melanophages) (Fig. 7.1k). Integrating all information, the diagnosis is melanoma in situ. Some parts of the melanoma mimic an acquired junctional nevus ("dysplastic" nevus) and this is the reason why some pathologists would sign this out as melanoma in situ arising in a "dysplastic nevus" or as "severely dysplastic nevus" or as MPATH-Dx Class 3. Regardless of the difference in terminology, the preferred management would be re-excision with 5 mm margins. Even if one accepts the idea that this lesion developed in a pre-existing nevus, the pre-existing nevus must have been very small (smaller than 4 mm), which is not in line with the usual definition of the "dysplastic nevus."

Diagnosis: Melanoma in situ.

Alternative diagnosis according to the WHO Classification of Tumours 4th ed.: "Melanoma in situ melanoma in skin with low cumulative sun damage" or "Melanoma in situ melanoma in skin with low cumulative sun damage arising in a dysplastic nevus." Although the extensive freckling in the surrounding skin and the solar elastosis visible in the specimen point to high cumulative sun damage, the back is regarded as a site of low cumulative sun damage according to the WHO classification. The definition of high cumulative sun damage hinges on the presence of solar elastosis in the histopathologic specimen and not on clinical criteria. It is unclear how much solar elastosis is needed to qualify as high cumulative sun damage.

7.1.1.2 Example 2: Nests Mainly (Fig. 7.2)

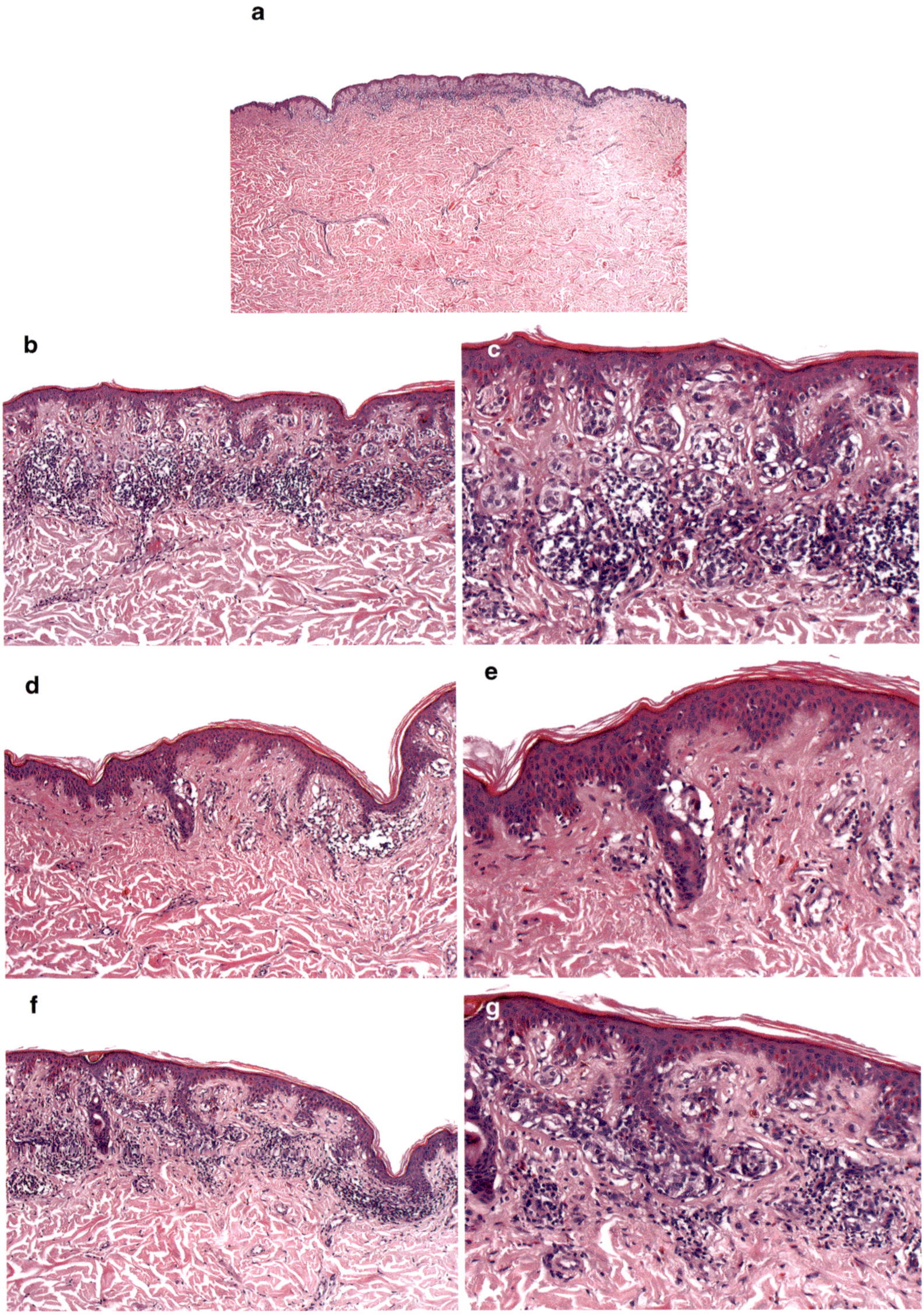

Fig. 7.2 (**a**–**i**) Junctional pattern, Example 2. (Courtesy of the Department of Dermatology, Medical University of Vienna)

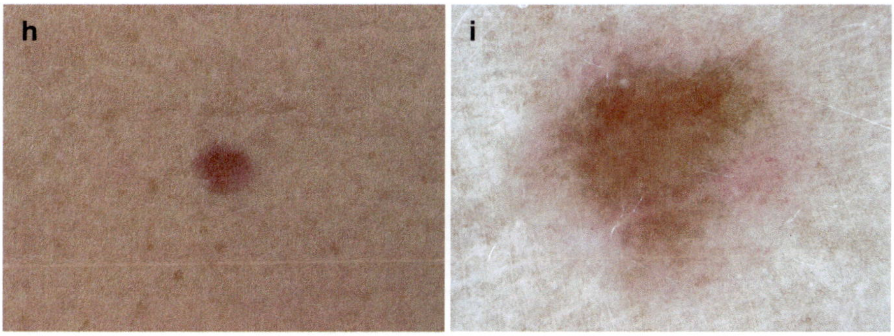

Fig. 7.2 (continued)

Overall Pattern: Nested, Epidermal and Dermal, Symmetric

Detailed Description

Silhouette

- Symmetric
- Well circumscribed
- Epidermal and dermal

Patterns

Epidermis

- Nested at the junction.
- Nests are similar in size and shape.
- Some horizontal confluence of nests.
- Melanocytes are found along the acrosyringium.
- Only a few melanocytes in suprabasal layers.

Dermis

- Nests in the papillary dermis

Cytology

- Most melanocytes are small and round, some epidermal melanocytes are enlarged, and some even multinuclear.

Other Changes

- Elongated rete ridges
- Fibroplasia around elongated rete ridges
- Melanophages in the papillary dermis
- Patchy infiltrate of lymphocytes in the papillary dermis

Integration

Pathologically, the diagnosis is most likely "compound nevus." (Fig. 7.2a–g). Clinically, this is a flat lesion of a male adult older than 50 years on the abdomen, which is surrounded by small pigmented freckles (solar lentigines) (Fig. 7.2h). The dermatoscopy shows a symmetric lesion with a reticular pattern that is uniformly pigmented (Fig. 7.2i). Integrating all information, the diagnosis is "compound nevus." The major differences between this lesion and the one shown in Example 1 are:

- This lesion is symmetric and well circumscribed on both sides; the lesion in Example 1 is asymmetric and poorly circumscribed.
- This lesion is mostly nested, the lesion in Example 1 shows parts with single cells.
- In this lesion the nests are equidistant, while the nests of the lesion in Example 1 are not equidistant, especially in the parts with the flattened epidermis.
- Although there are some occasional multinuclear cells in the epidermis, the melanocytes of this lesion are rather monomorphic, whereas the melanocytes of the lesion in Example 1 are polymorphic.
- The epidermal silhouette of this lesion is regular with preserved rete ridges, while the lesion shown in Example 1 has a flattened epidermis in some parts.
- This lesion has small nests of monomorphic melanocytes in the papillary dermis, the lesions shown in Example 1 have not.
- When viewed by dermatoscopy this lesion is symmetric and uniformly pigmented; the lesion in Example 1 is chaotic with regard to pattern and color.
- The chronic sun damage in the surrounding skin of this lesion is less than in the lesion shown in Example 1.

Diagnosis: (Acquired) compound nevus.

Alternative diagnosis according to the WHO Classification of Tumours 4th ed.: "Dysplastic nevus."

7.1.1.3 Example 3: Nests and Single Cells (Fig. 7.3)

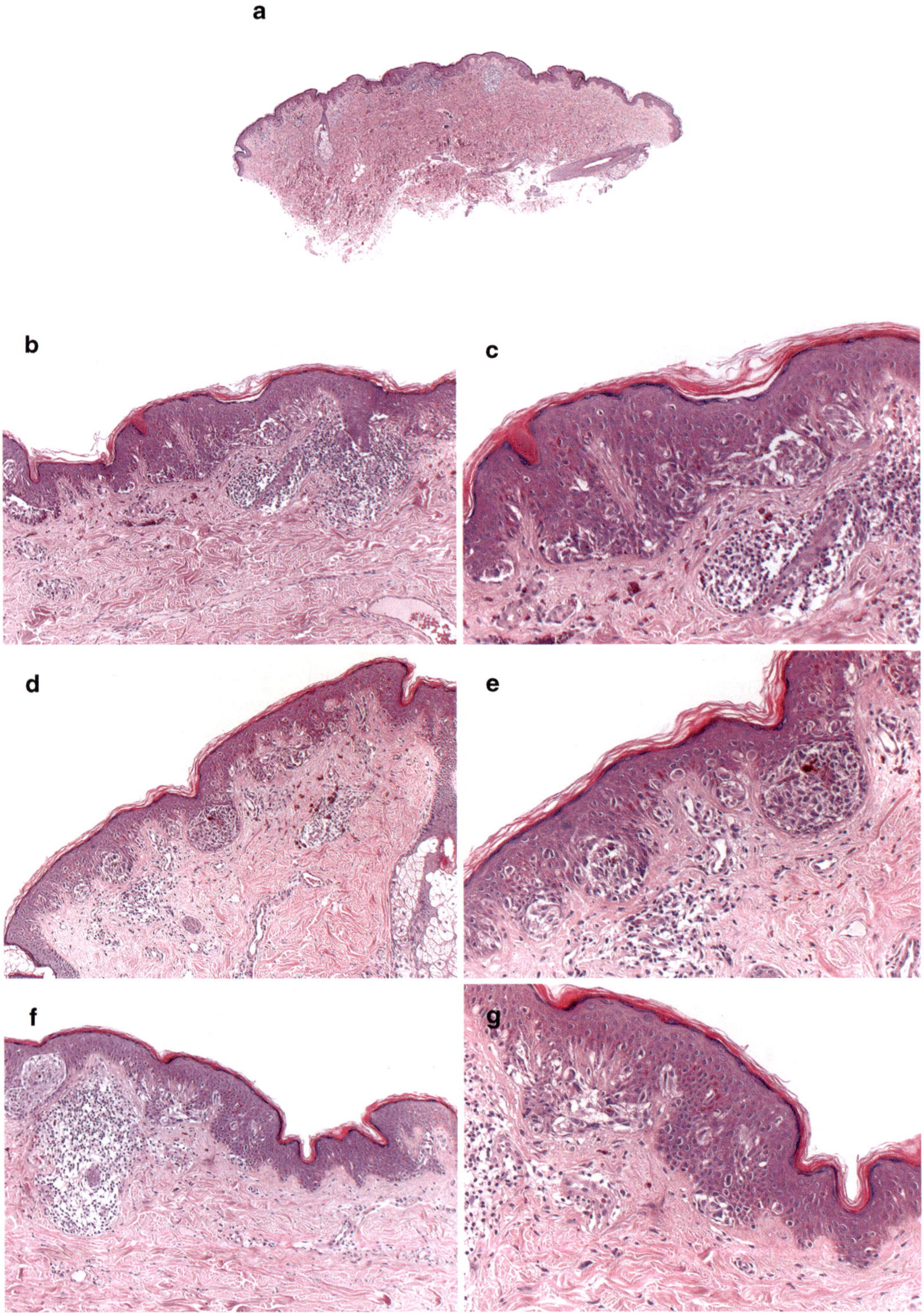

Fig. 7.3 (**a–i**) Junctional pattern, Example 3. (Courtesy of the Department of Dermatology, Medical University of Vienna)

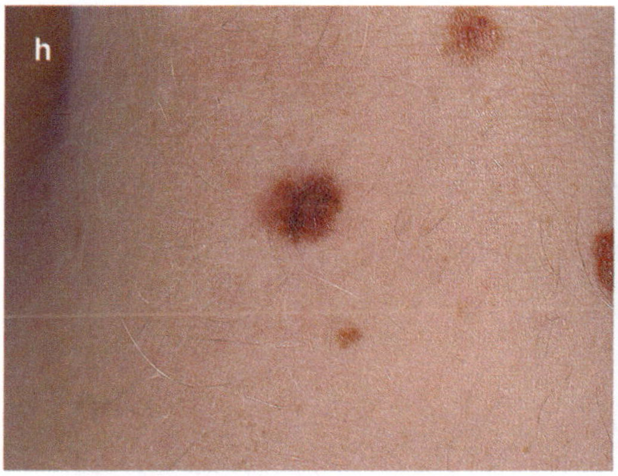

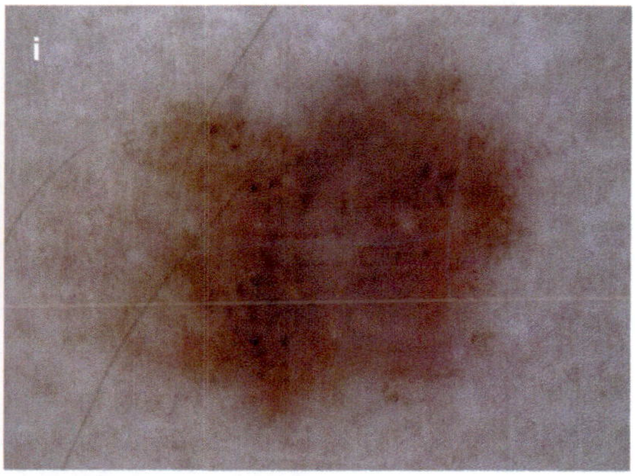

Fig. 7.3 (continued)

Overall Pattern: Epidermal, Asymmetric, Poorly Circumscribed

Detailed Description

Silhouette

- Asymmetric
- Poorly circumscribed
- Epidermal

Patterns

Epidermis

- Nests, unequal in size and shape, not equidistant
- Single melanocytes increased, unevenly distributed, also in suprapapillary arches of the epidermis
- Suprabasal single melanocytes

Cytology

- Mainly small, round melanocytes, some are enlarged and spindle.

Other Changes

- Patchy infiltrate of lymphocytes in the papillary dermis
- Melanophages in the papillary dermis

Integration

The epidermal melanocytic lesion is asymmetric and poorly circumscribed (Fig. 7.3a). Single cells predominate over nests in some parts of the lesions (Fig. 7.3b, d, f). Nests of melanocytes are not equal in size and shape and are not equidistant and single melanocytes can be found in higher layers of the epidermis (Fig. 7.3c, e, g). Clinically, this is a flat lesion with multiple shades of brown on intermittently sun-exposed skin in an adult (Fig. 7.3h). On dermatoscopy the lesion is chaotic, with multiple patterns, including brown and black dots that correspond to the nests of melanocytes in the epidermis (Fig. 7.3i). There is also slight erythema and gray dots, which correlate with inflammation and melanophages in the papillary dermis. Clinically, dermatoscopically, and pathologically the lesion shows features of melanoma. There is no associated nevus.

Diagnosis: Melanoma in situ.

Alternative diagnosis according to the WHO Classification of Tumours 4th ed.: Superficial spreading melanoma, in situ, melanoma in skin with low cumulative sun damage.

7.1.1.4 Example 4: Nests and Single Cells, Chronic Sun Damage (Fig. 7.4)

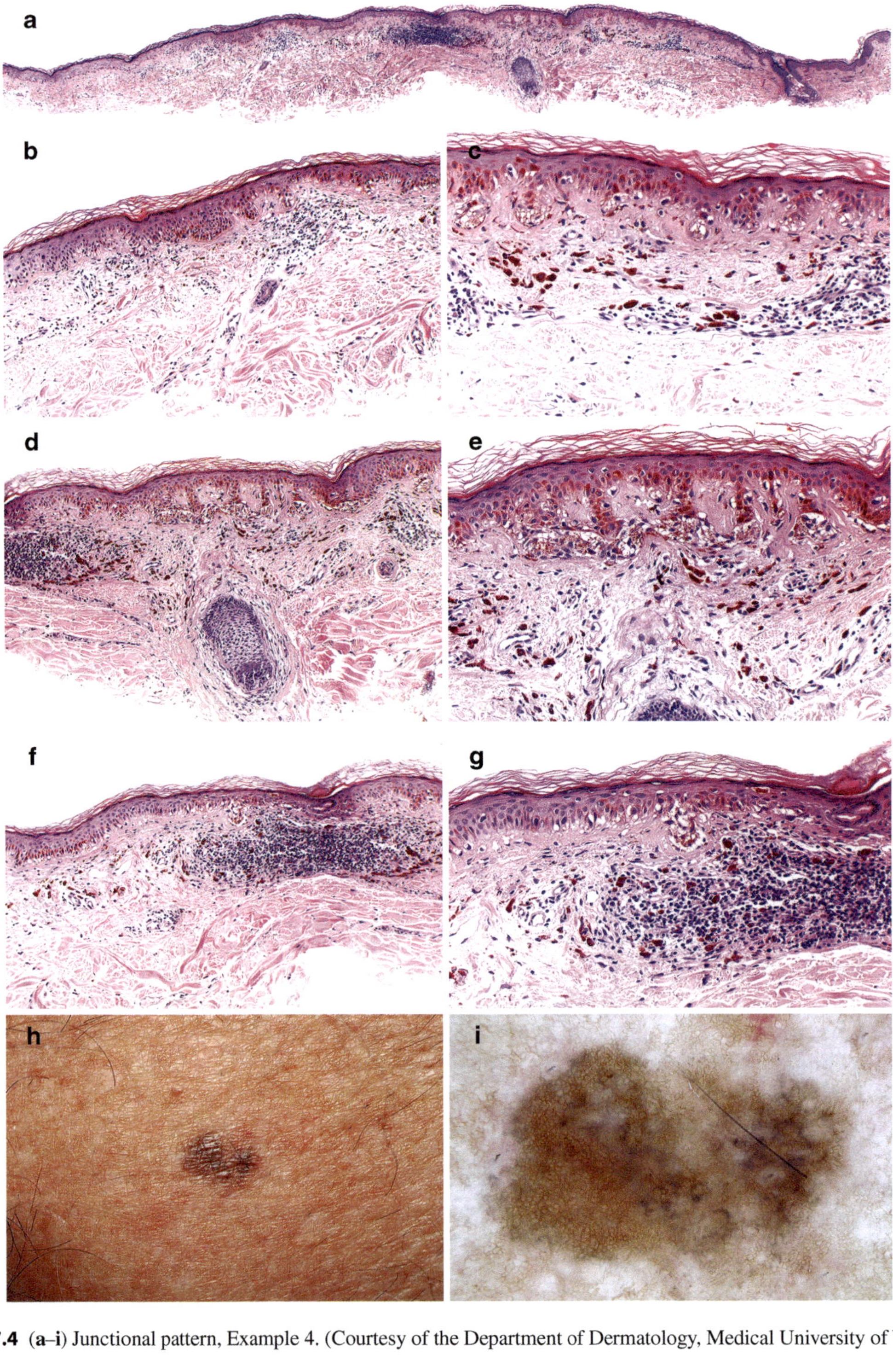

Fig. 7.4 (**a**–**i**) Junctional pattern, Example 4. (Courtesy of the Department of Dermatology, Medical University of Vienna)

Overall Pattern: Epidermal, Asymmetric, Poorly Circumscribed

Detailed Description

Silhouette

- Asymmetric
- Poorly circumscribed
- Epidermal

Patterns

Epidermis

- Small nests in bases of rete ridges, with horizontal confluence
- Single melanocytes increased between nests, unevenly distributed, on sides of rete ridges and suprapapillary arches of epidermis

Cytology

- Mainly small and round with melanin pigment

Other Changes

- Patchy infiltrate of lymphocytes in the papillary dermis.
- Melanophages in the papillary dermis.
- Epidermis is flattened in some parts.
- Dermal fibrosis.

Integration

Pathologically, the differential diagnosis is melanoma in situ versus junctional nevus versus melanoma in association with a nevus (Fig. 7.4a–g). Clinically, this is a flat, irregularly pigmented lesion surrounded by severe sun-damage on the back of an older male (Fig. 7.4h). Dermatoscopically, the lesion is chaotic with a reticular pattern and gray dots that may indicate regression (Fig. 7.4i). Adding it up gives the diagnosis of melanoma in situ. Similar to the lesion shown in Fig. 7.1 of this chapter, some parts of this melanoma mimic an acquired junctional nevus ("dysplastic" nevus) and this is the reason why some pathologists would sign this out as melanoma in situ arising in a "dysplastic nevus" or as "severely dysplastic nevus" or as MPATH-Dx Class 3. For us there is no need and no strong evidence to invoke a precursor lesion here. Like "lentigo maligna," melanoma in situ on chronic sun-damaged non-facial skin usually develops de novo and not in a pre-existing nevus but may mimic a benign melanocytic proliferation in some areas. It is common to mistake a simulator for a precursor (to mistake parts of a melanoma that simulate a nevus as part of a nevus).

Diagnosis: Melanoma in situ.

Alternative diagnosis according to the WHO Classification of Tumours 4th ed.: "Melanoma in situ in skin with low cumulative sun damage" or "Melanoma in situ in skin with low cumulative sun damage arising in a dysplastic nevus." Although the extensive freckling in the surrounding skin points to high cumulative sun damage, the back is regarded as a site of low cumulative sun damage according to the WHO classification. The definition of high cumulative sun damage hinges on the presence of solar elastosis in the histopathologic specimen and not on clinical criteria. It is unclear how much solar elastosis is needed to qualify as high cumulative sun damage.

7.1.1.5 Example 5: Small Lesion with Nests (Fig. 7.5)

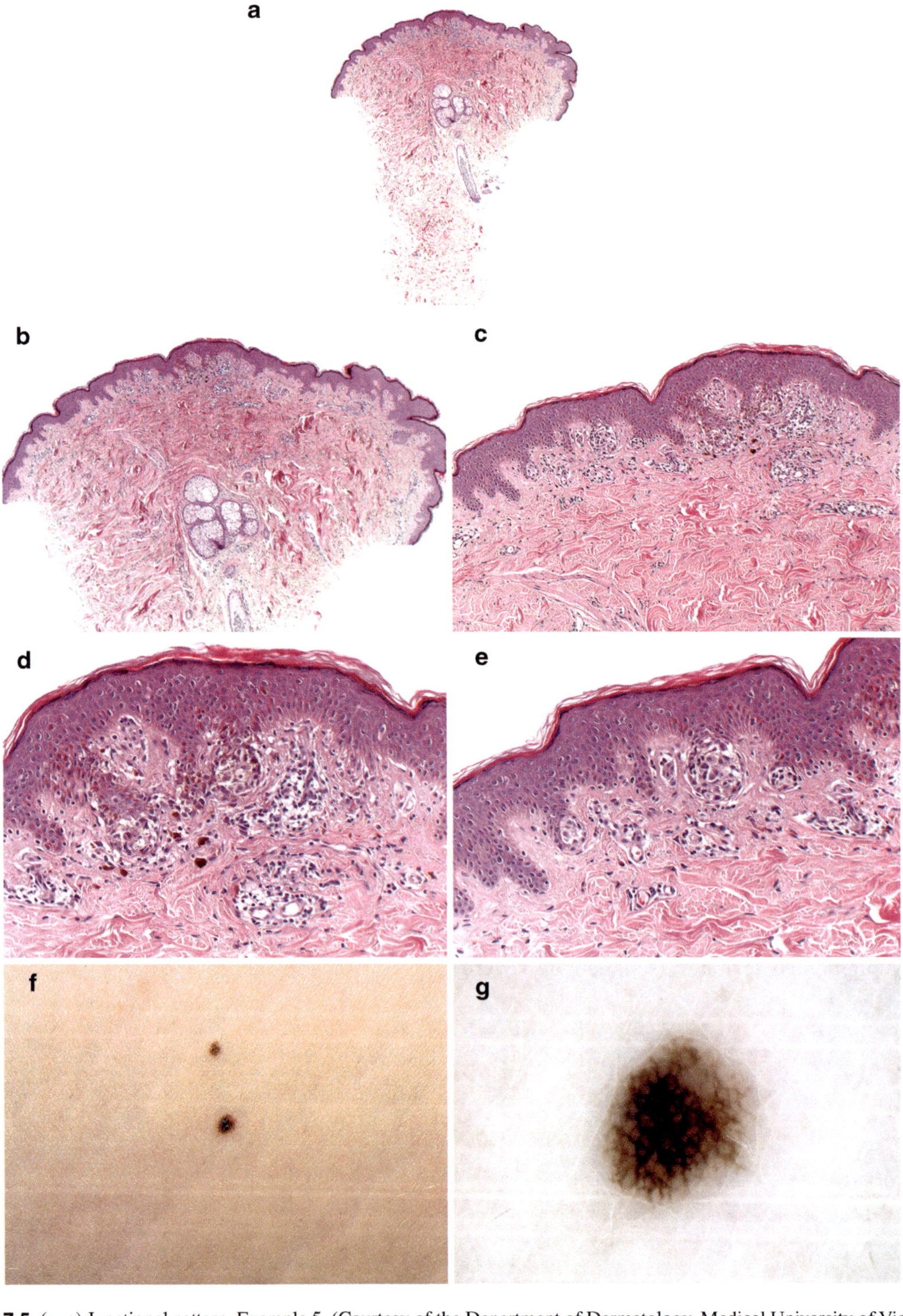

Fig. 7.5 (**a**–**g**) Junctional pattern, Example 5. (Courtesy of the Department of Dermatology, Medical University of Vienna)

Overall Pattern: Epidermal, Small, Nested, Symmetric

Detailed Description

Silhouette

- Small
- Symmetric
- Well circumscribed
- Epidermal

Patterns

Epidermis

- Nests, in bases of rete ridges
- Single melanocytes increased, unevenly distributed
- Suprabasal single melanocytes

Cytology

- Enlarged round melanocytes
- Fine melanin pigment in melanocytes

Other Changes

- Single melanophages in the papillary dermis

Integration

Clinically, this is a small dark brown macule (Fig. 7.5f). The surrounding skin does not show chronic sun damage. On dermatoscopy, the lesion is symmetric and consists of a pattern of reticular lines with dark brown color (Fig. 7.5g). The clinical and dermatoscopic appearance are in line with a small, hyperpigmented junctional nevus. These lesions are very common and frequently biopsied to rule out incipient melanoma.

Diagnosis: (Acquired) junctional nevus.

Alternative diagnosis according to the WHO Classification of Tumours 4th ed.: "Dysplastic nevus."

7.1.1.6 Example 6: Small Lesion with Nests, Heavily Pigmented (Fig. 7.6)

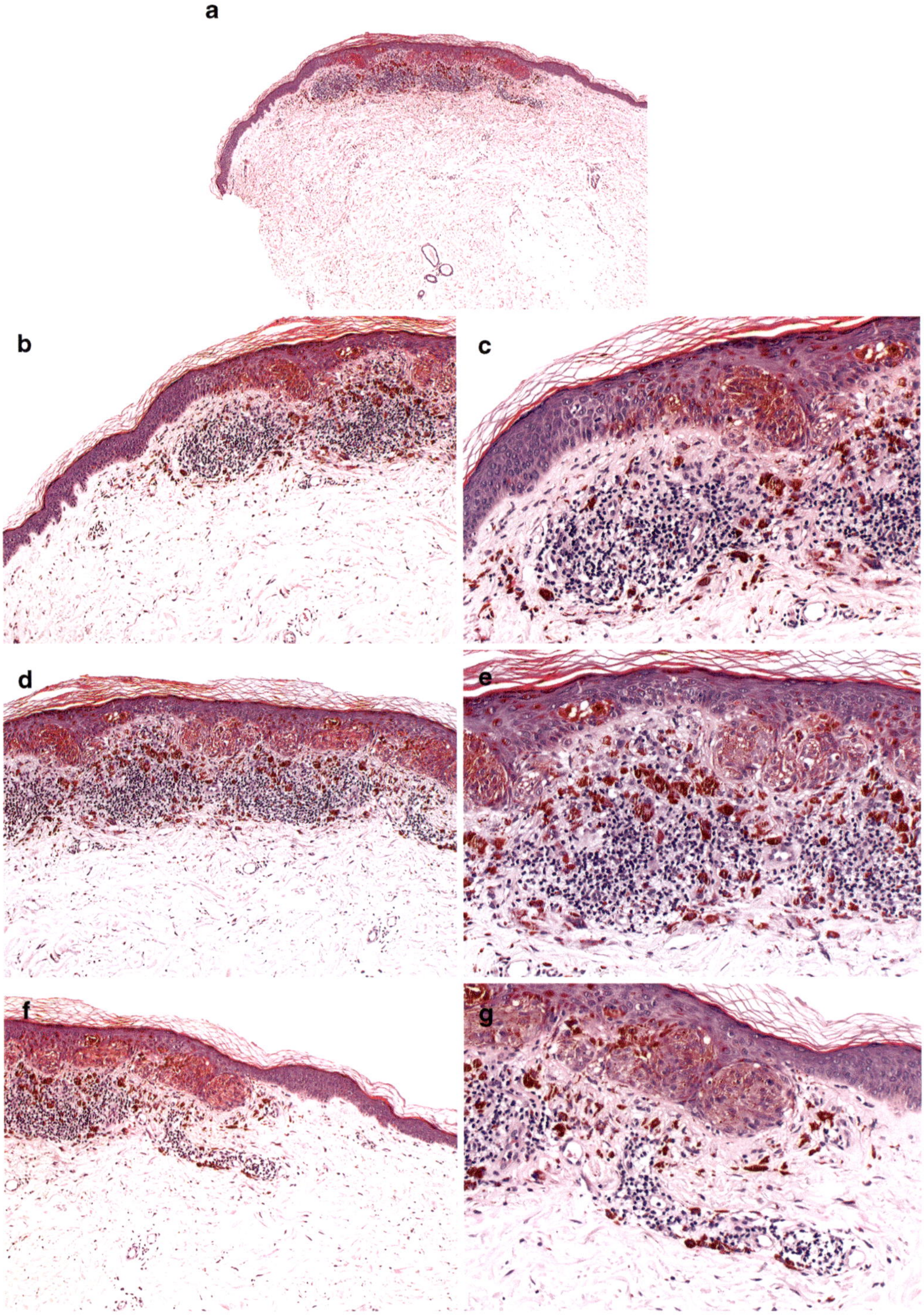

Fig. 7.6 (**a**–**i**) Junctional pattern, Example 6. (Courtesy of the Department of Dermatology, Medical University of Vienna)

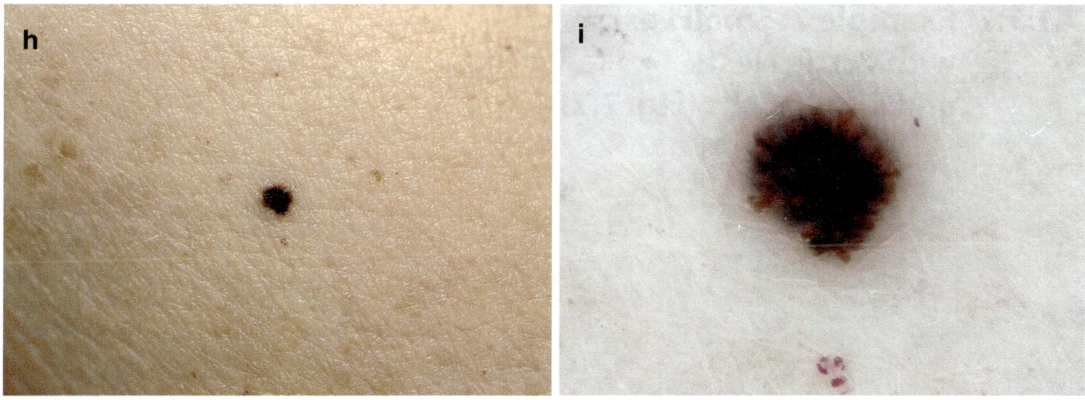

Fig. 7.6 (continued)

Overall Pattern: Epidermal, Small, Symmetric, Nested, Well Circumscribed

Detailed Description

Silhouette

- Symmetric
- Flat
- Well circumscribed
- Epidermal

Patterns

Epidermis

- Nests, equal in size and shape

Cytology

- Enlarged melanocytes, spindle melanocytes, heavily pigmented

Other Changes

- Patchy infiltrate of lymphocytes and melanophages in the papillary dermis

Integration

The epidermal melanocytic lesion is small, symmetric, and well circumscribed. Nests predominate (Fig. 7.6a–g). Clinically, it is a small black macule (Fig. 7.6h). Dermatoscopically, the lesion is structureless black in the center, and shows radial lines at the periphery *over the entire circumference*, which is typical of a pigmented spindle cell nevus (Fig. 7.6i). Note the absence of surrounding sun damage in the clinical and dermatoscopic image.

Diagnosis: Pigmented spindle cell nevus, junctional ("Reed nevus").

7.1.1.7 Example 7: Small Lesion with Large Nests and Single Cells (Fig. 7.7)

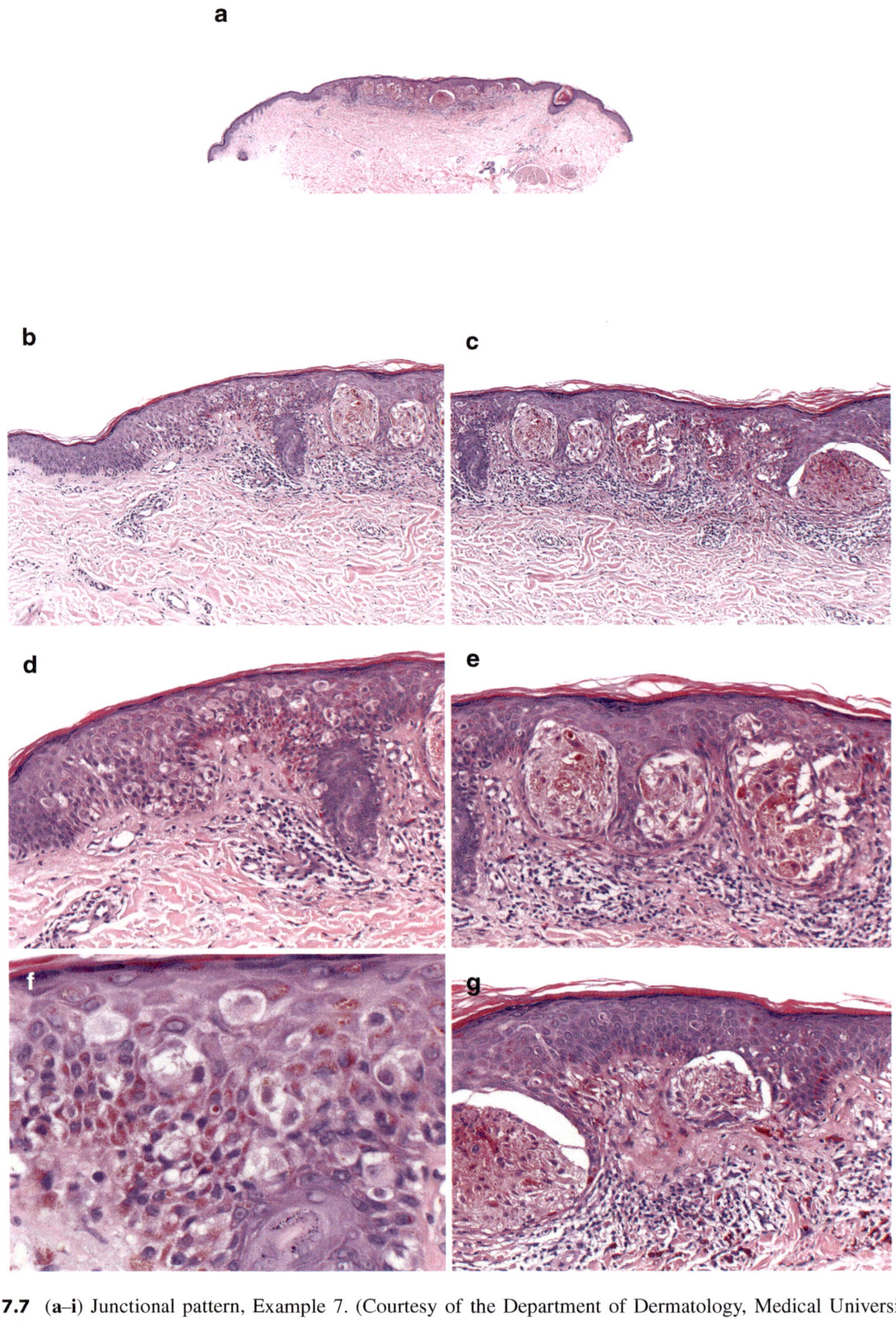

Fig. 7.7 (a–i) Junctional pattern, Example 7. (Courtesy of the Department of Dermatology, Medical University of Vienna)

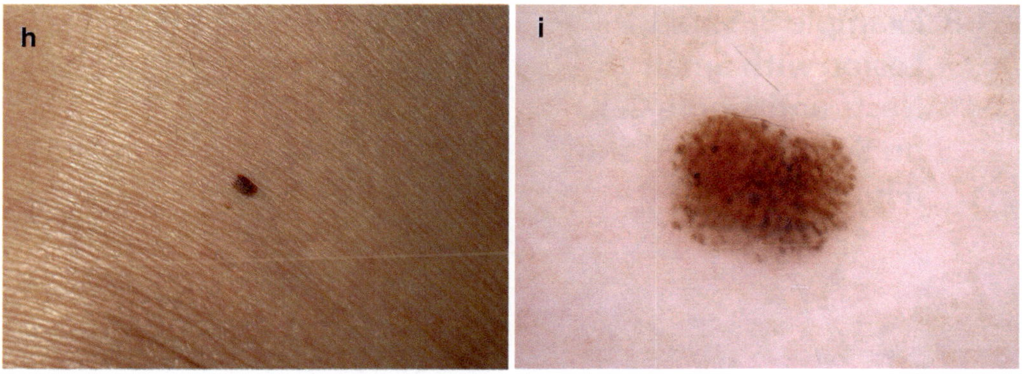

Fig. 7.7 (continued)

Overall Pattern: Epidermal, Asymmetric, Poorly Circumscribed

Detailed Description

Silhouette

- Asymmetric
- Poorly circumscribed
- Small
- Epidermal

Patterns

Epidermis

- Nests, uneven in size and shape, not equidistant
- Single melanocytes increased, unevenly distributed
- Suprabasal single melanocytes and nests

Cytology

- Epithelioid, spindled, and pagetoid melanocytes

Other Changes

- Patchy infiltrate of lymphocytes in the papillary dermis
- Melanophages in the papillary dermis

Integration

Clinically, this is a small brown papule that looks like a nevus. It is located on the thigh of a middle-aged woman. Dermatoscopically the lesion is chaotic with radial lines at the periphery and unevenly distributed black and brown dots. There is no associated nevus, neither clinically or dermatoscopically, nor pathologically. Although the lesion measures only 3 mm in diameter, the diagnosis of melanoma can be made with confidence.

Diagnosis: Melanoma in situ.

Alternative diagnosis according to the WHO Classification of Tumours 4th ed.: Superficial spreading melanoma, in situ, melanoma in situ in skin with low cumulative sun damage.

7.1.1.8 Example 8: Small Lesion with Small Nests and Single Cells on Sun-Damaged Skin (Fig. 7.8)

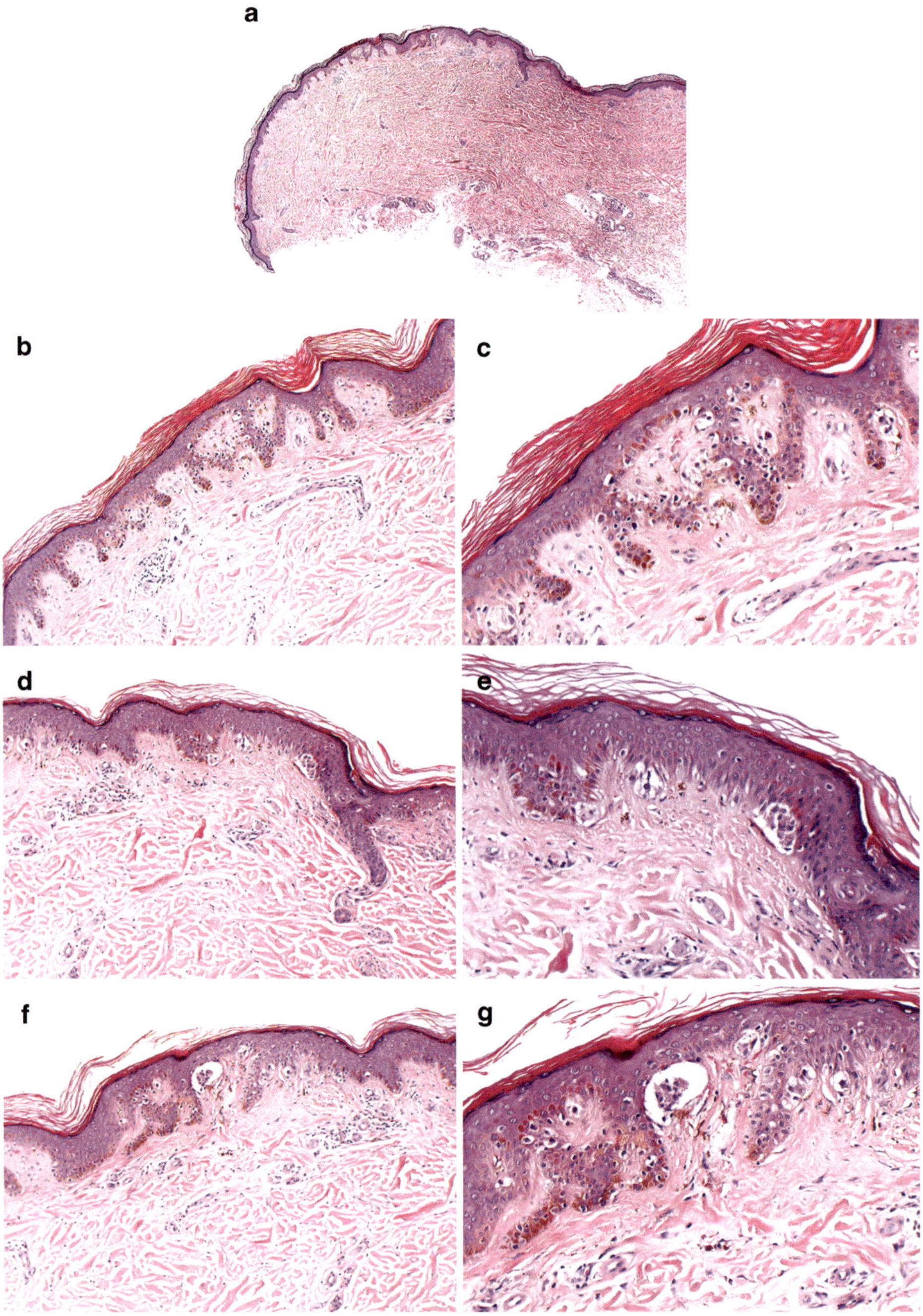

Fig. 7.8 (**a–i**) Junctional pattern, Example 8. (Courtesy of the Department of Dermatology, Medical University of Vienna)

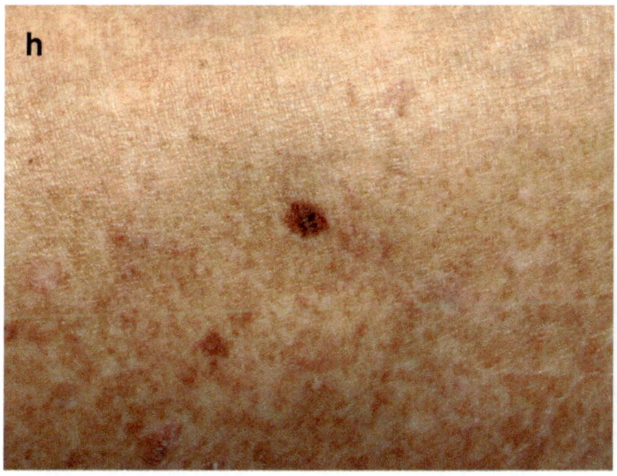
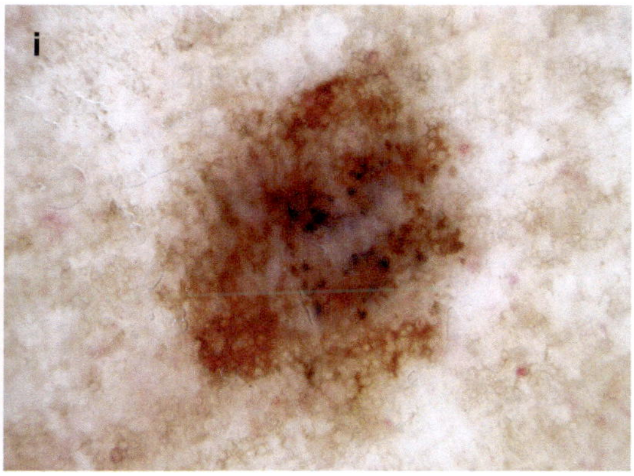

Fig. 7.8 (continued)

Overall Pattern: Epidermal, Asymmetric, Poorly Circumscribed

Detailed Description

Silhouette

- Asymmetric
- Poorly circumscribed
- Epidermal

Patterns

Epidermis

- Nests, unequal in size and shape, not equidistant
- Single melanocytes increased, unevenly distributed

Cytology

- Enlarged melanocytes

Other Changes

- Elongated rete ridges with basal pigmentation
- Clefting around nests
- Discrete lamellar fibroplasia of papillary dermis

Integration

Pathologically, the differential diagnosis is melanoma in situ versus junctional nevus (Fig. 7.8a–g). Clinically, it is a pigmented macule on the background of chronically sun-damaged skin (Fig. 7.8h). Dermatoscopically, the lesion is chaotic with reticular lines and unevenly distributed black dots (Fig. 7.8i). The lesion is located on the leg of an elderly woman, which increases the likelihood of melanoma. Adding it up, the only reasonable diagnosis is melanoma in situ.

Diagnosis: Melanoma in situ.

Alternative diagnosis according to the WHO Classification of Tumours 4th ed.: "Melanoma, in situ in skin with low cumulative sun damage." Although the extensive freckling in the surrounding skin points to high cumulative sun damage, the leg is regarded as a site of low cumulative sun damage according to the WHO classification. The definition of high cumulative sun damage hinges on the presence of solar elastosis in the histopathologic specimen and not on clinical criteria. It is unclear how much solar elastosis is needed to qualify as high cumulative sun damage.

7.1.1.9 Example 9: Small Lesion with Nests, Heavily Pigmented, Spitzoid (Fig. 7.9)

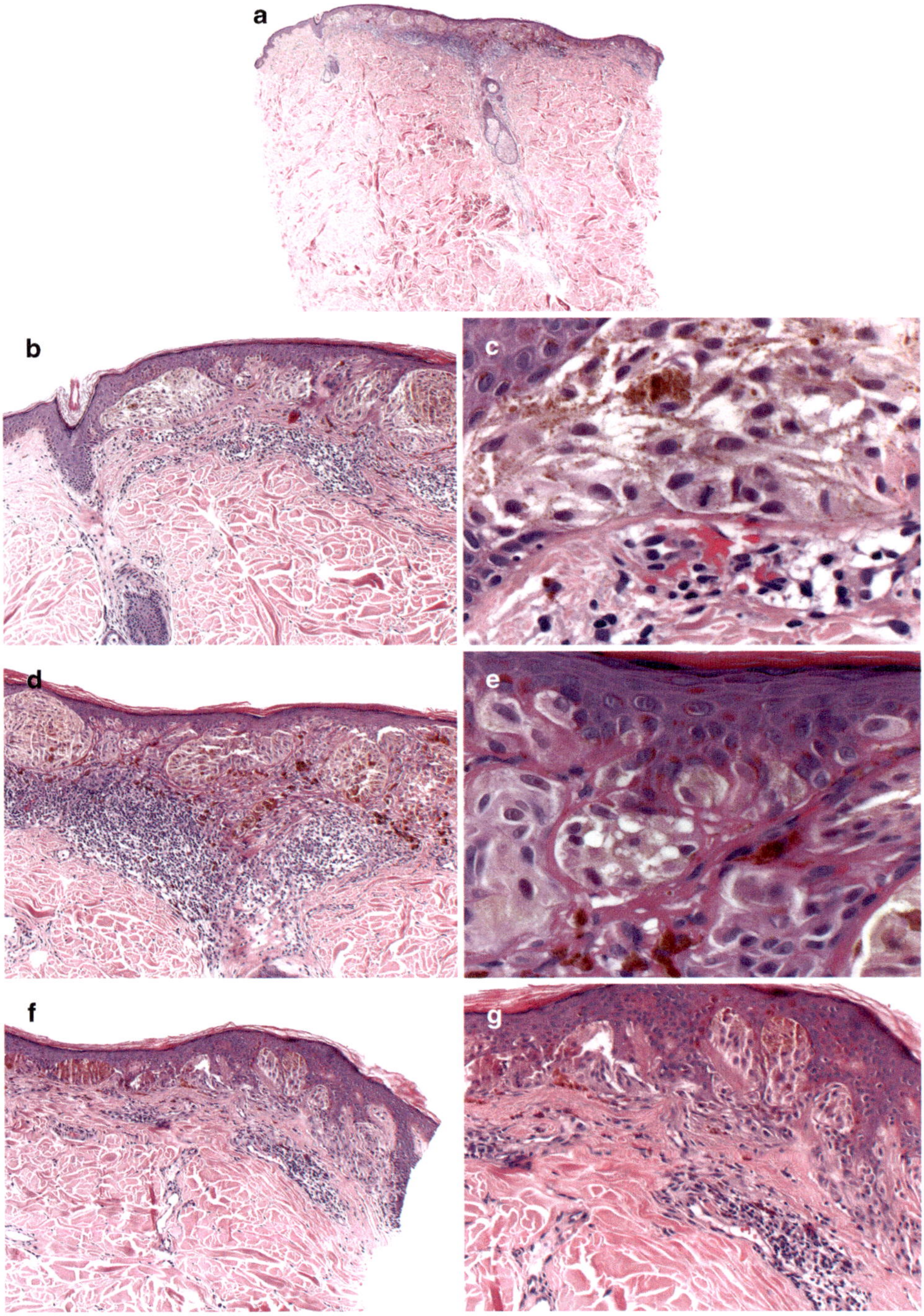

Fig. 7.9 (**a–i**) Junctional pattern, Example 9. (Courtesy of the Department of Dermatology, Medical University of Vienna)

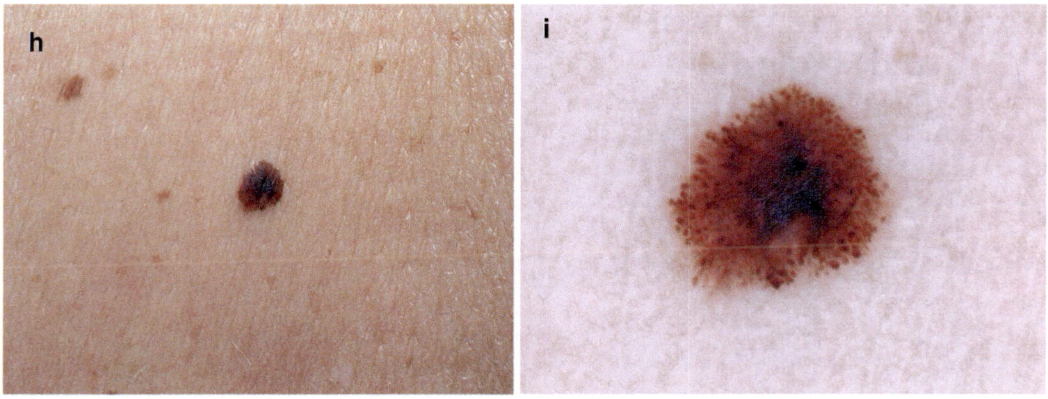

Fig. 7.9 (continued)

Overall Pattern: Epidermal, Asymmetric, Large Nests

Detailed Description

Silhouette

- Asymmetric
- Poorly circumscribed
- Epidermal

Patterns

Epidermis

- Nests, unequal in size and shape, not equidistant, some very large
- Few large single melanocytes

Cytology

- Enlarged melanocytes, epithelioid melanocytes, Pagetoid melanocytes
- Dusty melanin pigment
- Mitoses

Other Changes

- Lamellar stratum corneum
- Dense band-like and perifollicular infiltrate of lymphocytes in the papillary dermis

Already at scanning magnification it can be seen that the lesion consists of unequally sized nests with asymmetric distribution (Fig. 7.9a). Although only focal, proliferation of single large epithelioid cell melanocytes can be seen between the nests and in higher levels of the epidermis (Fig. 7.9b–g). Clinically, the small lesion is somewhat irregularly pigmented (Fig. 7.9h). The skin surrounding the lesion shows little evidence of sun damage. Dermatoscopically, the lesion has a pattern of brown clods at the periphery with a hyperpigmented center. The area in the center is not well circumscribed (Fig. 7.9i). Consistent with the clinical and dermoscopic differential diagnosis of a Spitz nevus versus an incipient melanoma, the adult patient reported that the lesion grew rapidly. There is no evidence of an associated nevus and although the lesion is small, the final diagnosis of melanoma in situ can be made with confidence.

Diagnosis: Melanoma in situ.

Alternative diagnosis according to the WHO Classification of Tumours 4th ed.: Superficial spreading melanoma, in situ, melanoma in skin with low cumulative sun damage.

7.1.1.10 Example 10: Nests and Single Cells (Fig. 7.10)

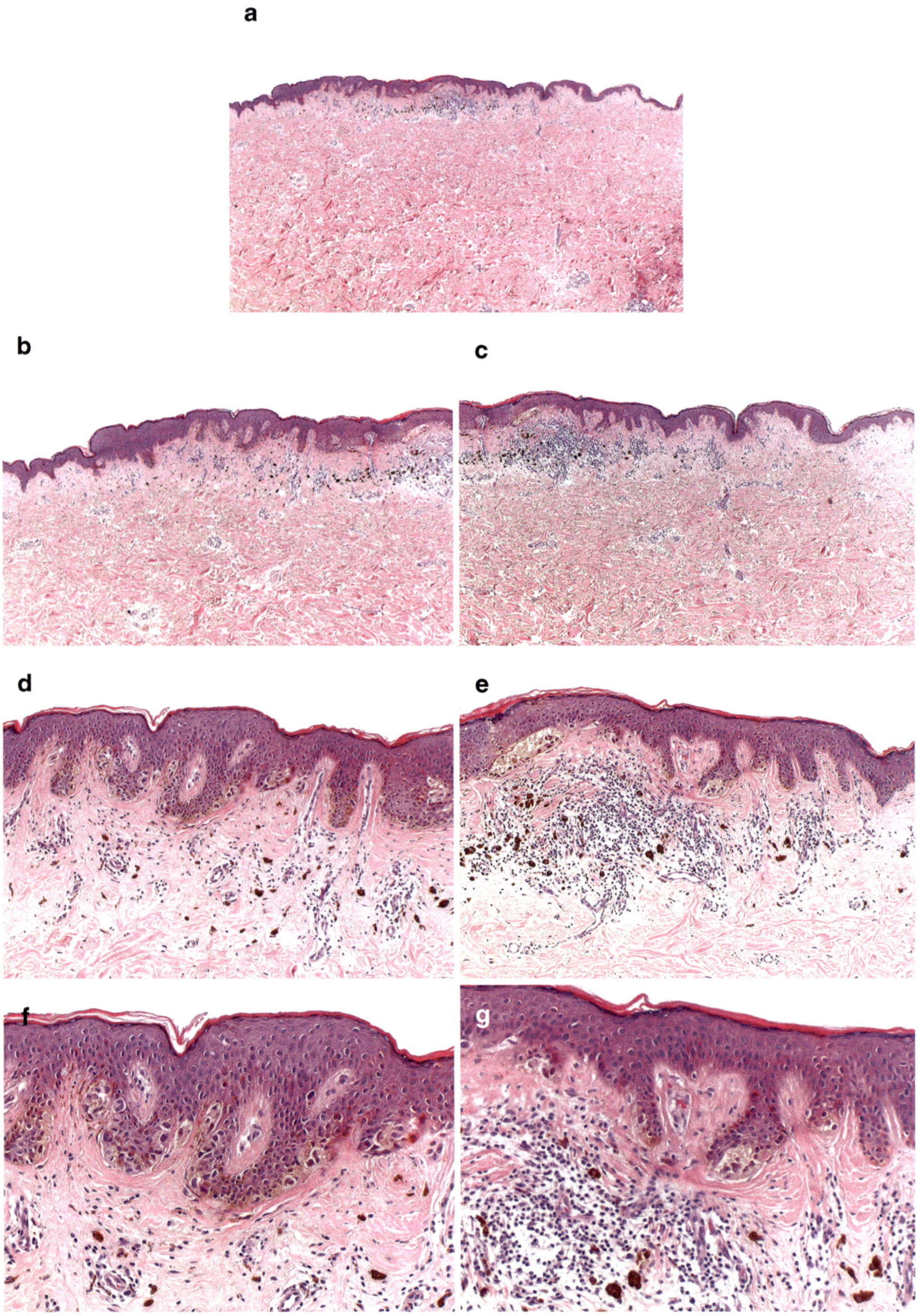

Fig. 7.10 (**a**–**i**) Junctional pattern, Example 10. (Courtesy of the Department of Dermatology, Medical University of Vienna)

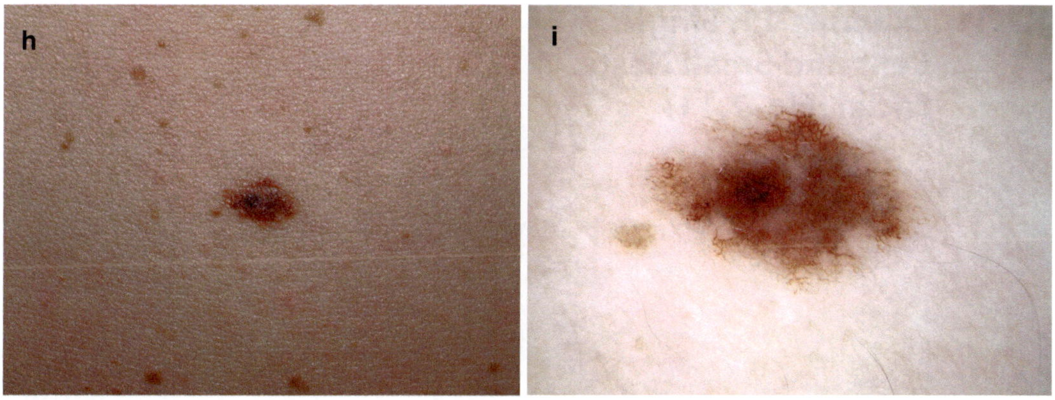

Fig. 7.10 (continued)

Overall Pattern: Epidermal, Asymmetric, Poorly Circumscribed

Detailed Description

Silhouette

- Asymmetric
- Poorly circumscribed
- Epidermal

Patterns

Epidermis

- Nests, unequal in size and shape, not equidistant
- Single melanocytes increased, unevenly distributed

Cytology

- Enlarged melanocytes

Other Changes

- Patchy infiltrate of lymphocytes in the papillary dermis
- Melanophages in the papillary dermis
- Prominent fibroplasia around rete ridges

Integration

The lesion is located on the trunk of a middle-aged male patient. Clinically, it shows multiple shades of brown (Fig. 7.10h). There is moderate sun-damage in the surrounding skin. Dermatoscopically, the pigmentation of the reticular lesion is chaotic (Fig. 7.10i). In sum, this is melanoma in situ. Note that suprabasal melanocytes are not evident (Fig. 7.10a–g). Because some parts of the melanoma look like an acquired junctional nevus and because features of melanomas are missing, some pathologists would sign this out as melanoma in situ arising in a "dysplastic nevus" or as "severely dysplastic nevus" or as MPATH-Dx Class 3. The management, however, would be the same.

Diagnosis: Melanoma in situ.

Alternative diagnosis according to the WHO Classification of Tumours 4th ed.: Superficial spreading melanoma, in situ, melanoma in skin with low cumulative sun damage or Superficial spreading melanoma, in situ, arising in a "dysplastic" nevus?

7.1.1.11 Example 11: Single Cells and Small Nests, Facial (Fig. 7.11)

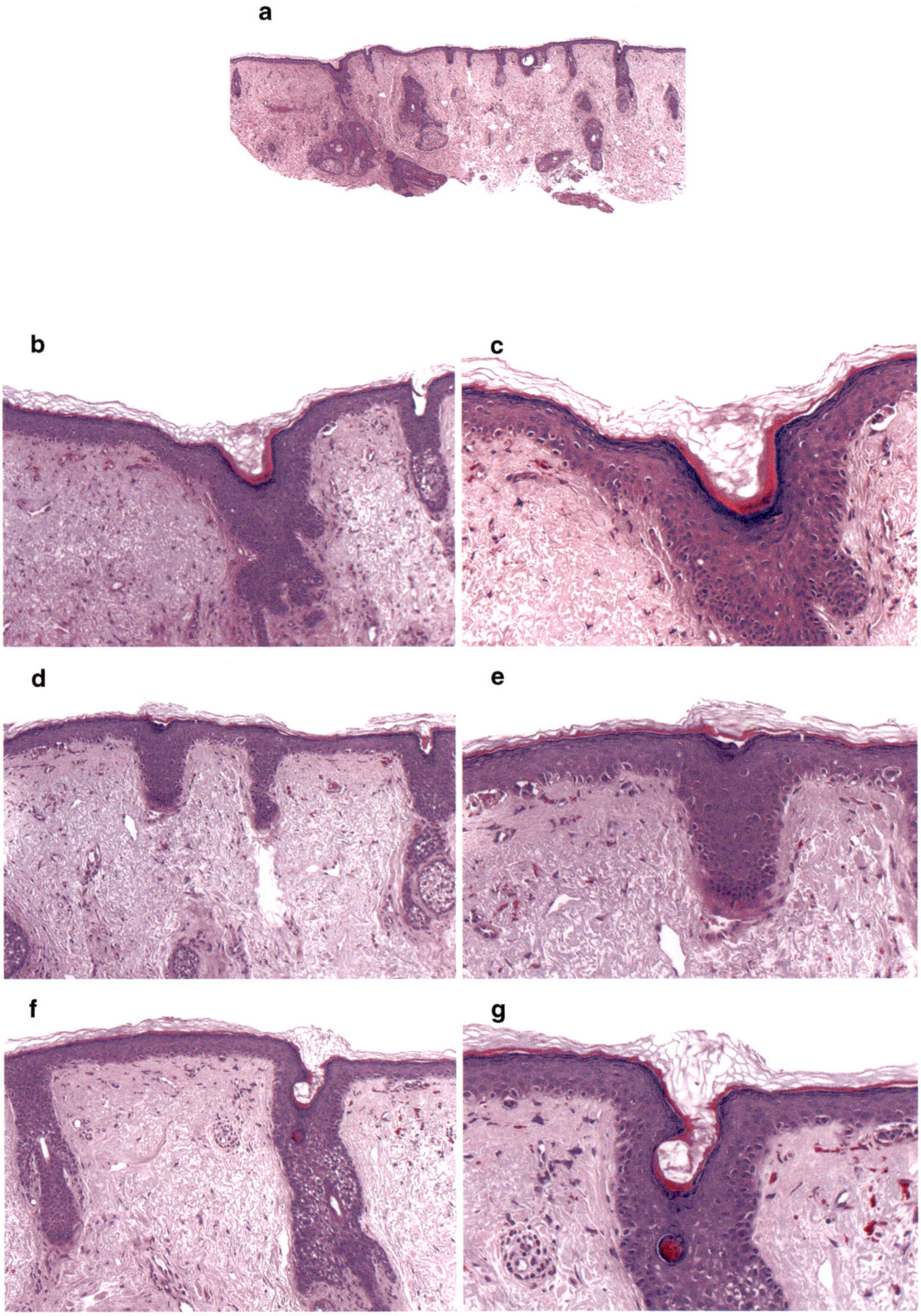

Fig. 7.11 (**a**–**i**) Junctional pattern, Example 11. (Courtesy of the Department of Dermatology, Medical University of Vienna)

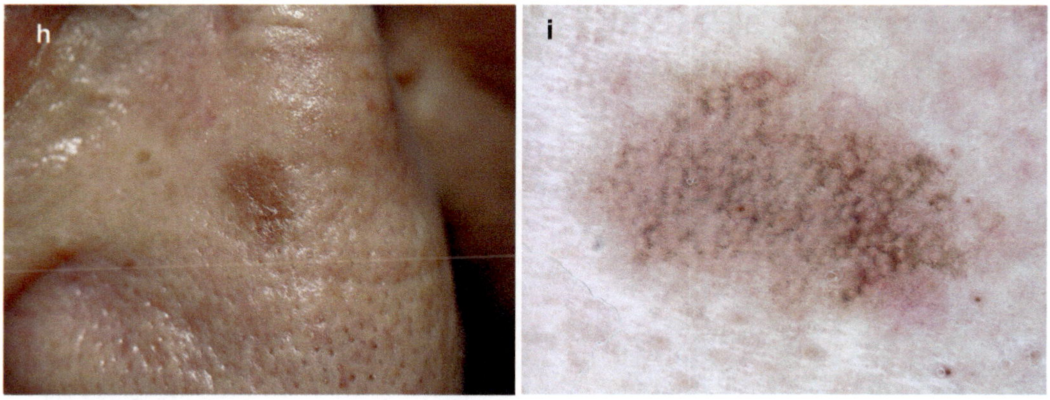

Fig. 7.11 (continued)

Overall Pattern: Epidermal, Asymmetric, Poorly Circumscribed

Detailed Description

Silhouette

- Asymmetric
- Poorly circumscribed
- Epidermal

Patterns

Epidermis

- Single melanocytes increased, unevenly distributed
- Small nests of melanocytes, unevenly distributed

Cytology

- Small melanocytes, enlarged melanocytes

Other Changes

- Abundant solar elastosis
- Melanophages in the papillary dermis

Integration

This is a flat pigmented lesion on the face of an elderly female. The pigmented macule is surrounded by severe chronic sun damage (Fig. 7.11h). Dermatoscopy shows gray pigmentation, which is a sensitive but not very specific indicator of melanoma in situ (Fig. 7.11i). Although the lesion is barely visible and there are only a few nests of neoplastic melanocytes in the epidermis, this can only be melanoma in situ (Fig. 7.11a–g). A junctional nevus is out of the question given the context. Historically, lesions like this have been designated "Hutchinson freckle" or "precancerous melanosis of Dubreuilh," terms that are now long forgotten, and rightly so. This is another example of how a mimic (a melanoma that mimics a benign proliferation) was confused with a precursor. Some researchers are terrified by the idea that a melanoma may develop without any precursor lesion. This is akin to the "horror vacui" of Aristotle who strongly believed that "nature abhors a vacuum" and it therefore cannot exist. A modern version of the precursor lesion of facial melanoma in situ is the so-called "unstable lentigo." Lentigines are often found in association with facial melanoma in situ because both are induced by high chronic sun exposure. The fact that a lentigo is found in the vicinity of a melanoma in situ does not make it unstable, only unlucky.

Diagnosis: Melanoma in situ.

Alternative diagnosis according to the WHO Classification of Tumours 4th ed.: melanoma in situ in skin with high cumulative sun damage (lentigo maligna).

7.1.1.12 Example 12: Nests and Single Melanocytes, Broad Lesion (Fig. 7.12)

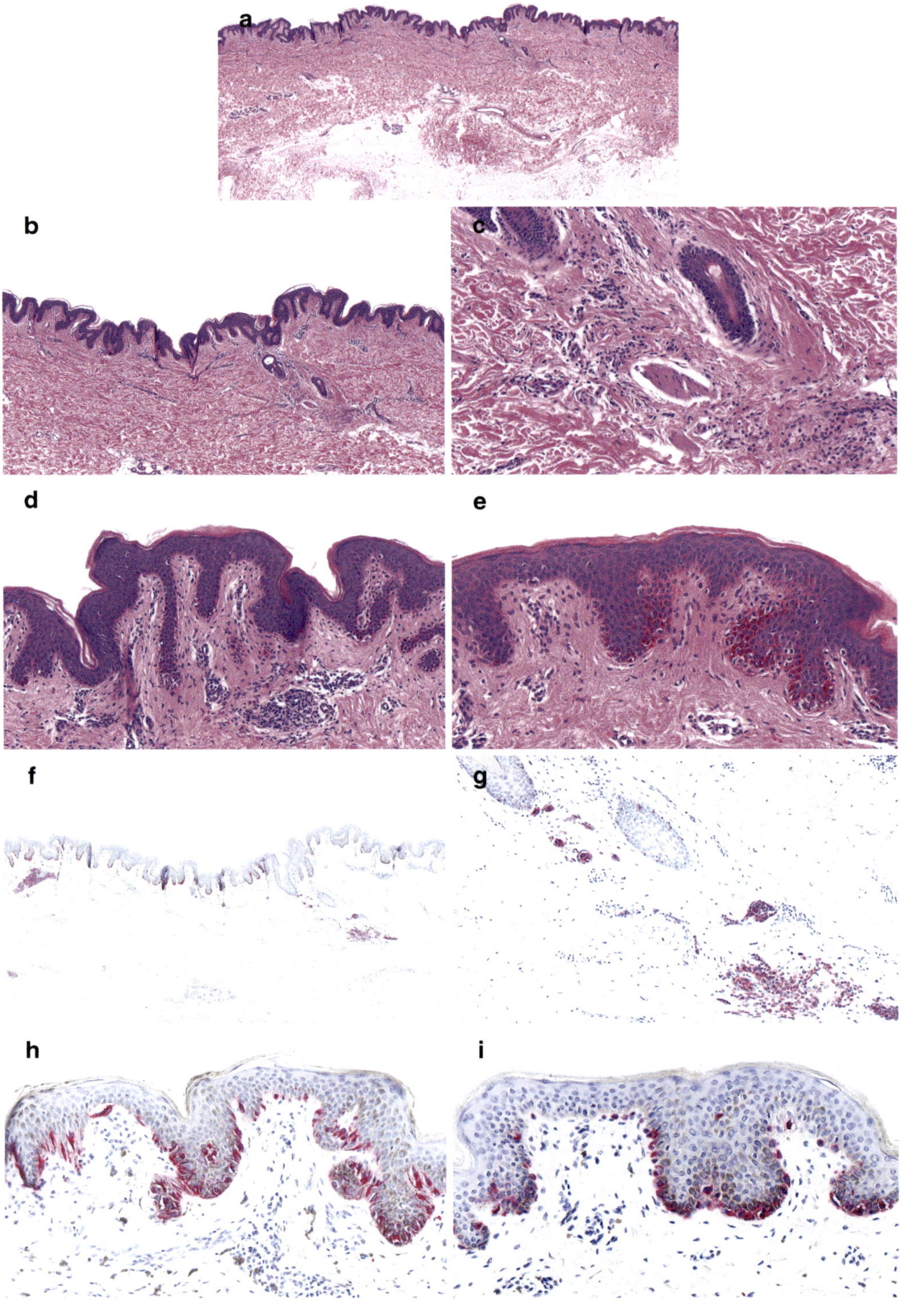

Fig. 7.12 (**a**–**k**) Junctional pattern, Example 12. (Courtesy of the Dermatologikum Hamburg)

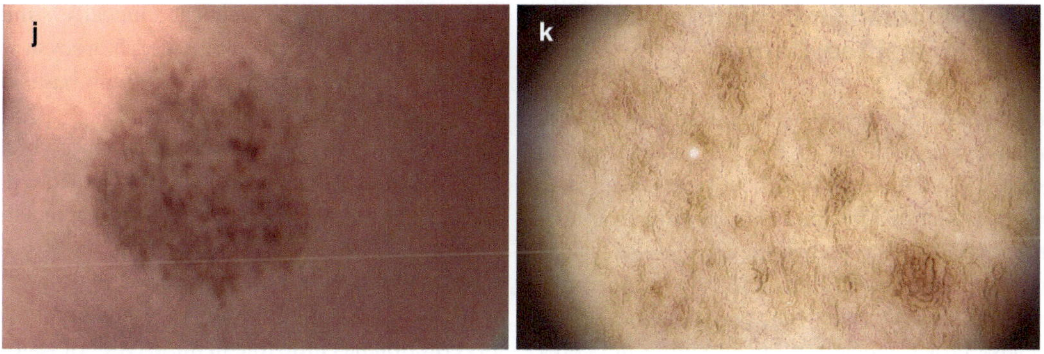

Fig. 7.12 (continued)

Overall Pattern: Epidermal and Dermal, Broad, Poorly Circumscribed

Detailed description

Silhouette

- Asymmetric
- Poorly circumscribed
- Epidermal and dermal

Patterns

Epidermis

- Single melanocytes increased at the base of rete ridges, evenly distributed
- Few nests at the junction

Dermis

- Nests of melanocytes in the superficial dermis and periadnexal
- Interstitial strands in periadnexal arrangement
- Maturation

Cytology

- Small, monomorphous

Other Changes

- Epidermal hyperplasia with elongated rete ridges
- Basal hyperpigmentation

Immunohistochemistry

- MelanA expressed at the junction, at the base of rete ridges in single melanocytes and nests
- MelanA expressed in nests and interstitial strands in the superficial dermis and around adnexa

Integration

At scanning magnification, epidermal hyperplasia with elongated rete ridges is the most impressive change in this section (Fig. 7.12a, b). At intermediate magnification, a broad melanocytic lesion is discernible (Fig. 7.12c–e). Large size and poor circumscription usually indicate melanoma, but the rete ridges pattern is well preserved and intraepidermal melanocytes are seen only in the basal layer and with even distribution (Fig. 7.12f, h, i). Dermal melanocytes have a nested and periadnexal arrangement with maturation just like it is seen in a conventional congenital nevus (Fig. 7.12f, g). These features are typical of a speckled lentiginous nevus, so-called nevus spilus. The clinical picture confirms the histopathologic diagnosis.

Diagnosis: Nevus spilus.

7.1.2 Spindled and/or Epithelioid Pigmented, Dermal

Prominently pigmented spindled and epithelioid melanocytes confined to the dermis and subcutis are the hallmark of blue nevi [128]. Why such lesions are termed *blue* may not be obvious immediately, as there is nothing *blue* about those lesions histologically. Rather, the clinician is seeing a lesion with homogenous blue pigmentation. This is because brown melanin pigment sitting in deeper portions of the skin, probably due to the Tyndall effect [129], is blue when viewed from the surface.

Clinically, the distinction of blue nevi to melanoma is often difficult based on morphologic assessment alone. With dermatoscopy one can gain a little more information [130], but eventually is of limited value regarding the decision to biopsy. In contrast to epidermal melanocytic proliferations, where the epidermal microanatomy causes specific dermatoscopic patterns, melanocytes in blue lesions are growing diffusely within the tissue, thus not giving rise to specific morphologic features. So without a convincing and reassuring patient history of longstanding presence without change, blue lesions are usually biopsied to rule out a melanoma. Other lesions that may appear clinically similar include dirt tattoos and pigmented hidrocystoma, albeit the latter is mostly confused with basal cell carcinoma clinically in our experience.

Histologically, melanoma as well as metastatic melanoma may be heavily pigmented either because of pigmented melanocytes or melanophages. Unfortunately, in contrast to most other melanocytic nevi with prominent dermal involvement, blue nevi often do not show maturation, so this criterion has little role in these types of lesions. Usually, it is the architectural and monomorphic cytologic pattern distinct to one of the known subtypes of blue nevi, which enables to make a clear-cut benign diagnosis with certainty. For some cases, certainly, insecurity will remain inevitably. If there is substantial suspicion of a melanoma arising within a blue nevus, this would be one of the selected situations where obtaining ancillary studies such as genetic analysis may be helpful.

7.1.2.1 Example 1: Pigmented Epithelioid, Dermal (Fig. 7.13)

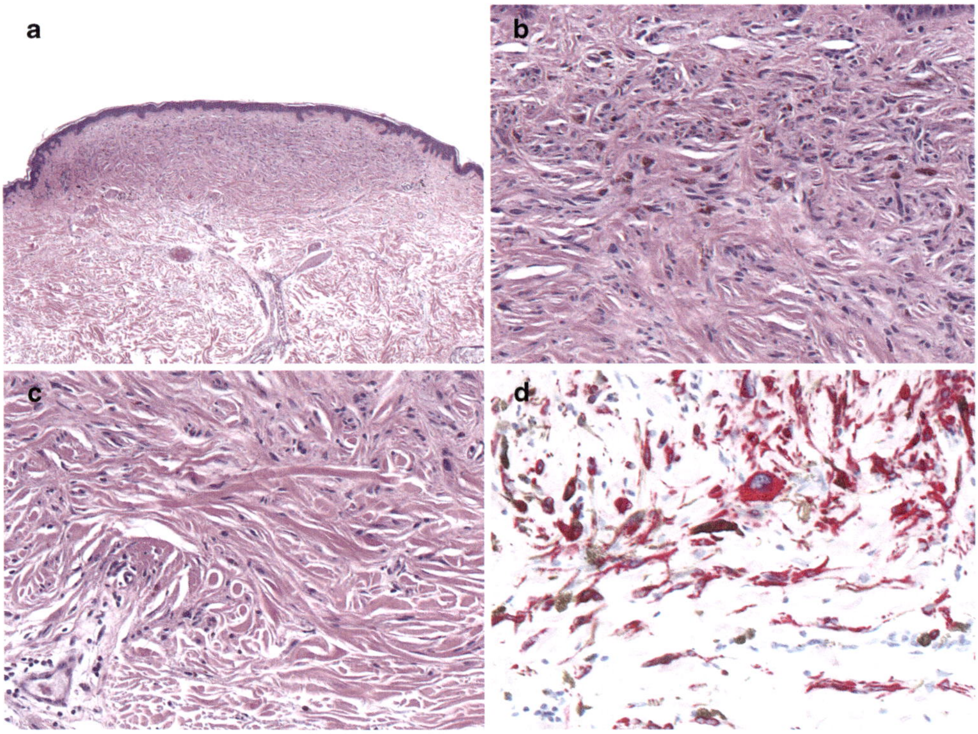

Fig. 7.13 (**a**–**d**) Spindled or epithelioid pigmented pattern, Example 1. (Courtesy of the Dermatologikum Hamburg)

Overall Pattern: Dermal, Well Circumscribed, Interstitial

Detailed Description

Silhouette

- Symmetric
- Well circumscribed
- Only dermal

Patterns

Epidermis

- None

Dermis

- Nests and fascicles in the upper part of the lesion
- Interstitial strands and fascicles in the lower part of the lesion
- Thickened, sclerotic collagen bundles

Cytology

- Bipolar and plump spindled
- Few plump dendritic melanocytes with enlarged nuclei
- No crowding, no mitoses, no necrotic cell

Other Changes

- Sclerosis

Integration

This lesion is well circumscribed, symmetrical, and confined to the upper dermis with no epidermal involvement (Fig. 7.13a). The good circumscription can better be appreciated in the MelanA immunostain, which also helps to differentiate melanocytes from melanophages (Fig. 7.13d). Apart from typical bipolar melanocytes, plump spindled and enlarged dendritic melanocytes are present here, a common finding in so-called "cellular" or "epithelioid" blue nevi (Fig. 7.12b, d). However, those melanocytes have inconspicuous nuclei and do not show a crowded arrangement. Sclerosis is prominent, simulating the keloidal collagen seen in dermatofibromas (Fig. 7.12c).

Diagnosis: Blue nevus, sclerosing.

7.1.2.2 Example 2: Pigmented Epithelioid, Dermal (Fig. 7.14)

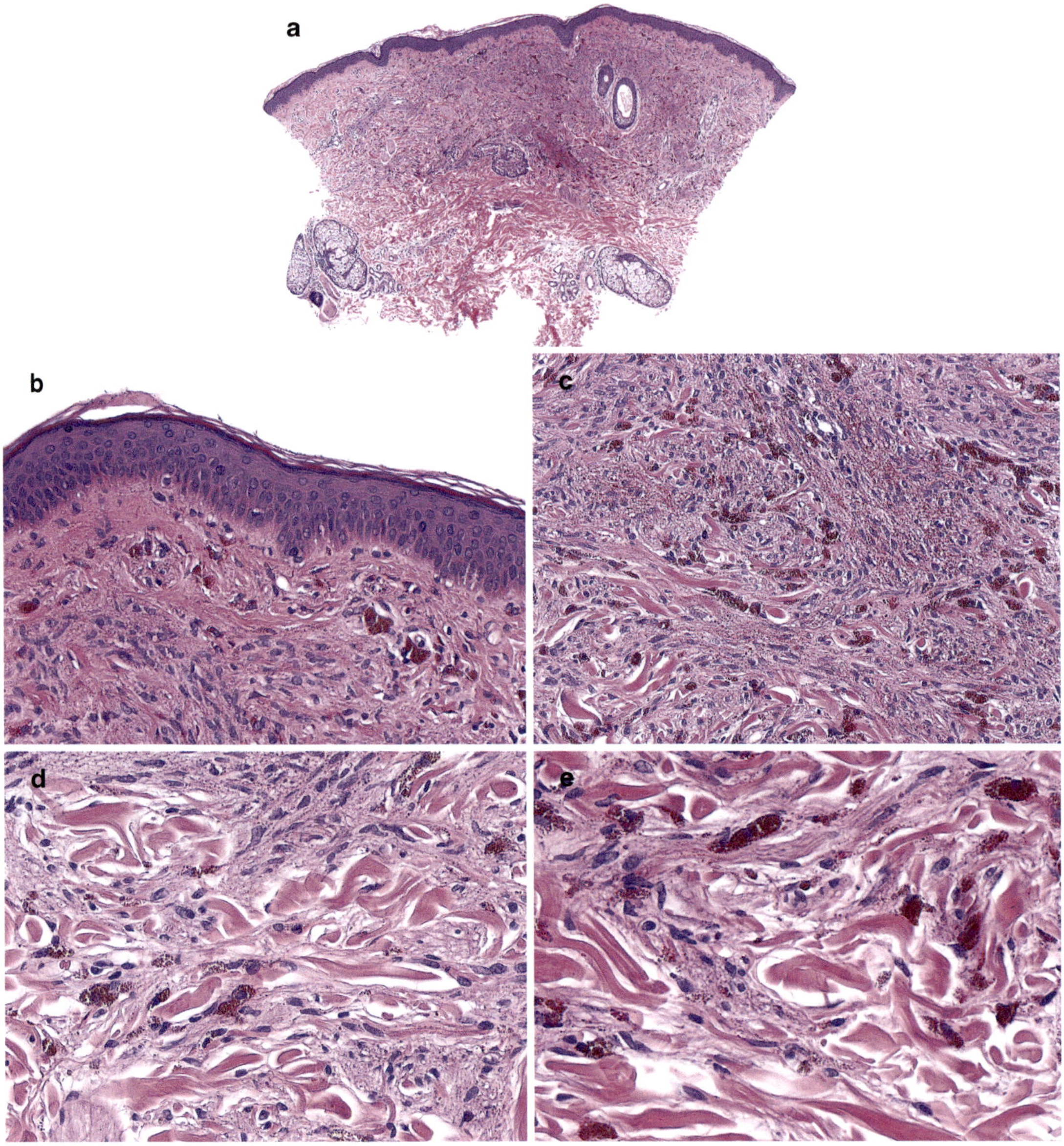

Fig. 7.14 (**a**–**e**) Spindled or epithelioid pigmented pattern, Example 2. (Courtesy of the Dermatologikum Hamburg)

Overall Pattern: Dermal, Plexiform, No Maturation

Detailed Description

Silhouette

- Symmetry cannot be assessed completely because the lesion extends to one margin.
- Circumscription difficult to determine.
- Dermal only.

Patterns

Epidermis

- None

Dermis

- Plexiform fascicles
- Interstitial strands and fascicles
- No maturation

Cytology

- Plump spindled and bipolar, with fine melanin granules
- Monomorphic
- No crowding
- No nucleoli, no mitoses

Other Changes

- Numerous melanophages with large melanin granules

Integration

Within the epidermis, there are only a few regularly distributed single melanocytes in the basal layer (Fig. 7.14b). The proliferation of melanocytes is situated only in the dermis in a fascicular and interstitial distribution, in which circumscription and symmetry are not obvious (Fig. 7.14a, c). The arrangement of fascicles and strands, however, is uniform throughout the lesion. Irregularity is only present in the degree of pigmentation, which varies throughout the lesion both, in regard to pigmentation of melanocytes and to accompanying melanophages (Fig. 7.14c, d). Large granules identify the heavily pigmented cells in the dermis as melanophages (Fig. 7.14e). The melanocytes have a spindled and bipolar cytology, some with wavy nuclei similar to that seen in neural cells, others with plump spindled nuclei and finely granular cytoplasm (Fig. 7.14e). No maturation is seen, but pleomorphism, mitoses, and necroses are absent. This combination of cytologic features is often seen in blue nevi and is referred to colloquially as "cellular blue nevus." The absence of maturation is not uncommon in blue nevi.

Diagnosis: Blue nevus.

7.1.2.3 Example 3: Asymmetric Pigmented Epithelioid, Dermal and Subcutaneous (Fig. 7.15)

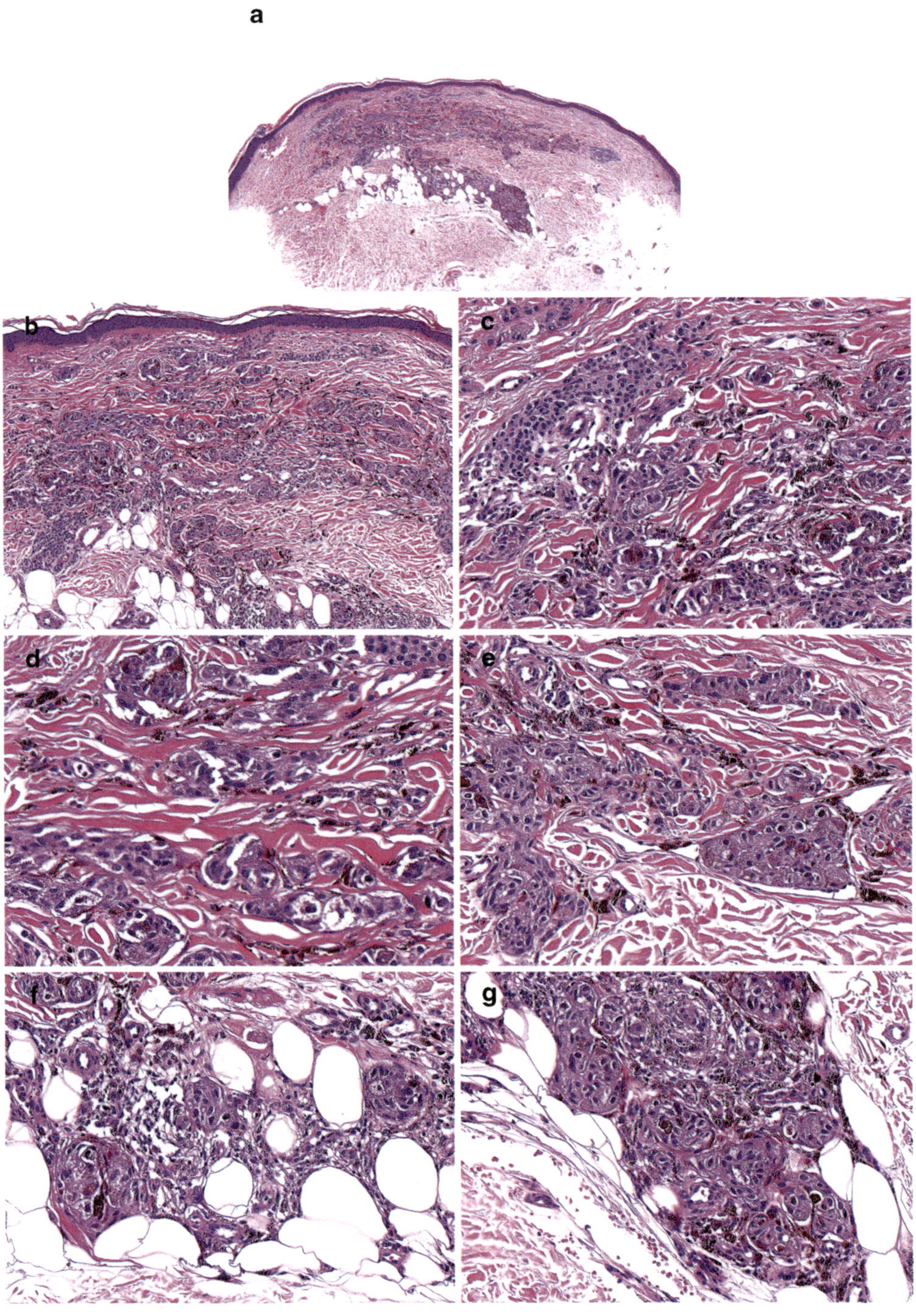

Fig. 7.15 (**a**–**g**) Spindled or epithelioid pigmented pattern, Example 3. (Courtesy of the Dermatologikum Hamburg)

Overall Pattern: Asymmetric, Nested and Plexiform, Dermal and Subcutaneous, No Maturation

Detailed Description

Silhouette

- Well circumscribed
- Asymmetric
- Dermal
- Extending into the superficial subcutis in the center

Patterns

Epidermis
- None

Dermis
- Nest in the upper dermis
- Fascicles throughout the reticular dermis
- No maturation

Subcutis
- Nests in superficial septa and lobules

Cytology

- Large, heavily pigmented melanocytes with enlarged but monomorphic nuclei
- Small second population of melanocytes with small nuclei devoid of cytoplasm in the upper left dermis
- No crowding, no nucleoli

Other Changes

- Numerous melanophages
- Some lymphocytic infiltrate

Integration

Even though this lesion is asymmetric, it is well circumscribed and has no epidermal component (Fig. 7.15a, b). The dermal proliferation in fact is made up of two different types of melanocytes, but each population is in itself monomorphic (Fig. 7.15c). The large, heavily pigmented melanocytes are typical of a so-called "deep penetrating nevus," which often involves superficial parts of the subcutis and shows a lack of maturation (Fig. 7.15d–g). Fascicular arrangement in the dermis is also quite characteristic. With these features, deep penetrating nevus represents a cytologically distinct variant with similarities to cellular blue nevi. While bipolar melanocytes are not seen in deep penetrating nevus, it commonly presents as a combined lesion with a second part being that of a conventional superficial congenital nevus, which is the case here (see upper left of the lesion in Fig. 7.15a, c).

Diagnosis: Deep penetrating nevus (combined with a superficial congenital nevus).

7.1.2.4 Example 4: Asymmetric Pigmented Epithelioid, Dermal and Subcutaneous (Fig. 7.16)

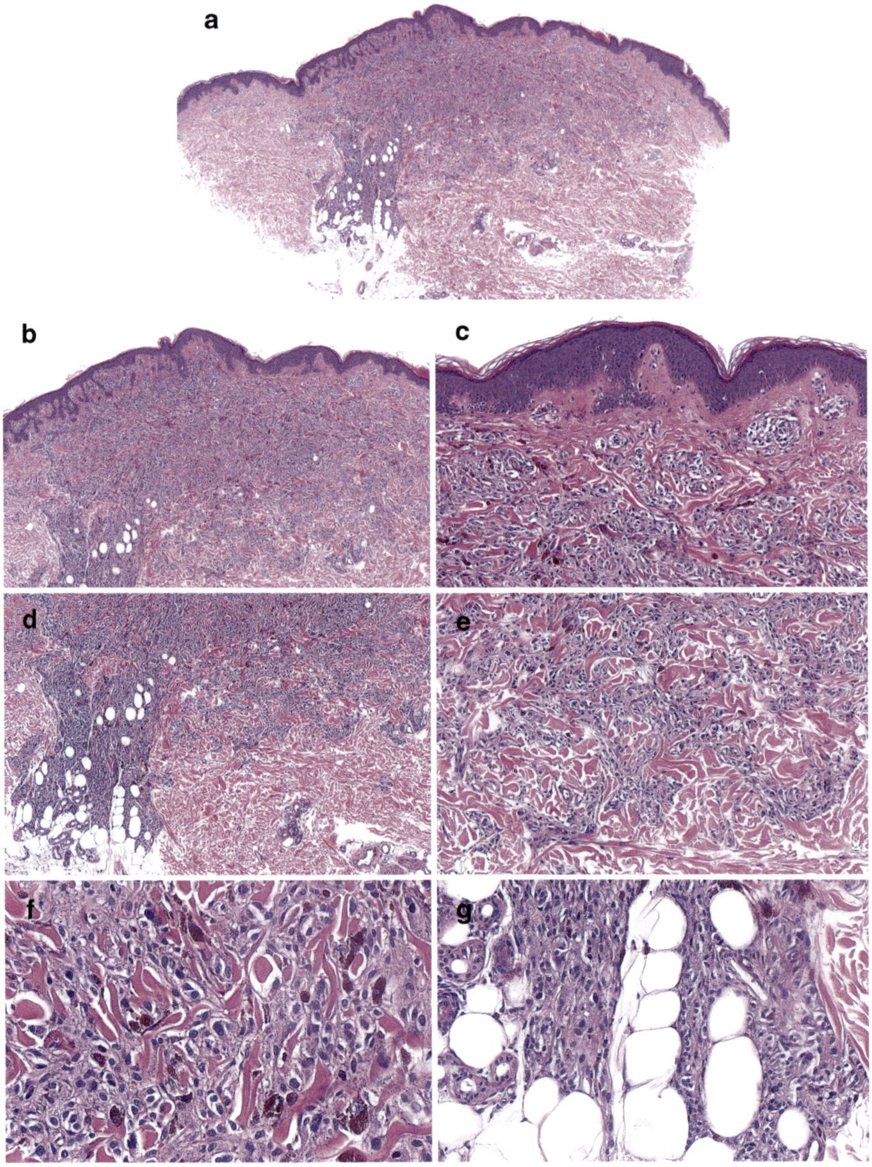

Fig. 7.16 (**a**–**k**) Spindled or epithelioid pigmented pattern, Example 4. (Courtesy of the Dermatologikum Hamburg)

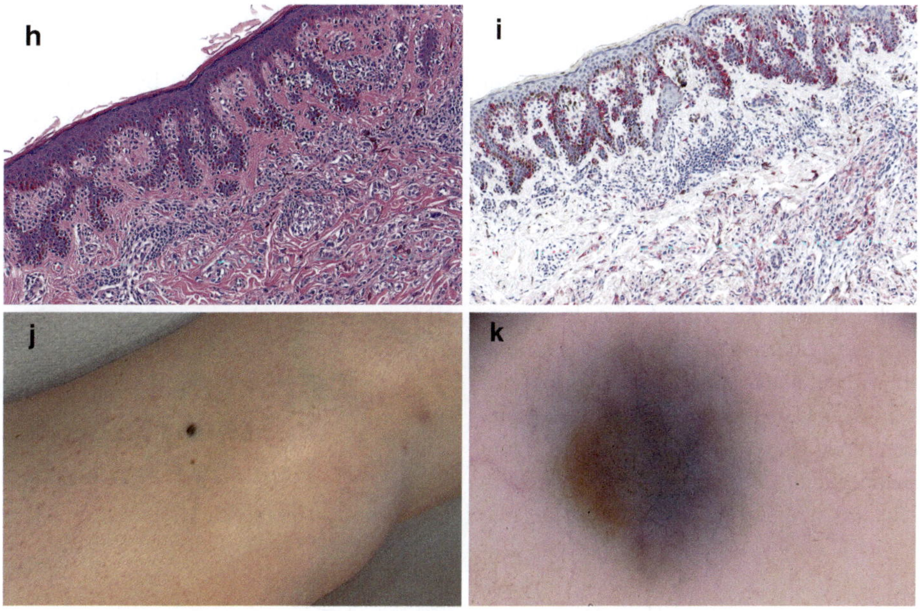

Fig. 7.16 (continued)

Overall Pattern: Asymmetric, Epidermal and Dermal, Well Circumscribed, No Maturation

Detailed Description

Silhouette

- Well circumscribed
- Asymmetric
- Epidermal and dermal
- Extending into the superficial subcutis

Patterns

Epidermis

- Small nests and single melanocytes, regularly distributed, at the base of rete ridges
- Elongated rete ridges

Dermis

- Nest and perivascular strands and columns in the upper dermis
- Interstitial strands and fascicles throughout the reticular dermis
- In the deeper dermis plexiform pattern
- No maturation

Subcutis

- Nests in superficial lobules

Cytology

- Large, heavily pigmented melanocytes with enlarged but monomorphic nuclei
- Small second population of melanocytes with small nuclei devoid of cytoplasm in the upper left dermis and epidermis
- No crowding, no nucleoli

Other Changes

- Elongated rete ridges on the left side of the lesion
- Numerous melanophages

Integration

Despite obvious asymmetry, the lesion is well circumscribed (Fig. 7.16a) with architectural and cytologic similarities to the previous example. The lesion is mainly made up of large melanocytes with finely granular pigmentation and slightly enlarged, but monomorphic nuclei (Fig. 7.16e–g). A small second component is situated in the upper left and shows epidermal involvement (Fig. 7.16b, h, i). Out of context, this second part fulfills all criteria of a small, superficial congenital nevus, given the epidermal hyperplasia and the nested and perivascular arrangement of small, round, monomorphic melanocytes. The large, heavily pigmented melanocytes in interstitial and plexiform distribution are typical of a deep penetrating nevus, which often involves superficial parts of the subcutis and shows a lack of maturation (Fig. 7.16f, g). Just as the previous example, this is a combined lesion with a second part being that of a superficial congenital nevus, but here the superficial congenital nevus has an epidermal part. From the histopathology it is obvious that this lesion must have been asymmetrical clinically, which is confirmed by the dermatoscopic photograph (Fig. 7.16j, k). It shows a large blue-gray structureless area and a small brown part with a reticular pattern corresponding very well to the two parts of the lesion.

Diagnosis: Combined nevus, deep penetrating nevus with a superficial congenital nevus.

7.1.2.5 Example 5: Nodular Reaching Subcutis, Heavily Pigmented (Fig. 7.17)

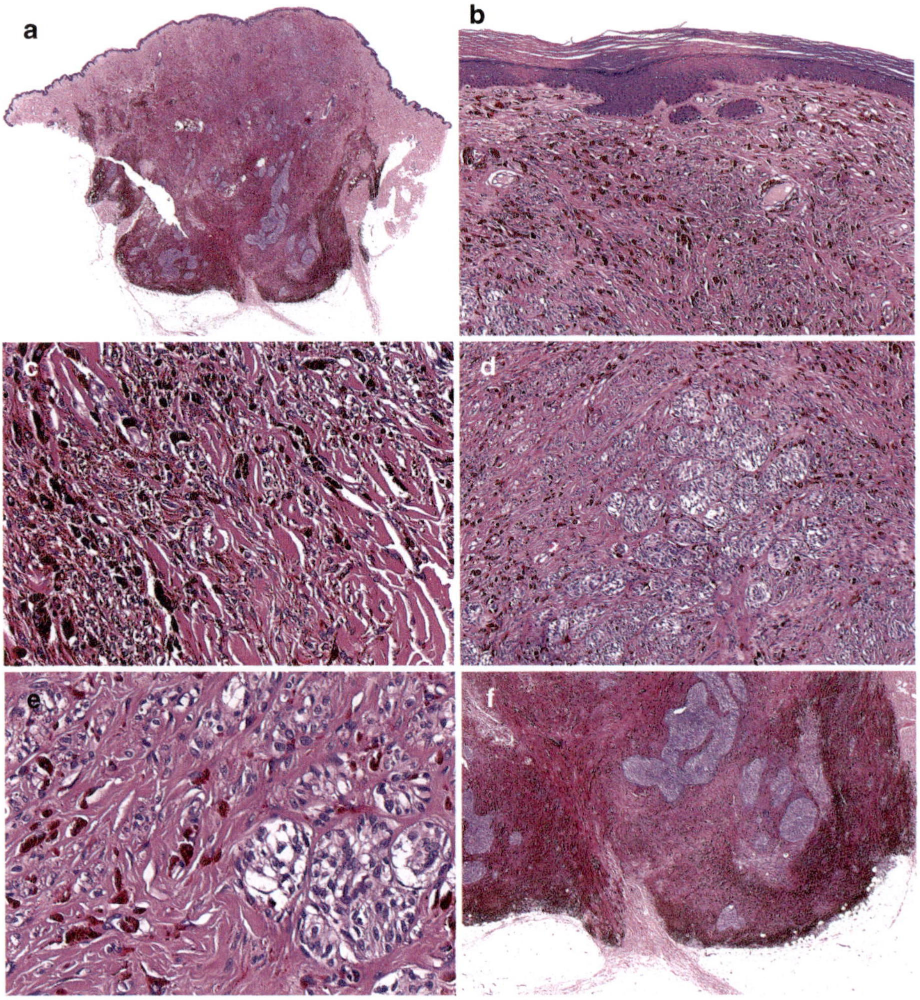

Fig. 7.17 (**a**–**h**) Spindled or epithelioid pigmented pattern, Example 5. (Courtesy of the Dermatologikum Hamburg)

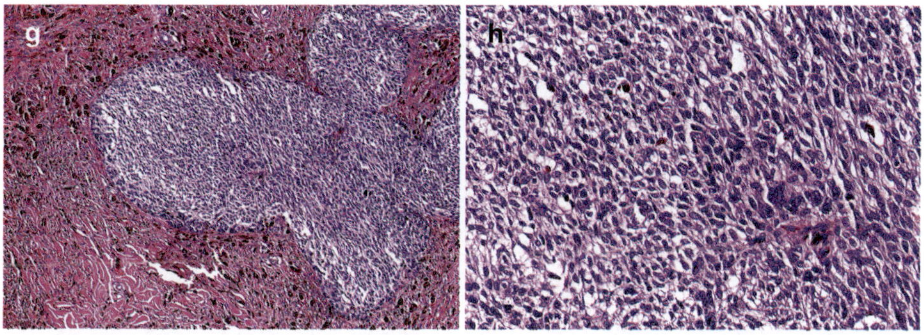

Fig. 7.17 (continued)

Overall Pattern: Nodular, Well Circumscribed, Dermal and Subcutaneous, Heavily Pigmented

Detailed Description

Silhouette

- Large, nodular lesion
- Well circumscribed
- Dermal and subcutaneous
- Heavy and heterogenous pigmentation

Patterns

Epidermis

- None

Dermis

- Interstitial strands and fascicles
- Small nests in the upper dermis

Subcutis

- Thick fascicles in plexiform arrangement
- Nodular protrusions of dermal sclerotic collagen with interstitial strands of melanocytes

Cytology

- Bipolar with fine melanin granules in the interstitial pattern
- Plump epithelioid with fine melanin granules in the nested pattern
- Plump spindled and epithelioid in the plexiform pattern
- Some variation in size and shape of nuclei in the plump spindled melanocytes
- No crowding, but some multinucleated melanocytes
- Small nucleoli, no mitoses

Other Changes

- Sclerotic collagen
- Numerous melanophages with large melanin granules

Integration

This lesion, which came from the right buttock of a young man, is impressive because of its size and irregular pigmentation (Fig. 7.17a). However, the combination of features of a sclerosing blue nevus with a plexiform proliferation of plump spindled melanocytes (Fig. 7.17f–h) is typical of a variant of blue nevus which is historically named Masson's neuronevus and which is often encountered on the buttock region. The absence of an epidermal proliferation (Fig. 7.17b) and the presence of interstitial bipolar melanocytes (Fig. 7.17c, e) are two strong features indicating a diagnosis of a blue nevus. The lack of maturation is expected in blue nevi. Multinucleated melanocytes should not be mistaken for crowding of nuclei and do not indicate malignancy. Despite its size, this lesion is completely benign.

Diagnosis: Blue nevus, so-called Neuronevus Masson.

7.1.2.6 Example 6: Heavily Pigmented Dermal Nodule with Junctional Component (Fig. 7.18)

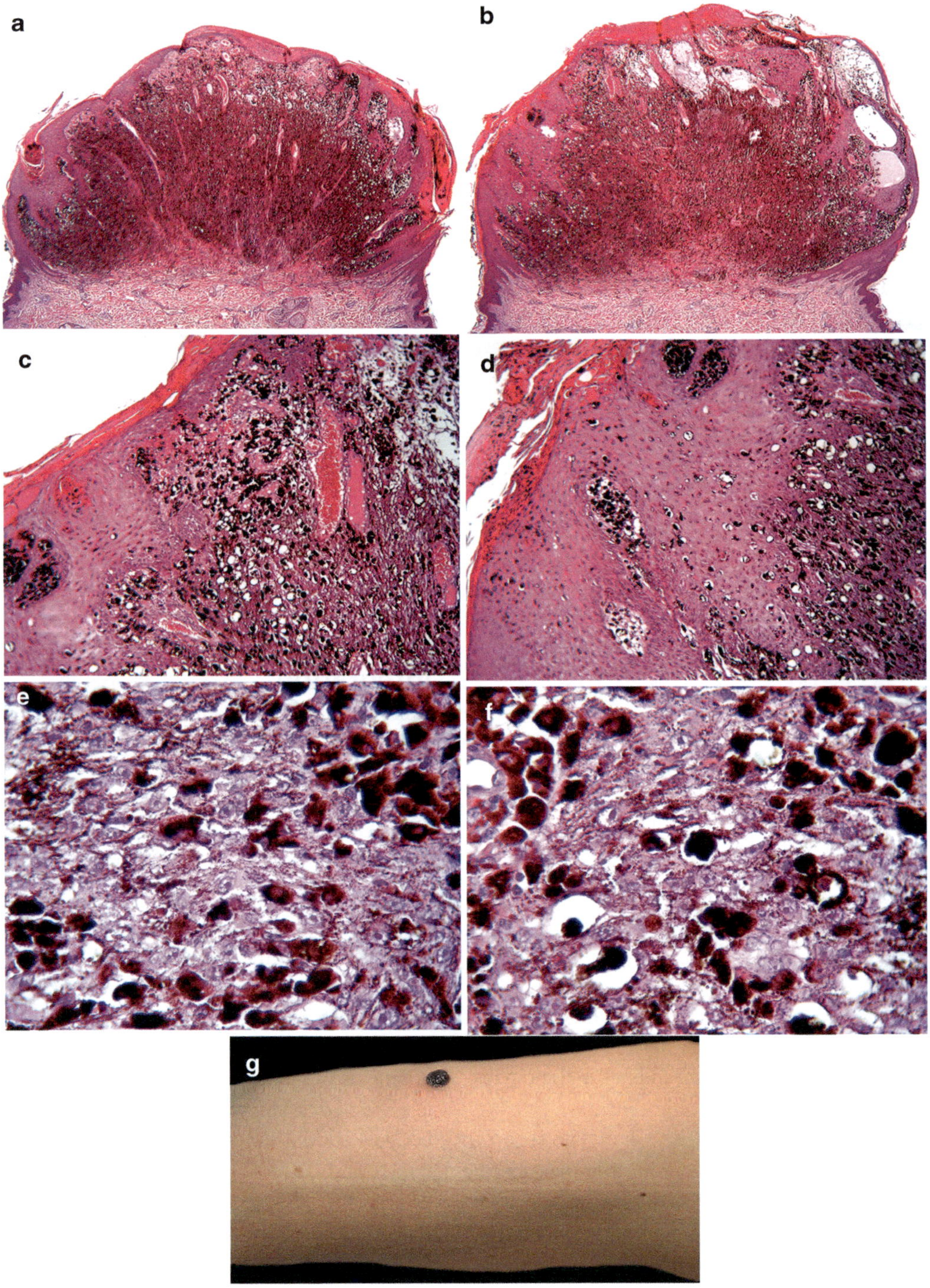

Fig. 7.18 (**a**–**f**) Spindled or epithelioid pigmented pattern, Example 6. (Courtesy of Gerardo Ferrara)

Overall Pattern: Epidermal and Dermal, Asymmetric, Relatively Well Circumscribed

Detailed Description

Silhouette

- Asymmetric
- Relatively well circumscribed
- Exophytic nodule

Patterns

Epidermis

- Single melanocytes increased, unevenly distributed
- Suprabasal single melanocytes

Dermis

- Sheets of melanocytes

Cytology

- Heavily pigmented epithelioid melanocytes

Other Changes

- Acanthosis and spongiosis of epidermis
- Hyper- and parakeratosis
- Ulceration
- Abundant melanophages in the dermis

Integration

This heavily pigmented ulcerated nodule is typified by sheets of epithelioid melanocytes in the dermis that are accompanied by numerous melanophages (Fig. 7.18a–f). Clinically, this is a pigmented nodule on the leg (Fig. 7.18g). There is no evidence of chronic sun damage in the surrounding skin. The differential diagnosis includes pigmented epithelioid melanocytoma (PEM) and melanoma. According to Zembovicz [131], "PEM may arise as a sporadic lesion or in patients with the Carney complex" and is a "borderline" lesion with metastatic potential limited to regional lymph nodes. This lesion depicted here has features that are in line with the description of PEM. Because of the epidermal component and the ulceration, some of the authors of this book favor PEM-like melanoma. Since we were not able to examine the original slide, we could not evaluate the presence and frequency of mitoses. The original diagnosis of this case, which was signed out nearly 20 years ago, was "animal type melanoma," a term that has been used as a synonym for PEM in the past but has been recently abandoned. Today we know that a subset of PEMs show loss of expression of the protein product of PRKAR1A [132–134], but this analysis was not available at the time the lesion was signed out. The patient had no evidence for metastatic disease 12 years after the diagnosis and was then lost to follow up.

Diagnosis: PEM or PEM-like melanoma.

7.1.2.7 Example 7: Small Superficial Dermal Nodule, Pigmented Epithelioid (Fig. 7.19)

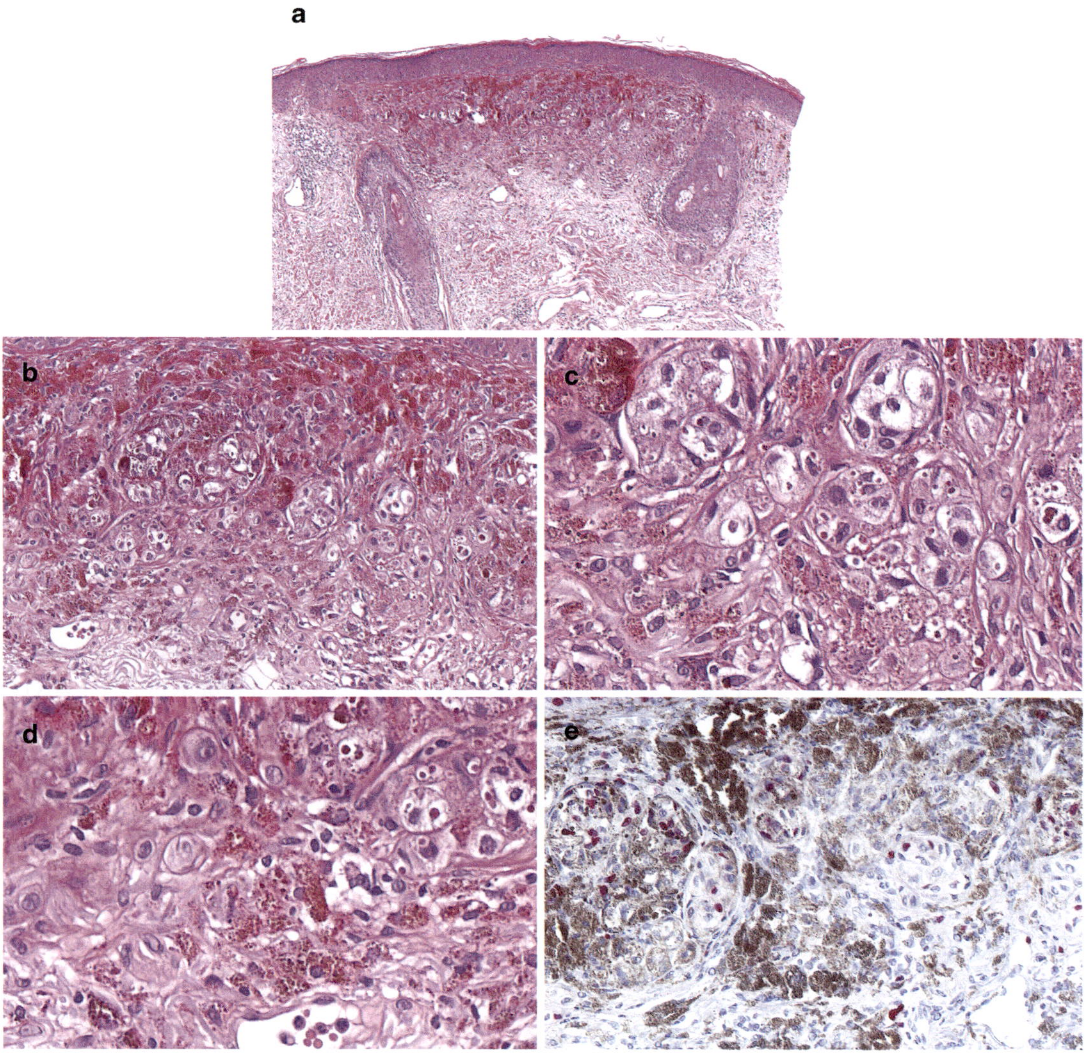

Fig. 7.19 (**a–e**) Spindled or epithelioid pigmented pattern, Example 7. (Courtesy of the Dermatologikum Hamburg)

Overall Pattern: Dermal, Nested, Well Circumscribed

Detailed Description

Silhouette

- Well circumscribed
- Slightly asymmetric
- Dermal only

Patterns

Epidermis

- None

Dermis

- Nested
- Some maturation
- Irregular melanophages

Cytology

- Epithelioid, but heavily pigmented
- Pagetoid
- Heterochromatic nuclei, some with large nucleoli

Other Changes

- Sun damage below the lesion

Immunohistochemistry

- Numerous nuclei positive on Ki67 (Fig. 7.19e).

Integration

A small and mostly nested dermal lesion usually is a dermal melanocytic nevus, but the sun damage below the lesion is suspicious and indicates that the lesion must have developed late in life, after the development of solar elastosis, which would be quite unusual for a dermal nevus (Fig. 7.19a, b). Even though there is some maturation, the cytology of the melanocytes is a strong indicator towards malignancy, because cells have partly a pagetoid appearance with abundant pigmented cytoplasm and heterochromatic nuclei (Fig. 7.19c, d). Some nuclei have enlarged nucleoli. In this constellation of findings, it is mandatory to search for mitoses and necrotic melanocytes which would strongly favor a diagnosis of a small melanoma metastasis. Because neither was obvious in this section, a Ki67 stain was performed and revealed numerous nuclei staining positively (Fig. 7.19e). This confirmed the diagnosis of melanoma metastasis in this small, nested lesion.

Diagnosis: Melanoma metastasis.

7.1.2.8 Example 8: Interstitial Dark Dermal Pigmentation (Fig. 7.20)

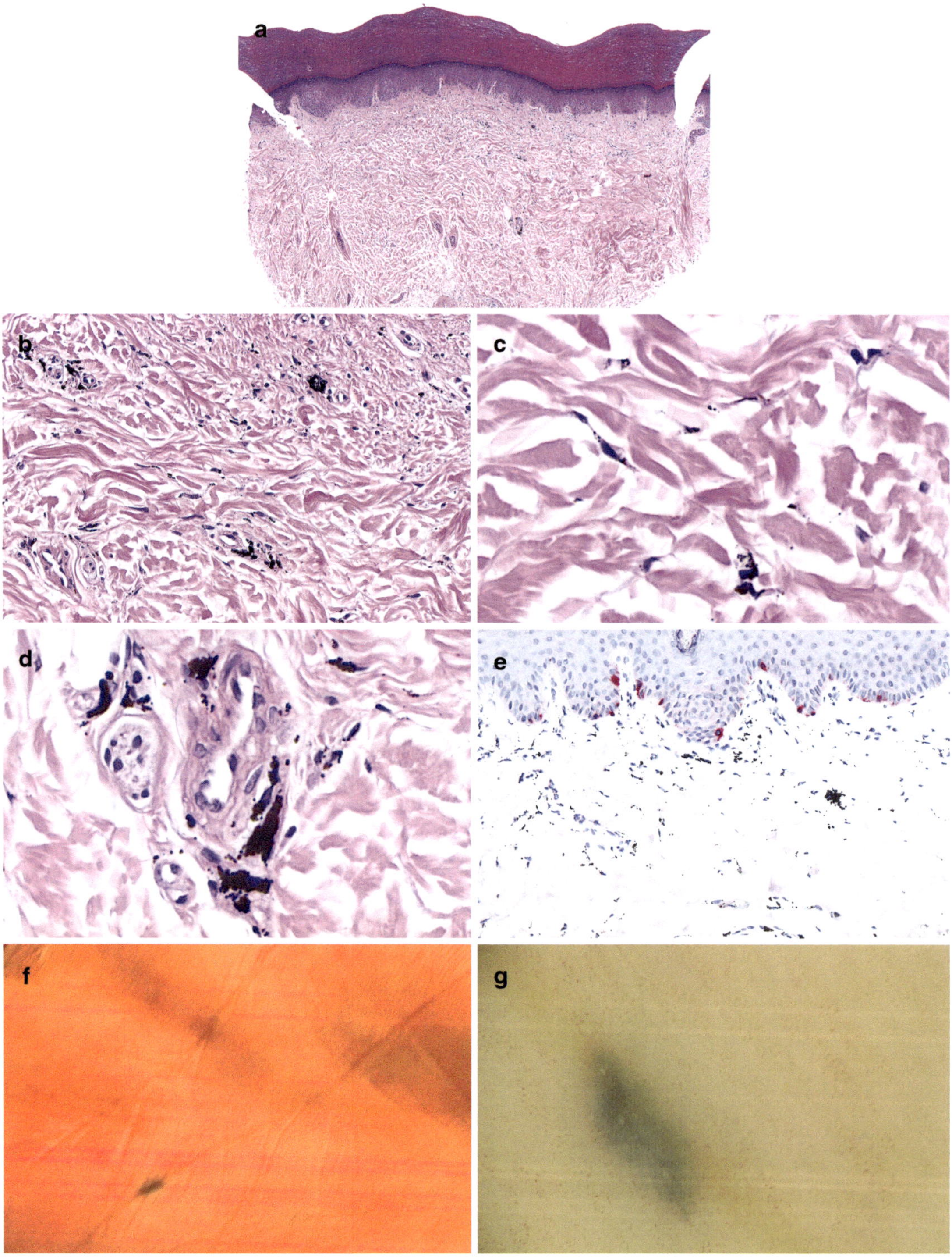

Fig. 7.20 (**a**–**g**) Spindled or epithelioid pigmented pattern, Example 8. (Courtesy of the Dermatologikum Hamburg)

Overall Pattern: Interstitial Pigmentation, Dermal

Detailed Description

Silhouette
- Poorly circumscribed
- Dermal only

Patterns

Epidermis
- None

Dermis
- Interstitial and perivascular pigmentation

Cytology
- Spindled and dendritic
- Large pigment granules

Immunohistochemistry
- MelanA stains normal melanocytes in the basal layer of the epidermis, but not the interstitial pigmented cells in the dermis (Fig. 7.20e).

Integration
This lesion on the palm imitates a common blue nevus clinically, dermatoscopically, and even histopathologically (Fig. 7.20a, c, f, g). However, the thin spindled pigmented cells in the dermis are not melanocytes (MelanA negative, Fig. 7.20e) but macrophages and the pigment is exogenous, namely, dirt from previous trauma.

Diagnosis: Dirt tattoo.

7.1.3 Epithelioid and/or Spindled Amphophilic

Large, epithelioid and pleomorphic melanocytes, so-called spitzoid melanocytes, are the hallmark of Spitz nevi, but they may be encountered also in other melanocytic nevi and in melanomas [16]. A classic Spitz nevus in a child is usually a straightforward diagnosis because of a symmetric silhouette, sharp circumscription with a predominantly nested pattern, presence of Kamino bodies, and epidermal hyperplasia with hypergranulosis and hyperkeratosis. However, Spitz nevi represent a spectrum of lesions including rare variants [135].

A. B. Ackerman and coworkers elaborated extensively on the histopathologic spectrum of Spitz nevi [63] and in recent research some patterns of Spitz nevi have been linked to specific genomic alterations [136–140]. While these works have enormously increased the knowledge about Spitz nevi and their pathogenesis, the everyday problem of differential diagnosis to spitzoid variants of melanoma remains.

Apart from a malignant-looking cytology, Spitz nevi also show classically a pagetoid pattern of intraepidermal melanocytes in between a mostly nested arrangement thereby voiding another important criterion for diagnosis of melanoma.

Melanocytic lesions with spitzoid cytology are especially challenging when classic criteria of a Spitz nevus such as Kamino bodies are absent or when a lesion is sampled incompletely, as it often is the case in shave specimens. Epithelioid melanocytes are also present in BAP1-inactivated naevi, which usually lack other features of Spitz nevi.

7.1.3.1 Example 1: Large Epidermal Nests and Epidermal Hyperplasia (Fig. 7.21)

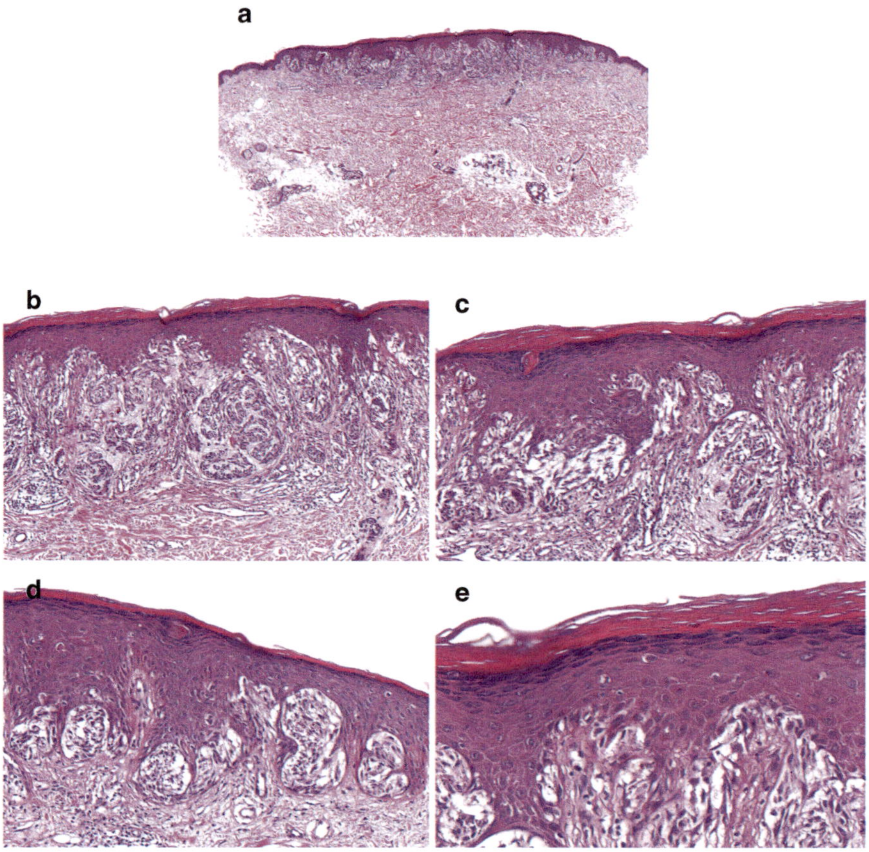

Fig. 7.21 (a–i) Epithelioid or spindled amphophilic pattern, Example 1. (Courtesy of the Dermatologikum Hamburg)

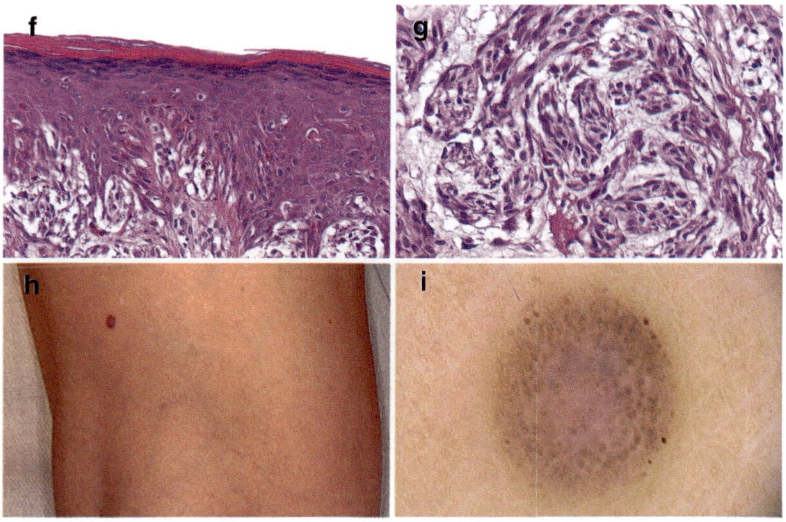

Fig. 7.21 (continued)

Overall Pattern: Symmetric, Epidermal and Dermal, Nested

Detailed Description

Silhouette

- Largely symmetrical
- Well circumscribed
- Epidermal and dermal

Patterns

Epidermis

- Nests predominate.
- Nests at the base of rete ridges.
- Nests vary in size and shape, some confluence of nests.
- Nests are mostly of large size.
- Some single melanocytes between the nests.
- Some single melanocytes in suprabasal layers.

Dermis

- Nests in the papillary and superficial reticular dermis in the center
- Some maturation

Cytology

- Large epithelioid and spindled
- Moderately pleomorphic nuclei
- No mitoses

Other Changes

- Acanthosis, hypergranulosis, and hyperkeratosis
- Band-like lymphocytic infiltrate, moderately dense
- Myxoid connective tissue

Integration

This lesion has the architecture of a nevus because it is symmetric and well circumscribed, the epidermis is evenly hyperplastic, intraepidermal melanocytes show a predominantly nested arrangement, and the dermal component is located in the center of the lesion with some maturation (Fig. 7.21a–c). The cytology is spitzoid with large epithelioid and spindled melanocytes (Fig. 7.21e–g). In a Spitz nevus, some confluence of nests and variation in size and shape is commonly seen and also the single melanocytes between the nests with some of them in suprabasal layers are an expected finding (Fig. 7.21e, f). However, even on several step sections this lesion did not show any Kamino bodies. It had a dyskeratotic keratinocyte which should not be mixed up with a Kamino body. Despite the absence of Kamino bodies, the best diagnosis in this lesion is Spitz nevus. While the presence of Kamino bodies is a helpful clue to the diagnosis of Spitz nevus, it is a fact that they are not always present and absence of them does not exclude the diagnosis of Spitz nevus.

This lesion comes from the thigh of a 54-year-old woman. Clinical appearance is rather inconspicuous (Fig. 7.21h, i).

Diagnosis: Spitz nevus (compound).

7.1.3.2 Example 2: Spindled and Epithelioid Cells in a Nodule in a Child (Fig. 7.22)

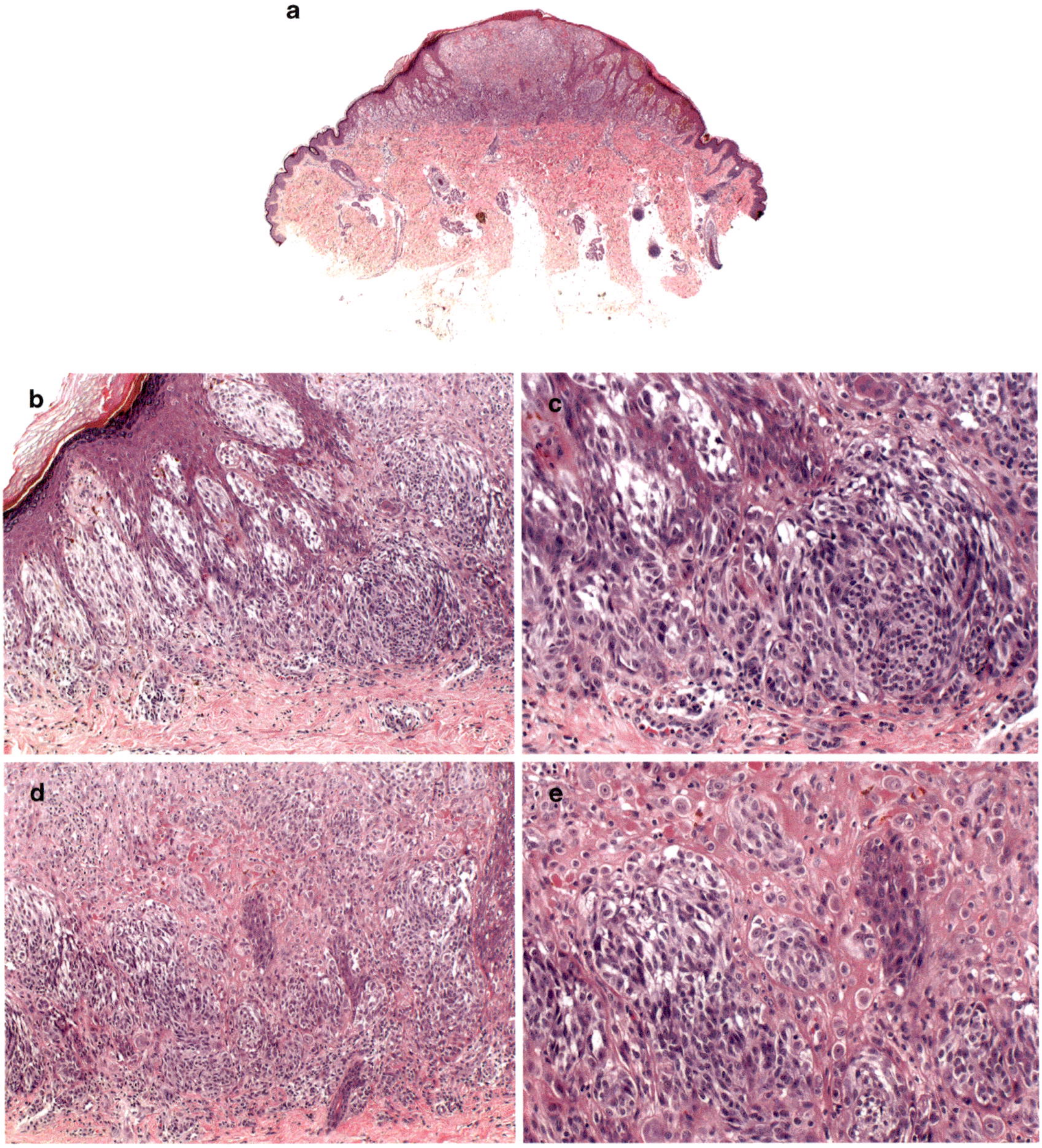

Fig. 7.22 (**a**–**i**) Epithelioid or spindled amphophilic pattern, Example 2. (Courtesy of the Department of Dermatology, Medical University of Vienna)

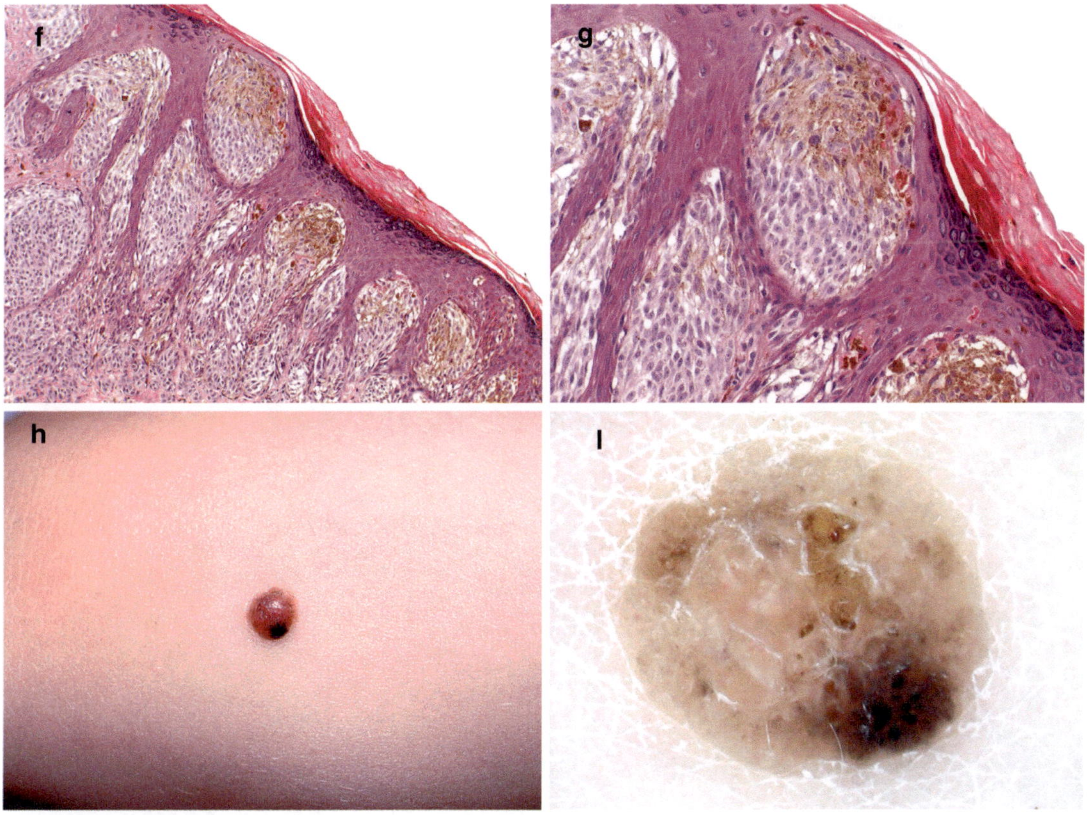

Fig. 7.22 (continued)

Overall Pattern: Epidermal and Dermal, Symmetric, Well Circumscribed

Detailed Description

Silhouette

- Symmetric
- Well circumscribed
- Epidermal and dermal

Patterns

Epidermis

- Large Nests

Dermis

- Nests, strands, fascicles, and single cells

Cytology

- Spindled and epithelioid melanocytes

Other Changes

- Acanthosis
- Hypergranulosis
- Melanophages in the dermis

Integration

Clinically, this is a quickly growing, partly pigmented nodule on the arm of a prepubescent child (Fig. 7.22h). Dermatoscopically, it is a chaotic lesion with brown clods between 3 and 6 o'clock (Fig. 7.22i). Together with the pathological findings (Fig. 7.22a–g), this is best interpreted as Spitz nevus.

Diagnosis: Spitz nevus (compound).

7.1.3.3 Example 3: Junctional, Epithelioid, with Kamino Bodies (Fig. 7.23)

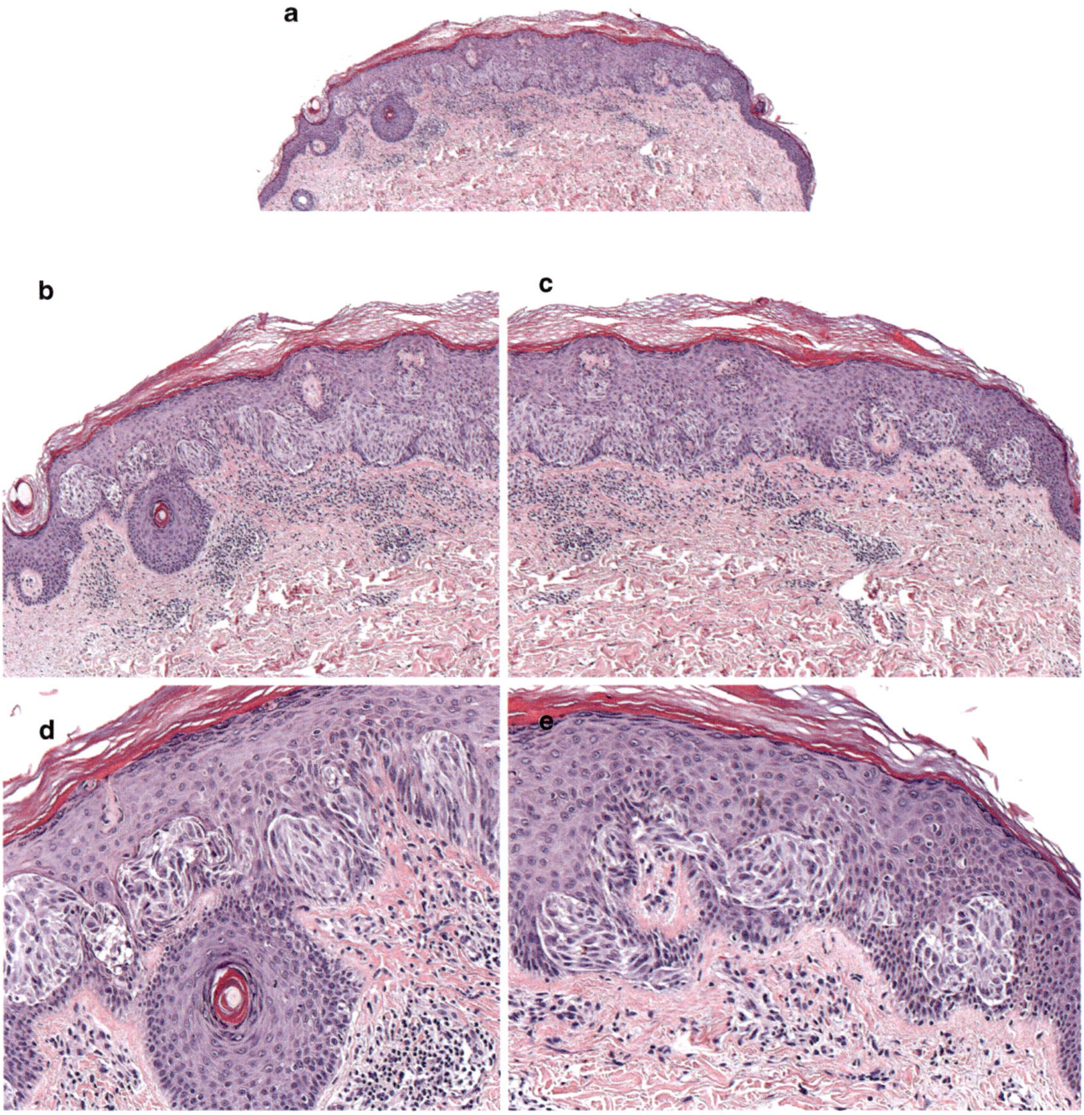

Fig. 7.23 (**a**–**i**) Epithelioid or spindled amphophilic pattern, Example 3. (Courtesy of the Department of Dermatology, Medical University of Vienna)

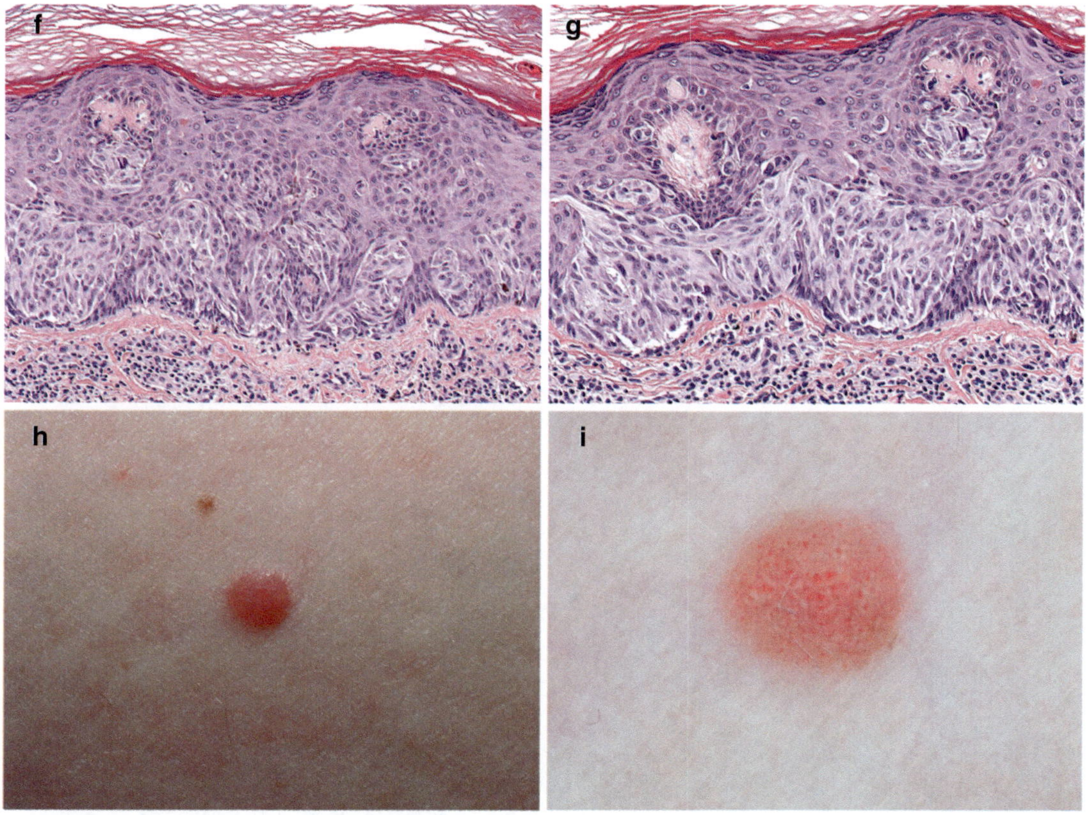

Fig. 7.23 (continued)

Overall Pattern: Epidermal, Symmetric, Well Circumscribed

Detailed Description

Silhouette

- Symmetric
- Well circumscribed
- Epidermal

Patterns

Epidermis

- Large Nests

Cytology

- Spindled and epithelioid melanocytes

Other Changes

- Acanthosis
- Hypergranulosis
- Kamino bodies (dull pink globules)
- Patchy lymphocytic infiltrate in the upper dermis

Integration

Clinically, this is a quickly growing, pink papule on the thigh of a 25-year-old female (Fig. 7.23h). Dermatoscopically, it is a pink lesion with vessels as dots and white lines (Fig. 7.23i). Together with the pathological findings, this is best interpreted as Spitz nevus (Fig. 7.23a–g).

Diagnosis: Spitz nevus.

7.1.3.4 Example 4: Dermal Nevus with Epithelioid Melanocytes (Fig. 7.24)

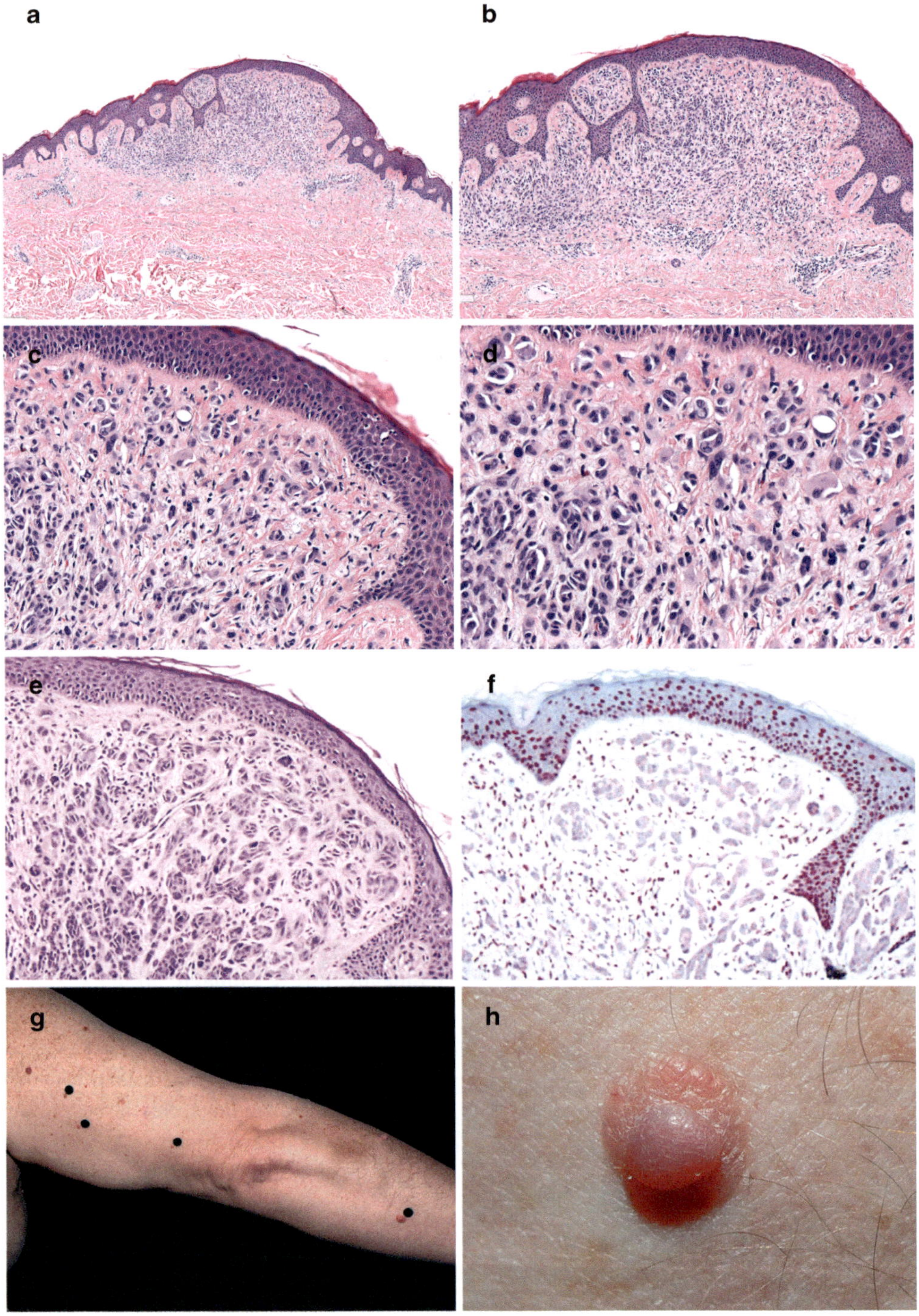

Fig. 7.24 (**a**–**h**) Epithelioid or spindled amphophilic pattern, Example 4. (Courtesy of the Department of Dermatology, Medical University of Vienna)

Overall Pattern: Symmetric, Dermal, Single Cells

Detailed Description

Silhouette
- Symmetrical
- Well circumscribed
- Dermal

Patterns

Dermis
- Nests, strands, and single cells in the papillary and superficial reticular dermis in the center
- Some maturation

Cytology
- Large epithelioid
- Moderately pleomorphic nuclei
- No mitoses

Other Changes
- Acanthosis

Integration
This lesion has the architecture of a nevus because it is symmetric and well circumscribed, the epidermis is evenly hyperplastic (Fig. 7.24a, b). The cytology of the dermal melanocytes is spitzoid with large epithelioid cells (Fig. 7.24c–e). The dermal melanocytes are mainly arranged as single cells and show some signs of maturation. No mitosis can be found. The BAP-1 immunostains show loss of BAP-1 expression in the dermal melanocytes, note that the nuclear BAP-1 expression in the keratinocytes serves as internal positive control (Fig. 7.24f). This lesion comes from the arm of a 50-year-old male with multiple similar lesions that look like dermal nevi, clinically (Fig. 7.24g, h). The patient also has a history of uveal melanoma and a family history of melanoma.

Diagnosis: BAP-1 inactivated nevus (BAPoma).

7.1.3.5 Example 5: Dermal Nodule of Pleomorphic Epithelioid Cells with Epidermal Hyperplasia (Fig. 7.25)

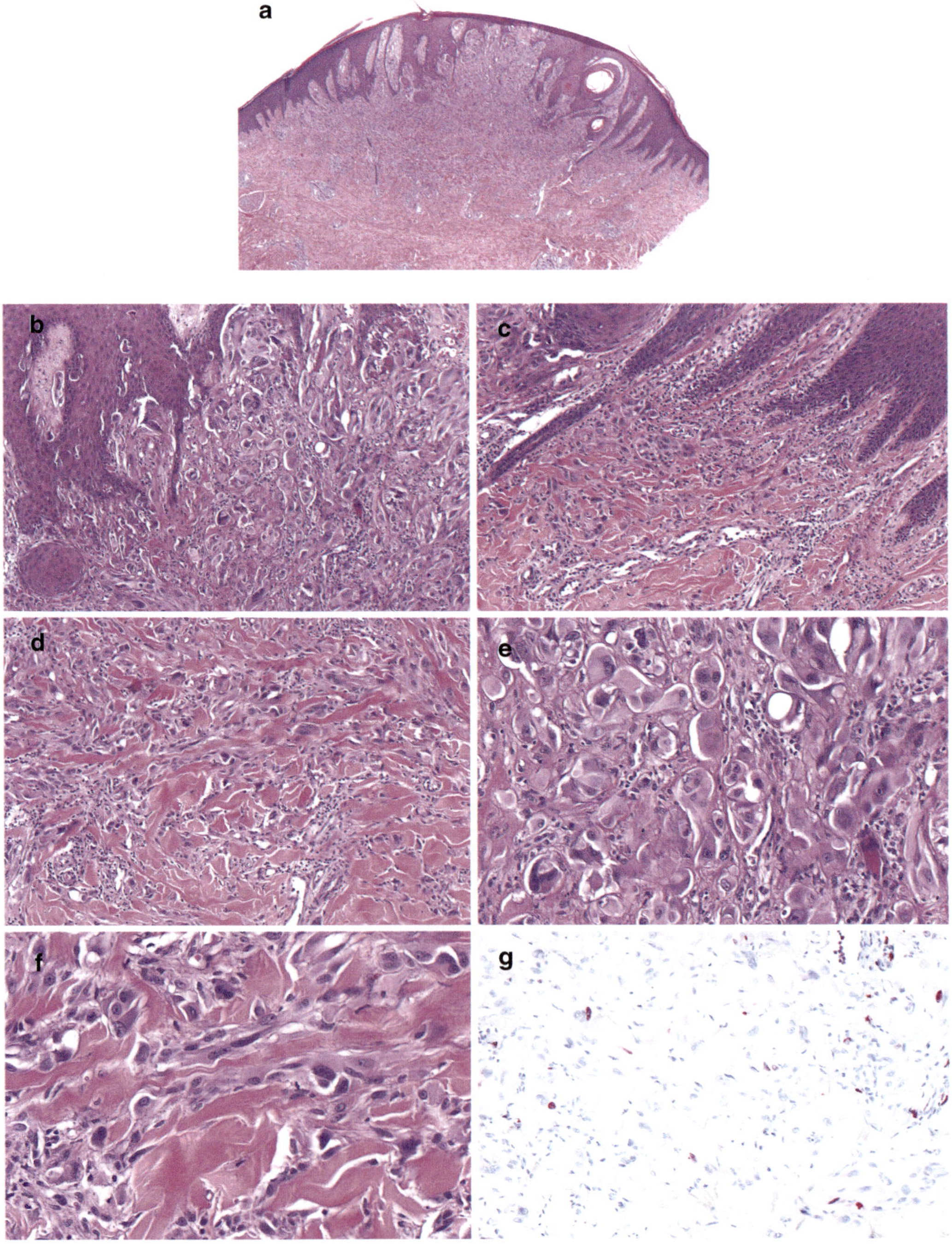

Fig. 7.25 (a–g) Epithelioid or spindled amphophilic pattern, Example 5. (Courtesy of the Dermatologikum Hamburg)

Overall Pattern: Largely Dermal, Well Circumscribed, Nested and Interstitial

Detailed Description

Silhouette

- Well circumscribed
- Symmetrical
- Epidermal and dermal

Patterns

Epidermis

- Nests of melanocytes at the base of rete ridges in the center of the lesion.
- Single melanocytes between nests, relatively regularly distributed.
- Some melanocytes in upper layers of the epidermis.
- Epidermal part does not extend over the dermal part.

Dermis

- Nests of melanocytes in the upper dermis
- Interstitial melanocytes in strands, cords, and columns
- Maturation

Cytology

- Large, epithelioid, amphophilic
- Obvious pleomorphism
- Few mitoses in the epidermal part of the lesion

Other Changes

- Epidermal hyperplasia with hypergranulosis and hyperkeratosis
- Epidermis thinned in the very center
- Adnexal epithelial hyperplasia
- Prominent and dilated vessels in the papillary dermis
- Thickened, sclerotic collagen in the reticular dermis

Immunohistochemistry

Expression of Ki67 in very few nuclei in the dermis (Fig. 7.25g)

Molecular Diagnostics

Sanger sequencing showed no BRAF or NRAS mutations.

Integration

This lesion, which came from the right leg of a 24-year-old woman with the clinical diagnosis of a dermatofibroma, has a benign-looking silhouette because it is largely symmetric and well circumscribed and shows maturation in the dermal part (Fig. 7.25a–c). The epidermis is hyperplastic with a very small focus of thinning, which can be due to outside irritation. The cytology, however, is strikingly pleomorphic (Fig. 7.25e, f) and no Kamino bodies are seen, which opens the differential diagnostic possibility of a spitzoid melanoma. In the dermis, the sclerosis is typical for a sclerosing type of a Spitz nevus (Fig. 7.25f), and no mitoses are found in the dermal part. Even Ki67-stain demonstrates only very few positive nuclei in the dermis (Fig. 7.25g). Because a melanoma of this thickness would have consequences for the patient, it is reasonable to make sure that the lesion is excised completely, which is accomplished in this excision. A molecular diagnostic for BRAF mutations can be of additional help, because Spitz nevi classically do not have BRAF mutations, while spitzoid melanomas often have. In this lesion, no BRAF mutation was found in Sanger Sequencing.

Diagnosis: Sclerosing Spitz nevus (so-called desmoplastic Spitz nevus), irritated in the center.

7.1.3.6 Example 6: Ill-Defined Dermal Nodule of Epithelioid Pleomorphic Cells with Heavy Inflammatory Infiltrate (Fig. 7.26)

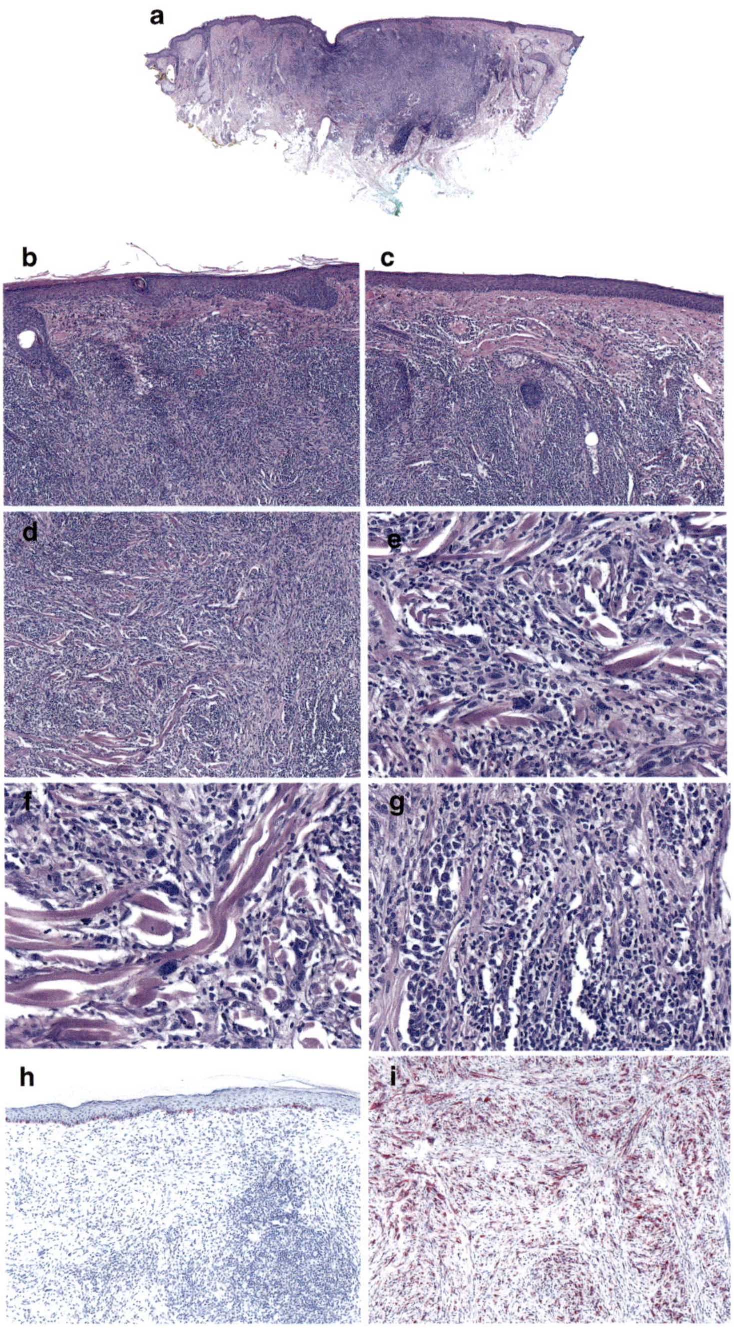

Fig. 7.26 (**a**–**k**) Epithelioid or spindled amphophilic pattern, Example 6. (Courtesy of the Dermatologikum Hamburg)

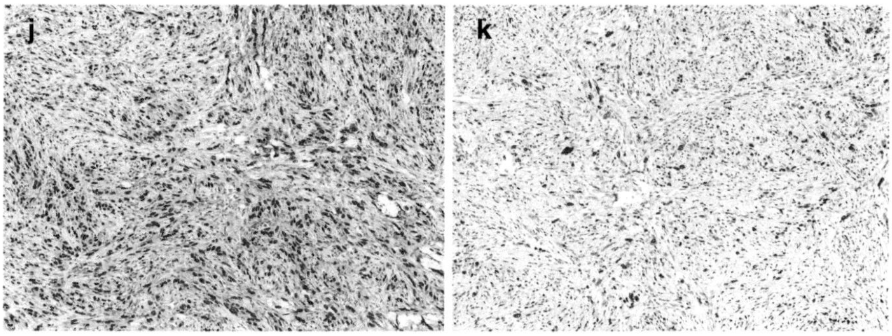

Fig. 7.26 (continued)

Overall Pattern: Dermal Only, Interstitial, Asymmetric, and Poorly Circumscribed

Detailed Description

Silhouette

- Dermal
- Interstitial, poorly circumscribed
- Asymmetric

Patterns

Epidermis
- Regularly distributed single melanocytes

Dermis
- Interstitial strands and fascicles
- Plexiform fascicles
- No maturation

Cytology
- Spindled and epithelioid
- Striking pleomorphism with enlarged and heterochromatic nuclei
- Prominent nucleoli
- Multinucleated cells

Other Changes
- Lymphoplasmacytic infiltrates throughout the lesion
- Patchy increase in density of the infiltrate
- Focal melanophages
- Solar elastosis

Immunohistochemistry
- Expression of MelanA only in single melanocytes in the basal layer (Fig. 7.26i)
- Pleomorphic cells express Sox 10 (Fig. 7.26j) and S100 (Fig. 7.26i)
- Approximately 80% of the melanocytes express Ki67 (Fig. 7.26k)

Integration
A dense lymphocytic infiltrate fills the entire dermis diffusely (Fig. 7.26a). No melanocytic proliferation is seen in the epidermis (Fig. 7.26b, c), but the rete ridges are flattened and some solar elastosis is seen in the dermis. At intermediate and high magnification, a pleomorphic spindle cell proliferation can be identified (Fig. 7.26d–f), which is obscured by the infiltrate which contains lymphocyte and plasma cells (Fig. 7.26g). The cells have enlarged cytoplasm and enlarged and irregular nuclei, many of them with prominent nucleoli and several of them with multiple nuclei. There is no hint to the biological nature of the pleomorphic cell proliferation so that immunohistochemistry (Fig. 7.26h–k) is mandatory. The proliferation is negative with MelanA (Fig. 7.26h) but expresses S100 and SOX10 (Fig. 7.26i, j) which is very compatible with desmoplastic melanoma. Within the epidermis, just a few regularly distributed melanocytes are seen on MelanA situated in the basal layer. Ki67 shows many positive nuclei in the proliferation (Fig. 7.26k).

Diagnosis: Desmoplastic melanoma.

7.1.3.7 Example 7: Asymmetric, Partly Plexiform Dermal Nodule (Fig. 7.27)

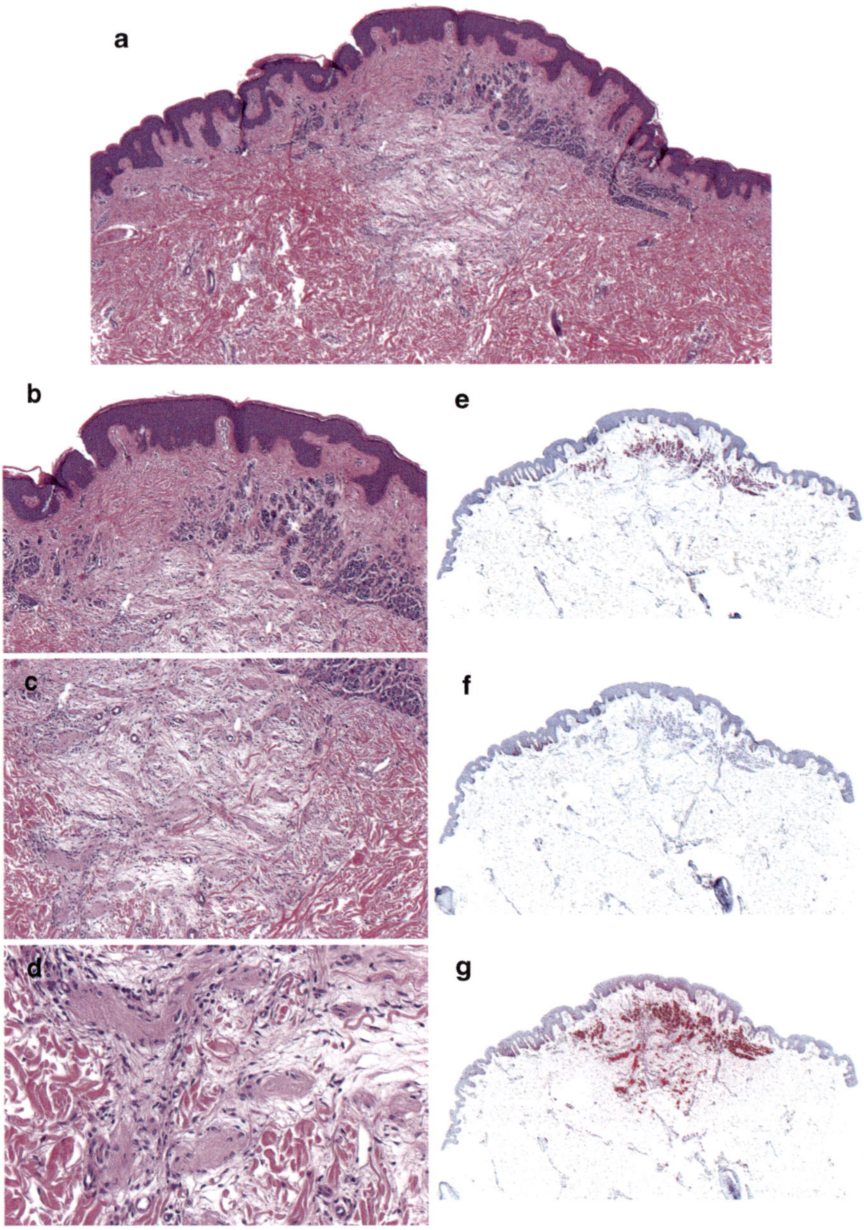

Fig. 7.27 (a–i) Epithelioid or spindled amphophilic pattern, Example 7. (Courtesy of the Dermatologikum Hamburg)

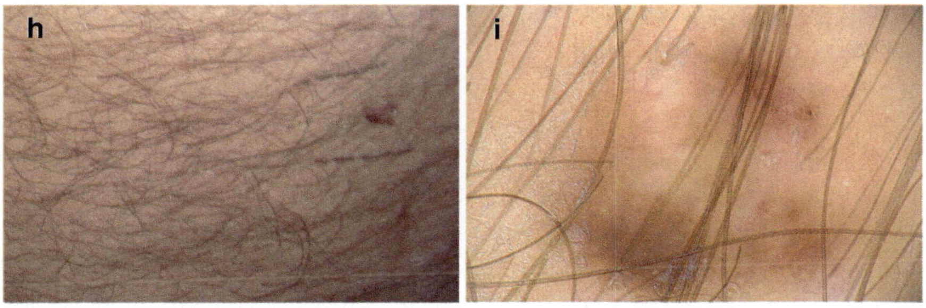

Fig. 7.27 (continued)

Overall Pattern: Asymmetric, Dermal, Nested, and Plexiform

Detailed Description

Silhouette

- Asymmetric
- Dermal

Patterns

Epidermis

- None

Dermis

- Nests in the upper part of the lesion
- Plexiform fascicles in the lower dermis
- Maturation

Cytology

- Small, with scant cytoplasm
- Spindled forming nerve-like fascicles

Other Changes

- Acanthosis and elongated rete ridges
- Hyperpigmentation of basal keratinocytes
- Mucin in the dermis between fascicles

Immunohistochemistry

- MelanA stains the nested part of the lesion (Fig. 7.27e)
- HMB45 is not expressed in the dermis, there is just focal expression in the basal epidermis (Fig. 7.27f)
- S100 stains the nested and the plexiform spindled part as well as Langerhans cells and dermal dendritic cells and nerves (Fig. 7.27g)

Integration

This lesion is asymmetric at scanning magnification, but it is restricted to the dermis and composed of two patterns, each of which is in itself homogenous (Fig. 7.27a, b). The spindled, plexiform and mucinous part simulates a plexiform neurofibroma and represents a rare variant of neural differentiation in a melanocytic nevus (Fig. 7.27c, d). Neural differentiation in the form of spindled melanocytes at the base of the proliferation is a common finding in congenital nevi. Less commonly it takes the form of nevic corpuscles which simulate Meissner corpuscles (often found in dermal nevi on the face). Even less frequently, neural differentiation is forming neural fascicles like it is seen here (Fig. 7.27d, g). All these variants also go under the designation "neurotization." Essentially, the lesion represents one manifestation of a combined congenital nevus. As is often the case in combined congenital nevi, the lesion is strikingly asymmetric clinically (Fig. 7.27h, i).

Diagnosis: Combined congenital nevus with neural differentiation ("Neurotized nevus").

7.1.4 Nevoid Melanoma and Melanoma Associated with Nevi

The term "nevoid melanoma" is used to designate a melanoma that closely simulates a nevus [62, 141, 142]. In fact, most melanomas simulate nevi to some extent, because both lesions are made up of melanocytes and share a common genetic background. That is precisely why the diagnosis of melanoma can be so challenging. "Nevoid melanoma" has been used to denote melanomas simulating congenital nevi, dermal nevi, blue nevi, Spitz nevi, and others and, therefore, it is not clearly defined as a specific entity. However, we would like to present here some examples of melanomas, which mimic melanocytic nevi by silhouette because of good circumscription, symmetry, predominance of nests, or cytology with lymphoid appearance. Such lesions are at risk to be misdiagnosed at scanning as a benign lesion and, once a diagnosis has already been made, closer inspection at intermediate and high magnifications may be missed. These examples should emphasize that any assessment made at scanning magnification should always be reconfirmed at higher magnification, even if the diagnosis seems simple at first glance.

Although most melanomas develop de novo, some may evolve in association with a nevus. When melanoma develops in a nevus, it is often a nevus with congenital features (monomorphic small melanocytes in the dermis that are distributed in an adnexocentric fashion). In these cases, the challenge may be to detect the melanoma at scanning magnification, especially if the lesion is so poorly sectioned that the melanoma is barely visible. Sometimes, multiple deeper sections are needed to spot the melanoma. If the diagnosis of the clinician was melanoma in a nevus, deeper levels should be cut by default. Ideally, the clinician also provides a clinical or dermatoscopic picture and the pathologist, who examines the slide, also performs the grossing. Unfortunately, this is rarely the case.

7.1.4.1 Example 1: Dense Dermal Sheets of Melanocytes (Fig. 7.28)

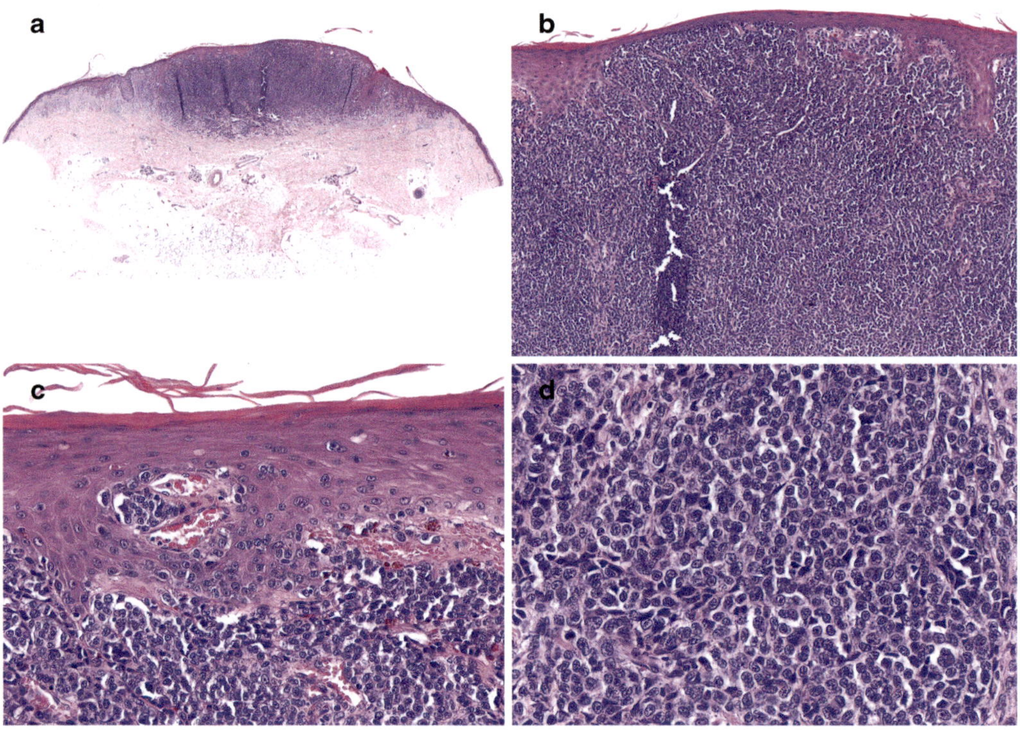

Fig. 7.28 (**a**–**h**) Nevoid melanoma and nevus-associated melanoma, Example 1. (Courtesy of the Dermatologikum Hamburg)

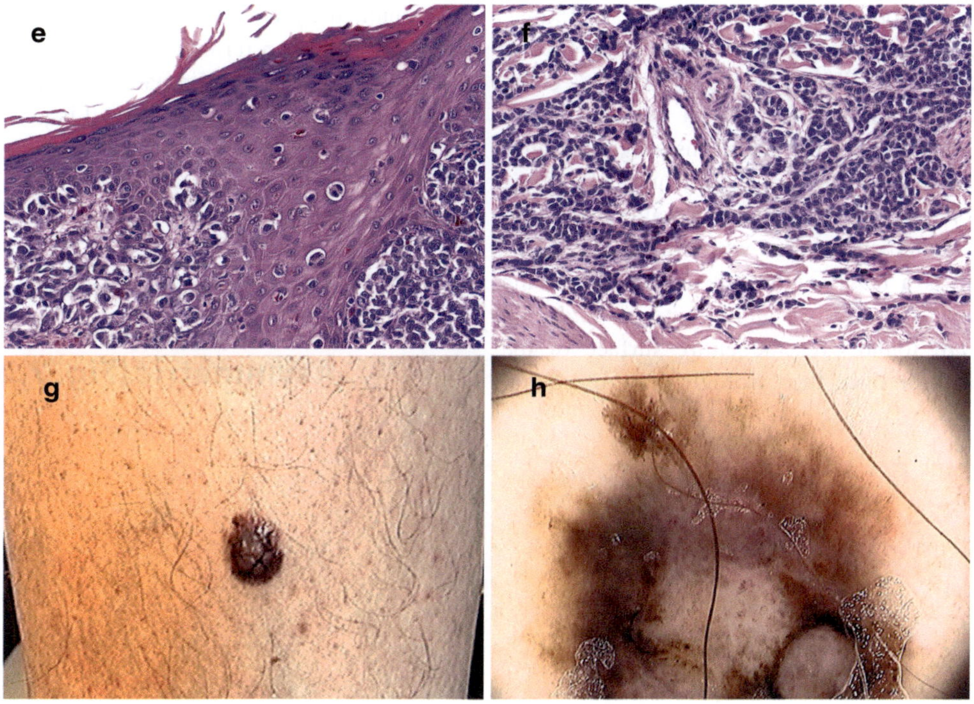

Fig. 7.28 (continued)

Overall Pattern: Symmetric, Epidermal and Dermal

Detailed Description

Silhouette
- Symmetrical
- Well circumscribed
- Epidermal and dermal

Patterns

Epidermis
- Nested at the base of rete ridges
- Some confluence of nests
- Single melanocytes between nests
- Some melanocytes in upper layers

Dermis
- Interstitial strands of melanocytes at the base
- Sheets of melanocytes in the upper dermis replacing collagen
- Little maturation

Cytology
- Oval with enlarged hyperchromatic nuclei and very little cytoplasm
- Some nuclei with irregular outlines
- Heterochromasia of nuclei
- Some nuclei with prominent nucleoli
- Few necrotic melanocytes

Other Changes
- Elongated rete ridges
- Some hypergranulosis, hyperkeratosis, parakeratosis
- Focally thinned epidermis

Integration
At scanning magnification this lesion seems symmetrical and well circumscribed with an interstitial distribution of melanocytes in the deep dermis reminiscent of a congenital nevus (Fig. 7.28a). However, in the upper dermis melanocytes form sheets largely replacing the dermal collagen (Fig. 7.28b, d). There is little if any maturation and melanocytes consist largely of nuclei with heterochromasia, irregular outlines,

and some prominent nucleoli (Fig. 7.28d–f). Melanocytic nuclei are crowded throughout the entire dermis. While the epidermis shows some hyperplasia, there is also focal thinning of the epidermis. Within the epidermis single melanocytes in upper layers are focally quite numerous (Fig. 7.28e). There is some parakeratosis and compact hyperkeratosis which could be interpreted as a result of outside irritation, but the amount of suprabasal melanocytes is high and they are found over the entire surface of the lesion. Moreover, the cytologic features cannot be explained by outside irritation. Lesions like this one have been termed "nevoid melanoma." Clinically, the lesion simulates the papillated surface of a congenital nevus, but it is asymmetric with multiple colors and irregular outline on dermatoscopy (Fig. 7.28g, h).

Diagnosis: Melanoma, invasive.

7.1.4.2 Example 2: Dermal Sheets and Nests, Asymmetric (Fig. 7.29)

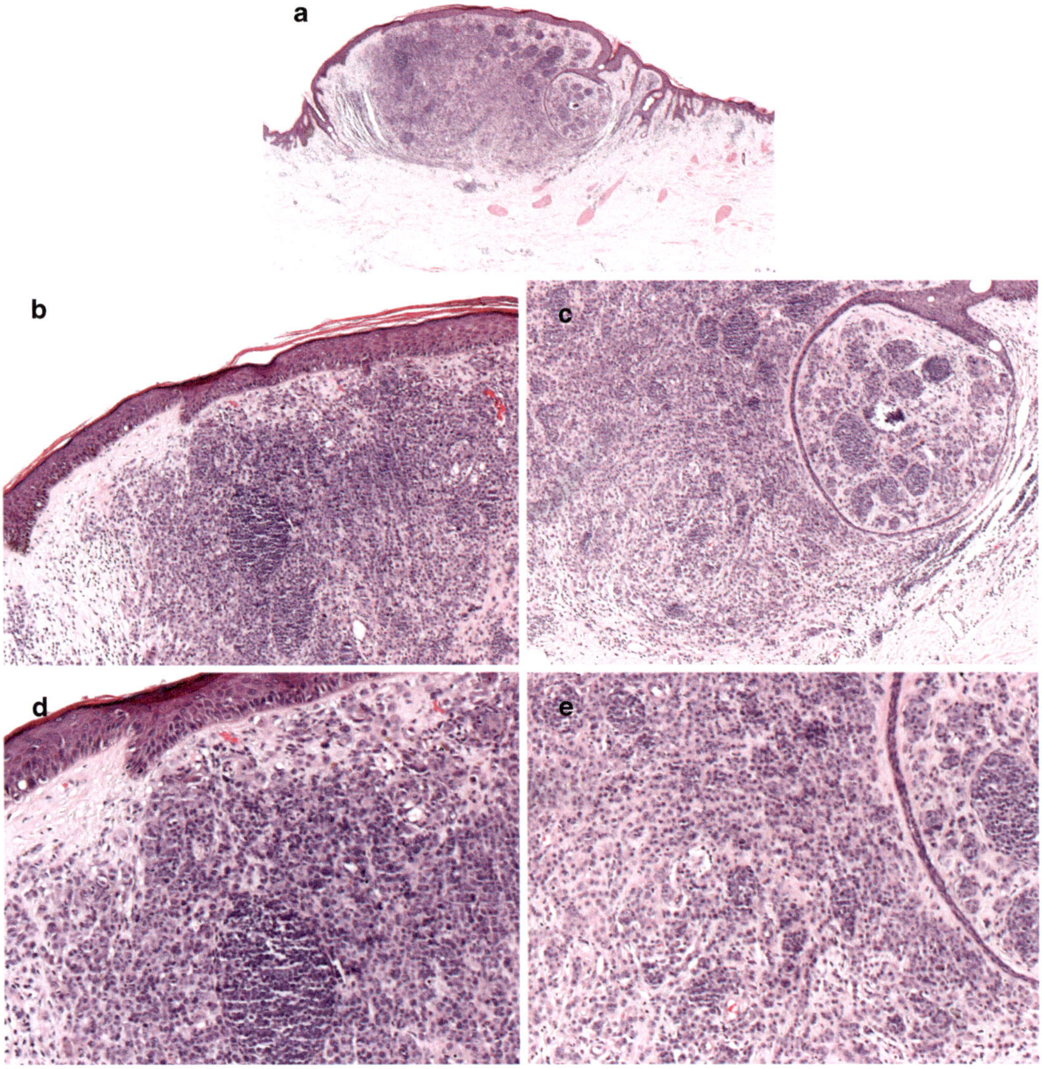

Fig. 7.29 (**a–j**) Nevoid melanoma and nevus-associated melanoma, Example 2. (Courtesy of the Department of Dermatology, Medical University of Vienna)

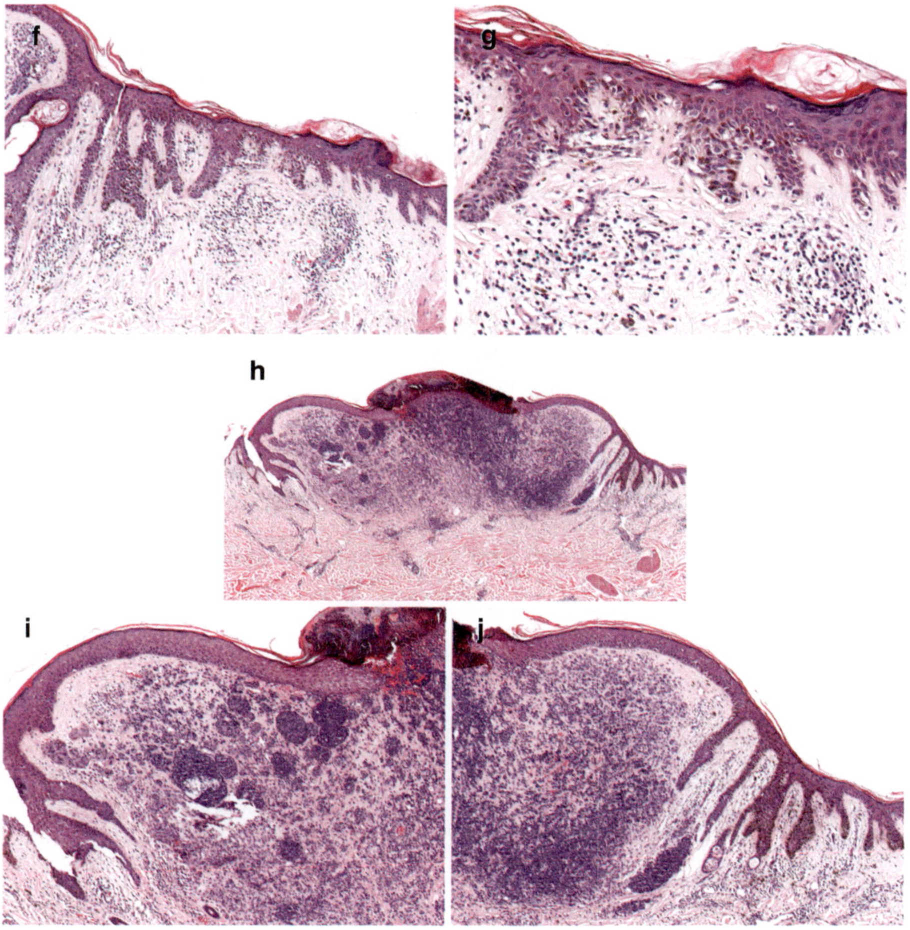

Fig. 7.29 (continued)

Overall Pattern: Mainly Dermal, Asymmetric Nests and Sheets

Detailed Description

Silhouette

- Symmetric
- Not well circumscribed
- Epidermal and dermal
- Exophytic and endophytic growth

Patterns

Epidermis

- Single cells, distributed asymmetrically, also in suprabasal layers
- Some nests at basal layers with confluence

Dermis

- Sheets of melanocytes in upper dermis, in parts replacing collagen
- Nests of melanocytes in upper dermis, varying in size and shape, distributed asymmetrically
- Crowding
- Little maturation

Cytology

- Partly small, hyperchromatic nuclei
- Partly large nuclei with prominent nucleoli, and abundant eosinophilic cytoplasm
- Few necrotic melanocytes

Other Changes

- Epidermis flattened
- Ulceration

Integration

The overall silhouette is symmetric, but the combination of dense dermal sheets of melanocytes with nests varying in size and shape reveal asymmetry within (Fig. 7.29a, h). And while the dermal part seems well circumscribed, the associated epidermal proliferation is not (Fig. 7.29f, g). The dense cellularity ("crowding") of the dermal proliferation can already be seen at scanning magnification due to abundant blue color, which we often call colloquially "too many cells," and is combined with a lack of maturation (Fig. 7.29b, d, i, j). All of these features combined lead to the diagnosis of an invasive melanoma. The visible ulceration is most probably not induced by external trauma, as there is a solid exophytic growth pattern with flattened epidermis, no reactive hyperplasia of surrounding epidermis, and almost no tissue reaction within the dermis such as fibrosis or inflammation.

Diagnosis: Melanoma, invasive.

Follow-up: The lesion developed on the trunk of a male, about 60 years old, patient. The sentinel lymph nodes were free of disease. Interestingly, he developed two further invasive melanomas and one in situ melanoma under close surveillance and was free of metastases 10 years thereafter.

7.1.4.3 Example 3: Very Large Nests, Epidermal (Fig. 7.30)

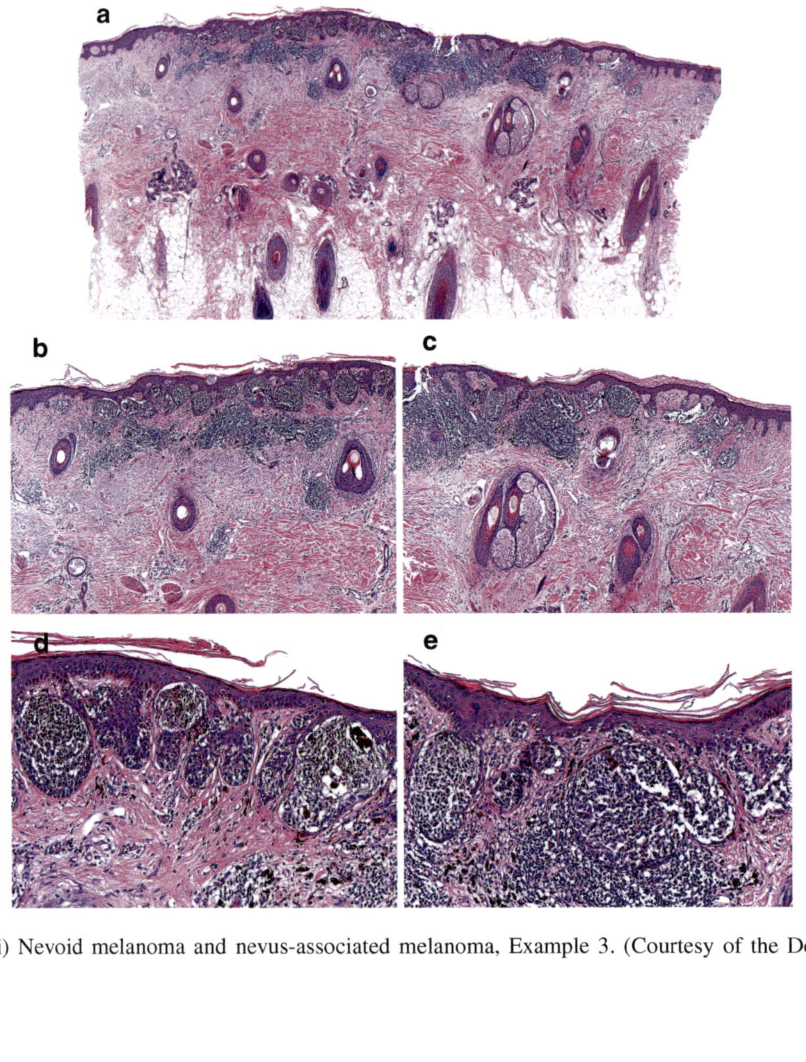

Fig. 7.30 (a–i) Nevoid melanoma and nevus-associated melanoma, Example 3. (Courtesy of the Dermatologikum Hamburg)

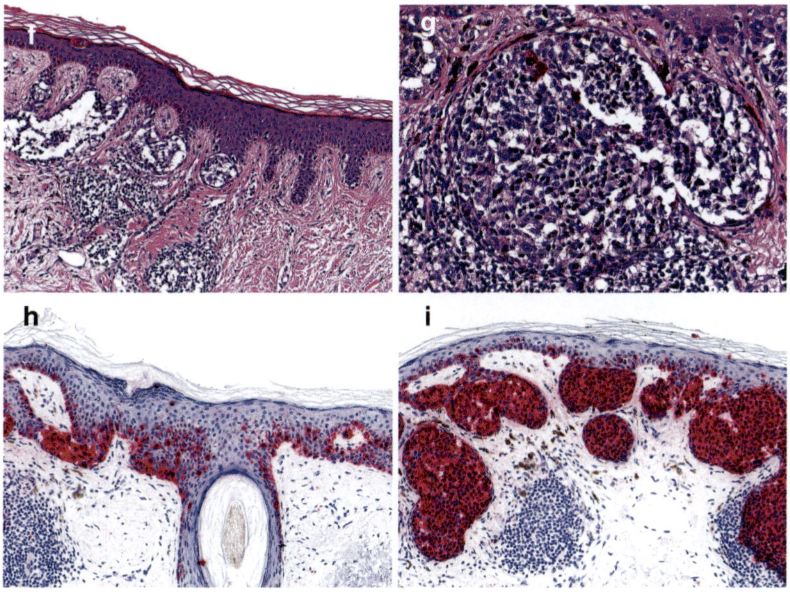

Fig. 7.30 (continued)

Overall Pattern: Nested, Epidermal

Detailed Description

Silhouette

- Well circumscribed
- Symmetric
- Only epidermal

Patterns

Epidermis

- Nests predominate
- Nests at the base of rete ridges
- Nests large and irregular
- Some single melanocytes between nests
- Some suprabasal melanocytes

Dermis

- None

Cytology

- Melanocytes with nuclear pleomorphism

Other Changes

- Prominent solar elastosis
- Prominent band-like lymphocytic infiltrate

Integration

This lesion has a predominantly nested pattern which seems arranged in a symmetric fashion (Fig. 7.30a–c). However, the proliferation developed on severely sun-damaged skin of the forehead and nests of melanocytes are irregular in size, some of them being very large (Fig. 7.30d–f). Higher magnification reveals single melanocytes between nests in irregular distribution, melanocytes in upper layers and also nuclear pleomorphism, which raises suspicion of a melanoma, especially because the lesion is located on severely sun-damaged skin. The number of single melanocytes between nests and the melanocytes in suprabasal layers can better be appreciated in the MelanA immunostain, which also demonstrates predominance of single melanocytes in adnexal ostia (Fig. 7.30h, i). Lesions like this one have been described in the literature under the term "nested melanoma of the elderly" [143, 144]. As a rule of thumb, any broad melanocytic lesion on severely sun-damaged skin should be regarded as a melanoma until proven otherwise. A pitfall in this lesion is also to misread irregular intraepithelial nests of melanocytes as dermal nests of melanocytes (Fig. 7.30g) and to interpret them either as a dermal part of a congenital nevus or as invasive melanoma. Serial sections or immunostaining with pan-cytokeratin can help to identify all the nests seen here to be in fact intraepithelial.

Diagnosis: Melanoma in situ.

7.1.4.4 Example 4: Biphasic Lesion (Fig. 7.31)

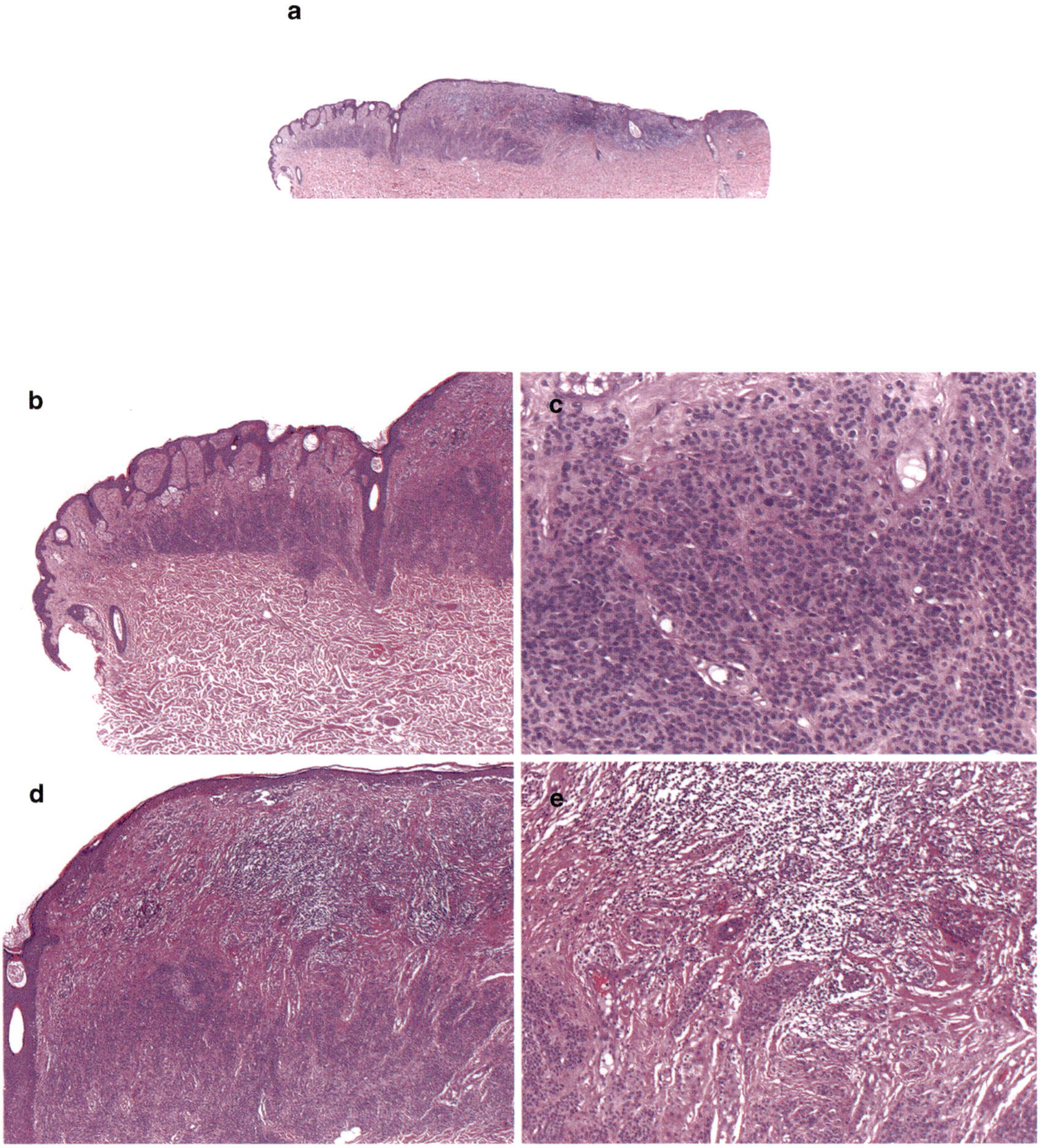

Fig. 7.31 (**a**–**i**) Nevoid melanoma and nevus-associated melanoma, Example 4. (Courtesy of the Department of Dermatology, Medical University of Vienna)

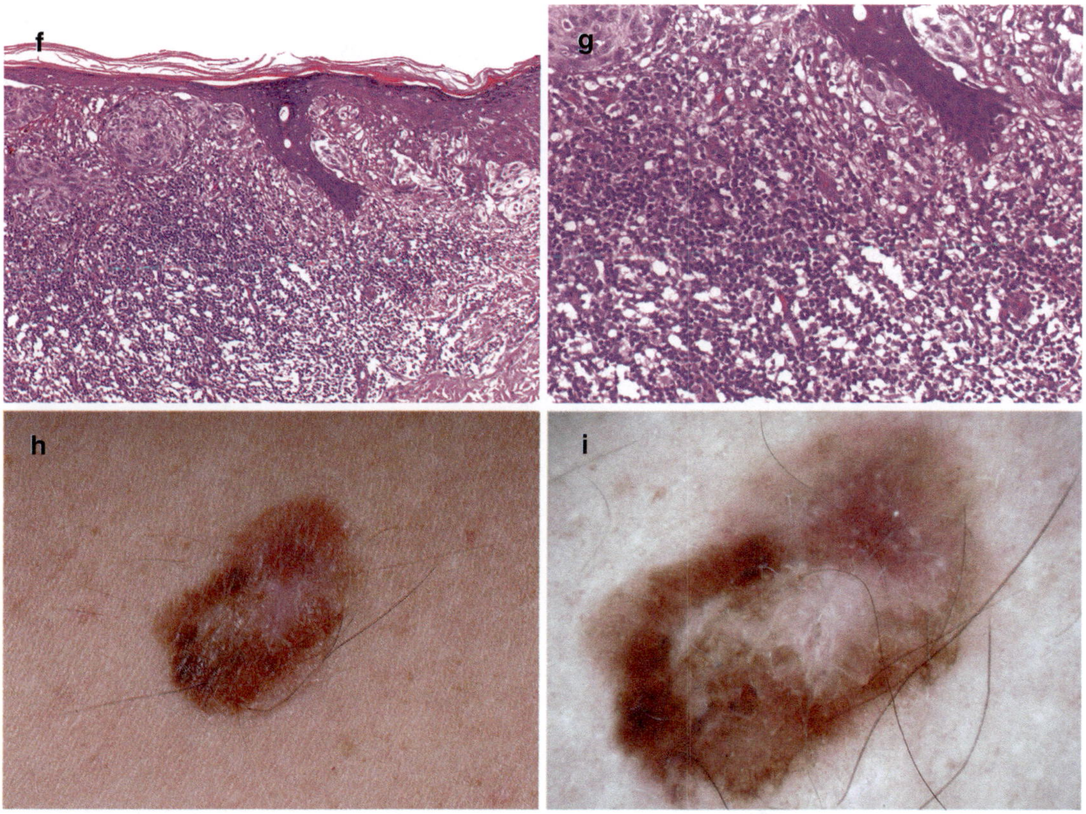

Fig. 7.31 (continued)

Overall Pattern: Epidermal and Dermal, Asymmetric, Poorly Circumscribed on One Site Well Circumscribed on the Other

Detailed Description

Silhouette

- Asymmetric
- Poorly circumscribed on one site, well circumscribed on the other
- Epidermal and dermal

Patterns

Epidermis

- Nests, unequal in size and shape, not equidistant
- Single melanocytes increased, unevenly distributed
- Suprabasal single melanocytes

Dermis

- Nests and strands of melanocytes

Cytology

- Small round melanocytes on one site enlarged and pleomorphic melanocytes on the other

Other Changes

- Infiltrate of lymphocytes in the upper dermis

Integration

Clinically, this is a pigmented papule with two parts and eccentric hyperpigmentation (Fig. 7.31h). The lower part of the lesion is replete with terminal hairs that indicate a congenital nevus. Dermatoscopically, the lesion is chaotic with white reticular lines, a feature that is commonly found in nevus-associated melanomas (Fig. 7.31i). Taken together, this is a melanoma that developed in association with a congenital nevus. Note that the nevus is mainly dermal and not "dysplastic" at all because it has no significant epidermal component (Fig. 7.31a–c). If a melanoma arises in a nevus, it may be in any type of nevus, "dysplastic" and "non-dysplastic." It is a common misconception to believe that a melanoma is more likely to develop in an "ugly" looking nevus (so-called "atypical" or "dysplastic") than in a banal nevus. This concept mistakes a mimic for a precursor. This fallacy is so common that it deserves its own name: the mimic-precursor confusion.

Diagnosis: Melanoma, in association with a congenital nevus.

Alternative diagnosis according to the WHO Classification of Tumours 4th ed.: Superficial spreading melanoma, melanoma in skin with low cumulative sun damage arising in a "dysplastic" nevus?

7.1.4.5 Example 5: Nodule in a Nevus Spilus (Fig. 7.32)

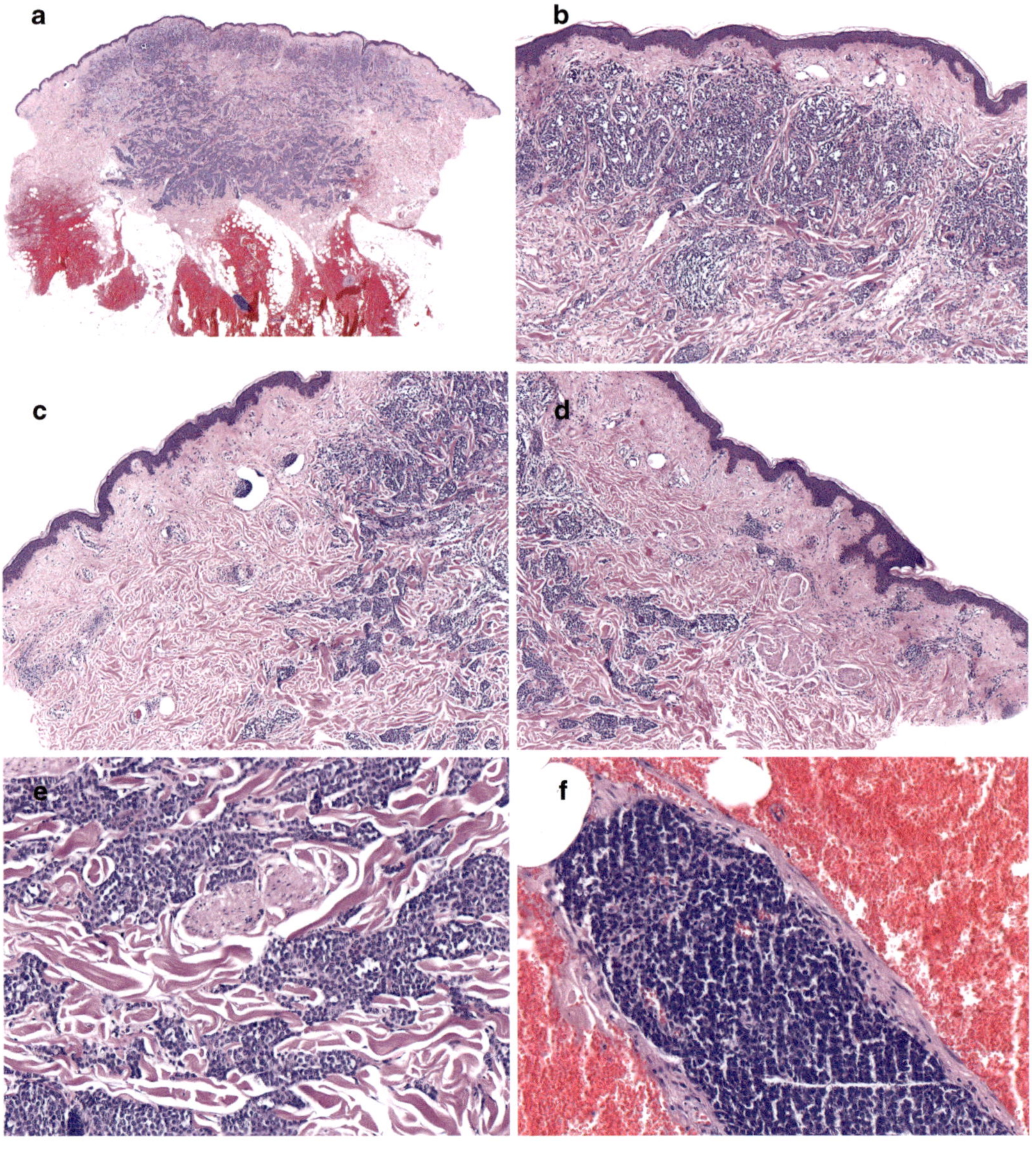

Fig. 7.32 (**a–j**) Nevoid melanoma and nevus-associated melanoma, Example 5. (Courtesy of the Dermatologikum Hamburg)

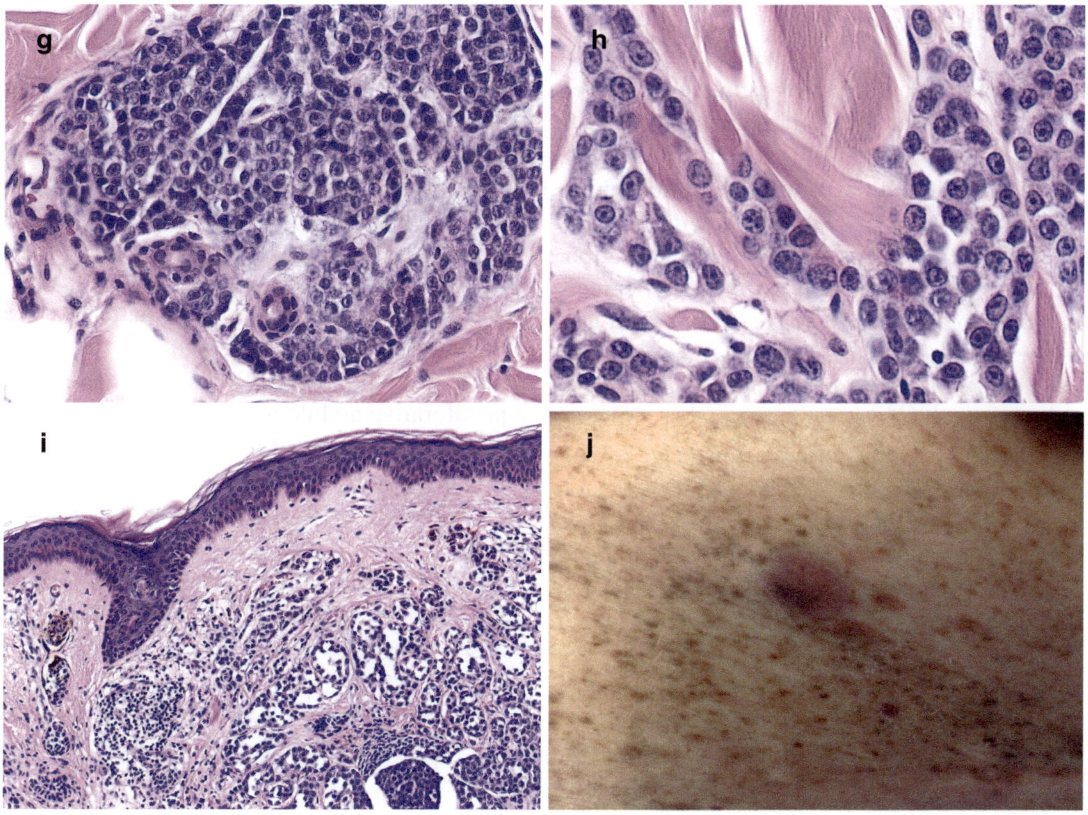

Fig. 7.32 (continued)

Overall Pattern: Interstitial Sheets Throughout the Dermis

Detailed Description

Silhouette

- Asymmetric
- Poorly circumscribed
- Dermal and focally subcutaneous

Patterns

Epidermis

- None

Dermis

- Interstitial strands and sheets filling the dermis, here no maturation
- In the superficial dermis foci of a second, nested periadnexal and interstitial proliferation with maturation

Subcutis

- Nodule in a subcutaneous septum

Cytology

- Large melanocytes with large nuclei with prominent nucleoli
- Crowding of nuclei
- Mitoses throughout the proliferation including the base of the lesion
- Second population of melanocytes in the superficial dermis with small melanocytes, pigmented in superficial nests, not pigmented below

Other Changes

- Vascular invasion: Nodule in the subcutis developed in a vessel
- Flattened rete ridges in the center, slight epidermal hyperplasia at the periphery

Integration

A large nodular growth developed in the context of a longstanding, congenital nevus, which clinically presented as a large nevus spilus on the trunk of a 73-year-old woman (Fig. 7.32j). The remnants of a nevus are seen in the superficial dermis with several foci showing features of a congenital nevus (nesting, maturation, umbrella of pigment, adnexocentricity, epidermal hyperplasia, Fig. 7.32a, c, d, i). The center of the specimen is filled with a relatively uniform appearing cell proliferation that is present with strands and sheets between collagen bundles and fills the entire dermis (Fig. 7.32a). No maturation is seen in this part of the lesion (Fig. 7.32e, g). On closer inspection, the cells are pleomorphic with strikingly enlarged nuclei, prominent nucleoli, hyperchromasia and heterochromasia as well as crowding of nuclei (Fig. 7.32g, h). Mitotic figures are present even at the base of the lesion. With some distance, a nodule with the same cytology is identified in a subcutaneous septum. This nodule is surrounded by a vascular lining (muscle layer discernible even on H&E) and therefore has to be interpreted as vascular invasion (Fig. 7.32f). This lesion is a nodular, amelanotic and purely dermal melanoma arising in a nevus spilus. It is important to note that purely dermal melanomas with no involvement of the epidermis are extremely rare. In such cases, all criteria for diagnosis of melanoma that are based on epidermal patterns are useless. Still the diagnosis can be made using dermal patterns (lack of maturation, sheets) and cytology (pleomorphism, mitoses). The differential diagnosis of a proliferative nodule in a congenital nevus can be ruled out because of the dermal arrangement in sheets, the pleomorphic cytology, the presence of vascular invasion and, not the least, the age of the patient. This lesion harbored an NRAS Q61K mutation which can be found in large speckled congenital nevi with and without associated melanoma, no BRAF mutation was identified.

Diagnosis: Nodular amelanotic melanoma with vascular invasion, arising in a Naevus spilus.

7.1.5 Regression, Sclerosis, Recurrence, and Inflammation

Connective tissue alterations are not uncommon in melanocytic lesions and they may develop for various reasons: (1) a specific type of melanocytic lesion always induces a characteristic alteration of the connective tissue as is the case in sclerosing blue nevus and sclerosing (desmoplastic) spitz nevus, (2) a lesion was traumatized and mechanisms of wound healing appear in the melanocytic lesion, (3) a lesion is recognized by the immune system and a specific type of inflammatory response develops in response to the melanocytic neoplasm as is seen in Halo nevus or in regression of melanoma. In the following we give examples for the latter two circumstances.

External trauma, which includes rubbing, scratching, partial removal by scalpel or ablative laser systems, will induce changes in a melanocytic lesion that increase difficulties in differential diagnosis of melanocytic nevi from melanoma. Acute trauma such as scratching or UV radiation may result in suprabasal melanocytes. Incomplete removal of a nevus with recurrence of the lesion in the scar may produce so-called "pseudomelanoma" changes, i.e., flattened rete ridges, irregular epidermal melanocytic proliferations with dominance of single melanocytes and suprabasal melanocytes [145, 146]. Moreover, dermal parts of a recurrent nevus may lack good maturation and may express HMB45 [147]. Unfortunately even PRAME expression can be observed in recurrent nevi, but in a minority of cases [97]. The situation is even more complicated by the fact that scratching or incomplete removal may also at times happen in a melanoma [148]. For histopathologic differentiation it is most important to study the architecture and cytology of the melanocytic lesion at the periphery of the connective tissue change. If suprabasal melanocytes and irregular arrangement of single melanocytes extend beyond the fibrosis, it is considered a sign of melanoma [149]. In a recurrent nevus, the "pseudomelanoma" changes should be restricted to the zone of trauma/fibrosis [149]. Interestingly, this histological observation correlates well with dermoscopy. In a multivariate analysis, pigmentation beyond the scar's edge was a strong clue for melanoma [150]. If the trauma to a lesion was a previous operation and the re-excision poses diagnostic difficulty, the original specimen should be reviewed to reassess the diagnosis [151].

Up to 35% of all melanomas show histologically areas with reduced tumor cells, flattened epidermis, variable degrees of inflammation and melanophages and fibrosis with neovascularization, which has been termed regression [152]. These microscopic features correlate with gray or white zones with dots of dark pigment and bizarre-shaped vessels clinically and dermatoscopically. Depending on the extent of histological inflammation and fibrosis, regression has been specified as early (inflammation), intermediate and late (fibrosis) [153]. As of today, it is a matter of controversy whether the histological finding of regression is a good or a bad prognostic sign [152, 154–157]. It is obvious, however, that the finding of regression increases doubts about the measurement of thickness as a reliable indicator of prognosis. It cannot be determined with surety, what the thickness of a melanoma was before it regressed. In most cases, regression is seen only in a focus of a lesion, but sometimes the question of complete regression arises. In that setting it may be impossible to determine the biological nature of the regressed lesion, because regressed areas in melanoma, in basal cell carcinoma, or in lichen planus-like keratosis/regressed seborrheic keratosis look essentially the same. A prominent band of melanophages and complete absence of melanocytes from the epidermis in the regressed lesion are used to suggest a regressed melanocytic lesion, but not beyond doubt.

Inflammatory infiltrates do not only occur in malignant melanoma or after trauma. In fact, many melanocytic nevi show some degree of inflammatory infiltrate. A specific type of inflammation is that seen in Halo nevi, which may be so dense that the melanocytic lesion is hardly discernible. It is well known that the inflammation in Halo nevi may lead, over years, to complete disappearance of the melanocytic lesion with a clinical appearance of a vitiligo-like depigmentation, meaning that not only melanocytes of the nevus but also normal epidermal melanocytes disappear [158].

7.1.5.1 Example 1: Irregular Epidermal Melanocytes with Underlying Scar (Fig. 7.33)

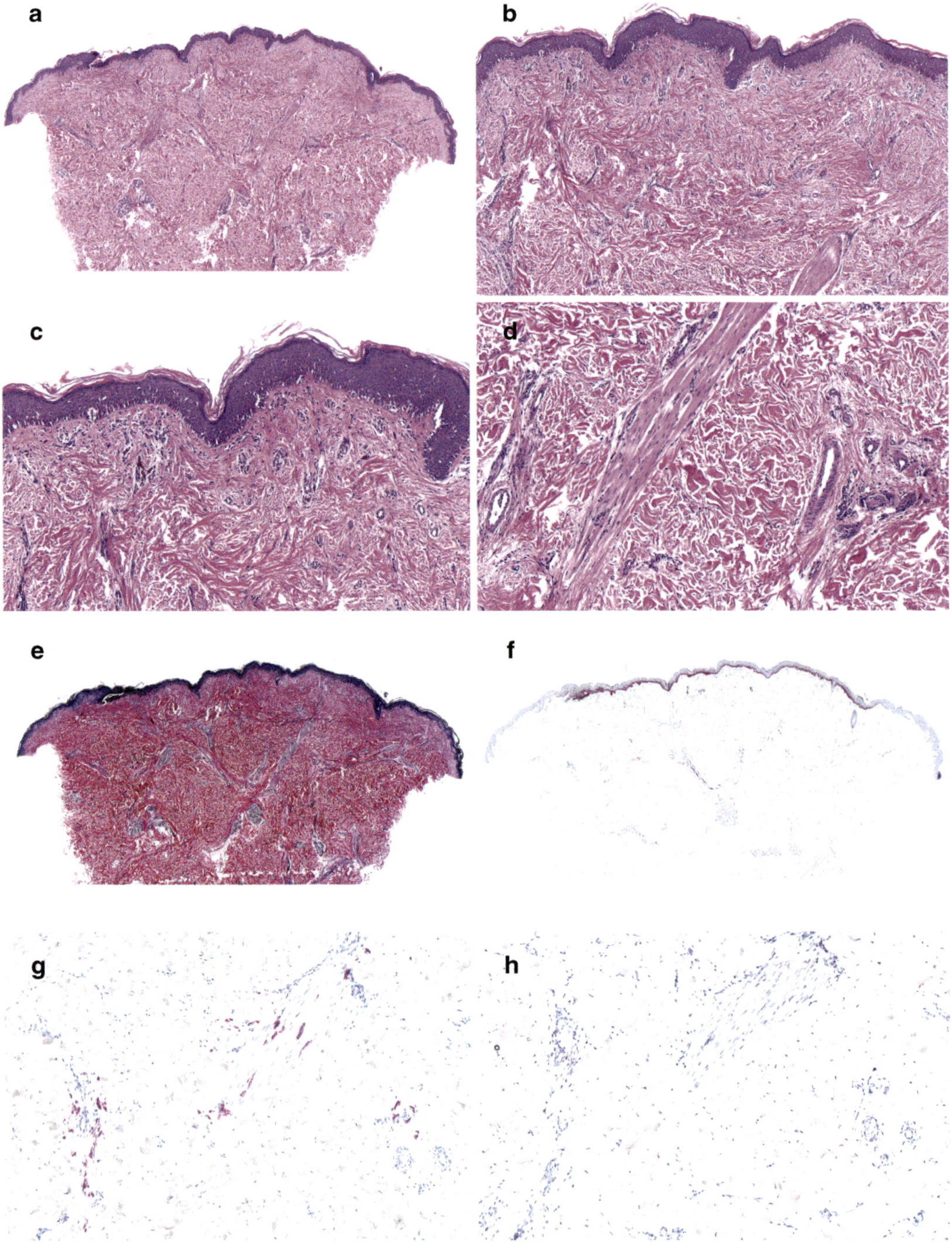

Fig. 7.33 (**a**–**h**) Regression, sclerosis, recurrence, and inflammation, Example 1. (Courtesy of the Dermatologikum Hamburg)

Overall Pattern: Broad, Single Melanocytes Predominate, Mostly Epidermal

Detailed Description

Silhouette

- Largely epidermal
- Broad lesion
- Poorly circumscribed

Patterns

Epidermis

- Single melanocytes, unevenly distributed
- Few nests
- Single melanocytes in suprabasal layers

Dermis

- Small nests of melanocytes around vessels
- Small nests of melanocytes within and around arrector pili muscle

Cytology

- Small melanocytes
- Monomorphic nuclei

Other Changes

- Flattened rete ridges
- Horizontal arrangement of collagen
- Slight increase of dermal fibroblasts

Elastica Stain

- Horizontal arrangement of collagen in the upper part of the dermis (Fig. 7.33e)
- Regular collagen below the horizontal arrangement (Fig. 7.33e)

Immunohistochemistry

- MelanA stain highlights the predominance of single melanocytes in the epidermis and suprabasal melanocytes (Fig. 7.33f, g).
- Melanocytes are present in the deep dermis around vessels and around and within muscle (MelanA) (Fig. 7.33g).
- HMB45 is not expressed in the dermal part of the lesion (Fig. 7.33h).

Integration

This lesion is broad, poorly circumscribed and dominated by single melanocytes with melanocytes in upper epidermal layers—all criteria for melanoma in situ (Fig. 7.33a–c). However, the dermis has a characteristic horizontal arrangement of collagen fibers with increased fibroblasts indicating a scar after previous trauma (Fig. 7.33b, c). The scar also explains the flattened rete ridges. Immunohistochemical staining with MelanA is very helpful here, because the perivascular and myotropic arrangement of melanocytes in the deep dermis is seen much easier than in H&E staining (Fig. 7.33g). The lack of expression of HMB45 is typical of a dermal part of a congenital nevus (Fig. 7.33h). This example shows how important it is to have a complete excision of the lesion. In a superficial shave, the findings shown here could easily be misinterpreted as those of a melanoma. These features of a recurrent nevus have been described as "pseudomelanoma after trauma" [145].

Diagnosis: Recurrence of a congenital nevus in a scar.

7.1.5.2 Example 2: Irregular Epidermal and Dermal Melanocytes with Underlying Scar (Fig. 7.34)

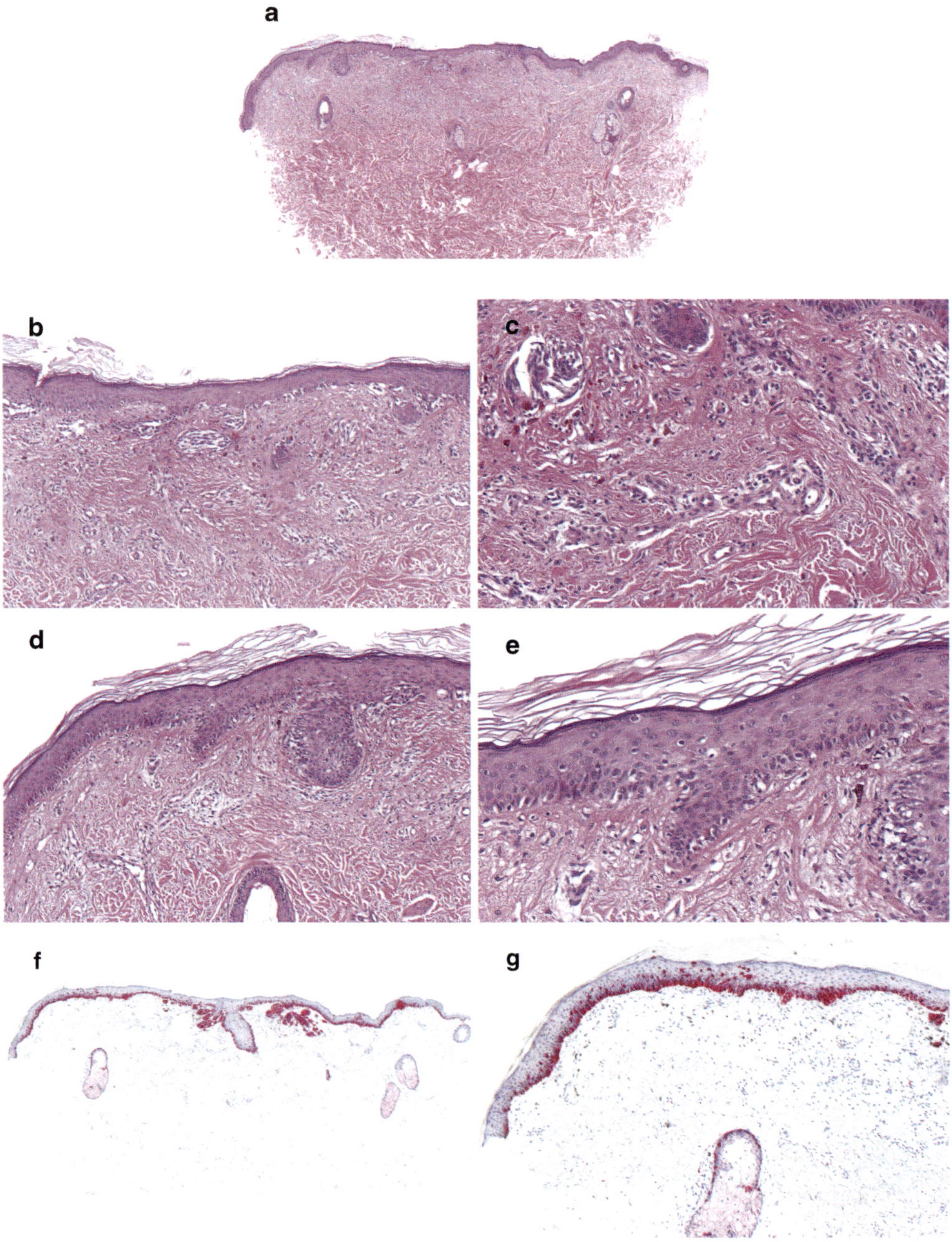

Fig. 7.34 (**a**–**i**) Regression, sclerosis, recurrence, and inflammation, Example 2. (Courtesy of the Dermatologikum Hamburg)

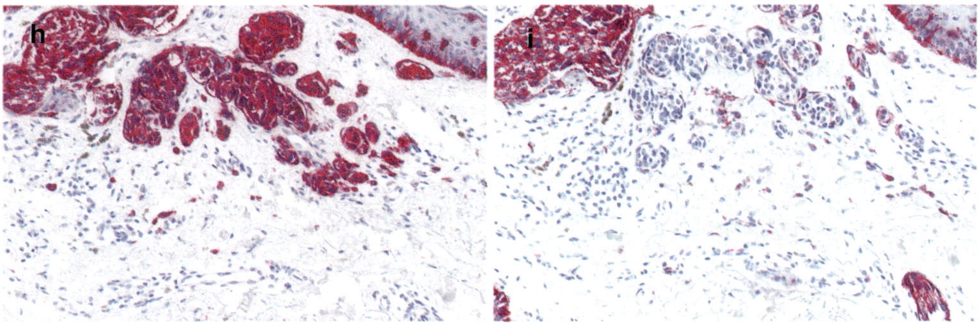

Fig. 7.34 (continued)

Overall Pattern: Asymmetric, Poorly Circumscribed, Epidermal and Dermal, Some Maturation

Detailed Description

Silhouette

- Epidermal and dermal
- Broad lesion
- Poorly circumscribed
- Asymmetric

Patterns

Epidermis

- Single melanocytes, unevenly distributed
- Few nests of variable size
- Single melanocytes in suprabasal layers

Adnexal Epithelium

- Single melanocytes in uneven distribution in follicular and eccrine epithelium
- Nests of variable sizes in adnexal epithelia

Dermis

- Nests of melanocytes with maturation and periadnexal arrangement
- Few irregularly shaped nests in the superficial dermis

Cytology

- Epithelioid melanocytes in the epidermis and in adnexal epithelia
- Epithelioid melanocytes in few superficial nests in the dermis
- Smaller melanocytes with less cytoplasm in periadnexal nests

Other Changes

- Horizontal collagen in one focus with slight increase of dermal fibroblasts
- Solar elastosis adjacent to fibrosis
- Flattened rete ridges

Immunohistochemistry

- MelanA stain highlights the predominance of single melanocytes in the epidermis, suprabasal melanocytes, and focal nests in the superficial dermis (Fig. 7.34f, g).
- HMB45 is expressed in the epidermal and adnexal epithelial part of the lesion and in irregularly shaped nests in the superficial dermis but not in those with periadnexal arrangement and maturation (Fig. 7.34h, i).

Integration

The differential diagnosis in this lesion is between a traumatized congenital nevus with features of a "pseudomelanoma" and a melanoma arising in a congenital nevus with signs of previous trauma. Single melanocytes and suprabasal melanocytes are present in the epidermis above the zone of fibrosis, but they also extend to involve epidermis above unaltered dermis with some solar elastosis where rete ridges are flattened, too (Fig. 7.34a–e). This is a strong hint to the diagnosis of melanoma. Nests of melanocytes in the dermis show two different cytologies with variable expression of HMB45. The nests with epithelioid cytology and expression of HMB45 are better interpreted as an invasive part of the melanoma while the periadnexal nests with maturation and lack of expression of HMB45 are likely those of a pre-existing congenital nevus (Fig. 7.34h, i).

Diagnosis: Melanoma, superficially invasive, arising in a congenital nevus with focal scar.

7.1.5.3 Example 3: Traumatized Nevus (Fig. 7.35)

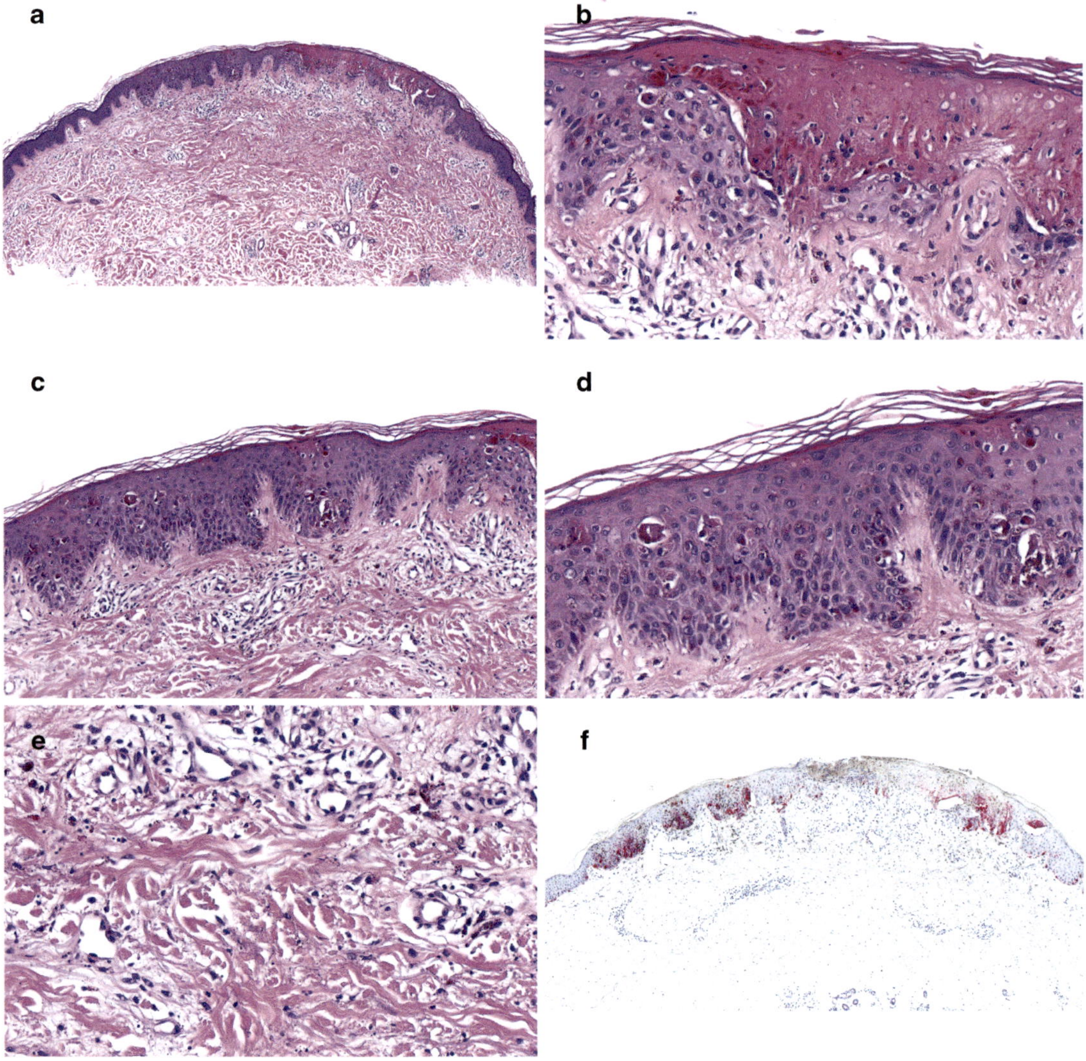

Fig. 7.35 (**a**–**f**) Regression, sclerosis, recurrence, and inflammation, Example 3. (Courtesy of the Dermatologikum Hamburg)

Overall Pattern: Small, Asymmetric, Epidermal Only, Single Cells, and Nests

Detailed Description

Silhouette

- Asymmetric, but small and well circumscribed
- Epidermal only

Patterns

Epidermis

- Single melanocytes and nests
- Irregular distribution
- Some melanocytes in suprabasal layers

Dermis

- None

Cytology

- Slightly epithelioid with fine pigmentation

Other Changes

- Extensive necrosis of the epidermis on the right
- Individual necrotic keratinocytes in upper layers throughout the lesion, some of them pigmented
- Heavy pigmentation of keratinocytes
- Numerous melanophages in the dermis
- Some lymphocytic infiltrate
- Subtle subepidermal fibrosis

Immunohistochemistry

- MelanA highlights the good circumscription of the lesion (Fig. 7.35f).
- Not all suprabasal pigmented cells are melanocytes, some are pigmented keratinocytes which do not express MelanA.

Integration

The asymmetry in this lesion is caused by the partial necrosis which is the result of acute trauma (Fig. 7.35a, b). Without immunohistochemistry it is easy to misread the pigmented necrotic keratinocytes in suprabasal layers as melanocytes (Fig. 7.35c, d). MelanA demonstrates that very few suprabasal melanocytes are present, which is compatible with the diagnosis of a traumatized nevus (Fig. 7.35f). Moreover, the lesion is small, partly nested and well circumscribed.

Diagnosis: Junctional melanocytic nevus with signs of recent trauma.

7.1.5.4 Example 4: Increased Epidermal Melanocytes in Melanoma Re-excision (Fig. 7.36)

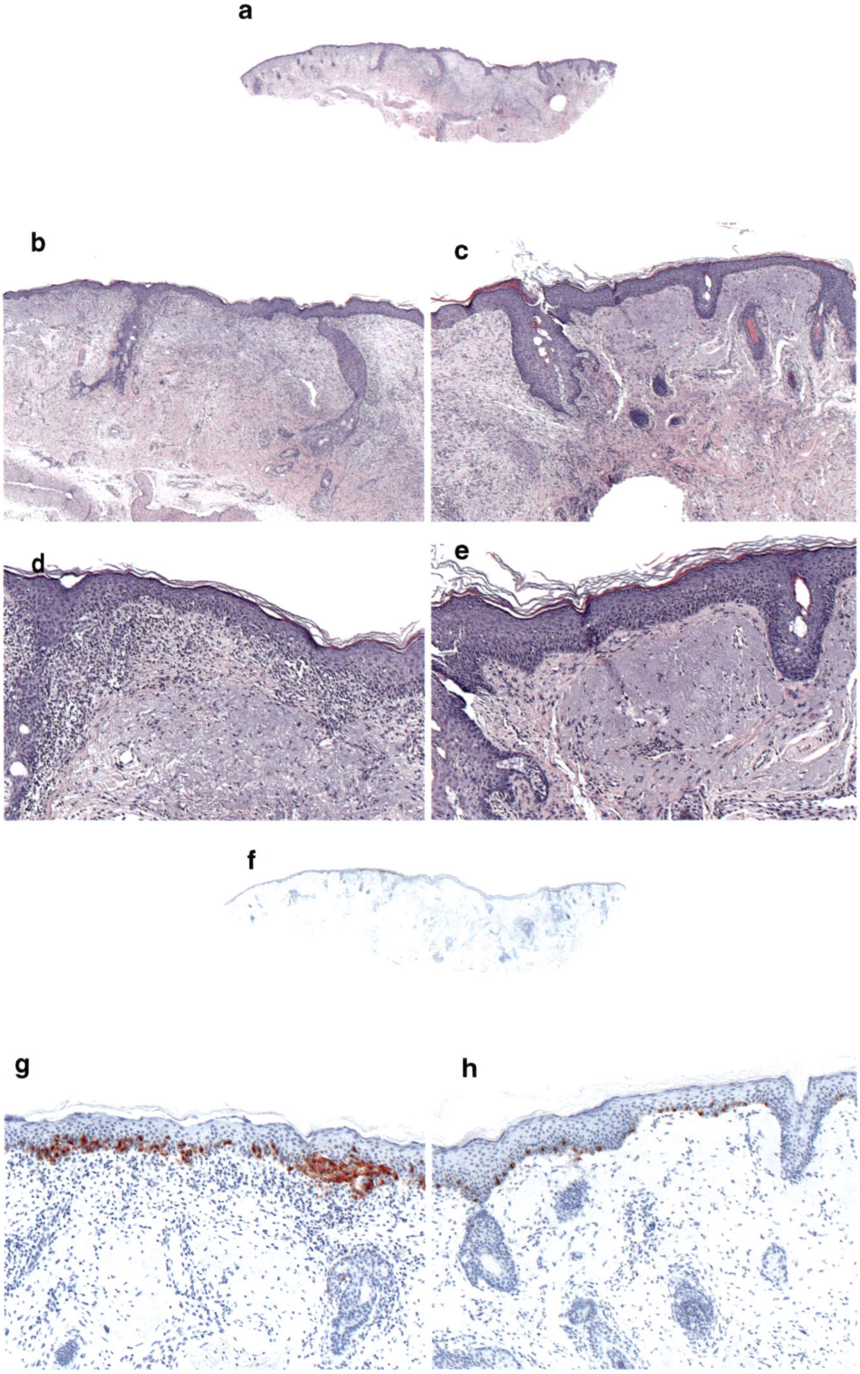

Fig. 7.36 (a–k) Regression, sclerosis, recurrence, and inflammation, Example 4. (Courtesy of the Department of Dermatology, Medical University of Vienna)

Fig. 7.36 (continued)

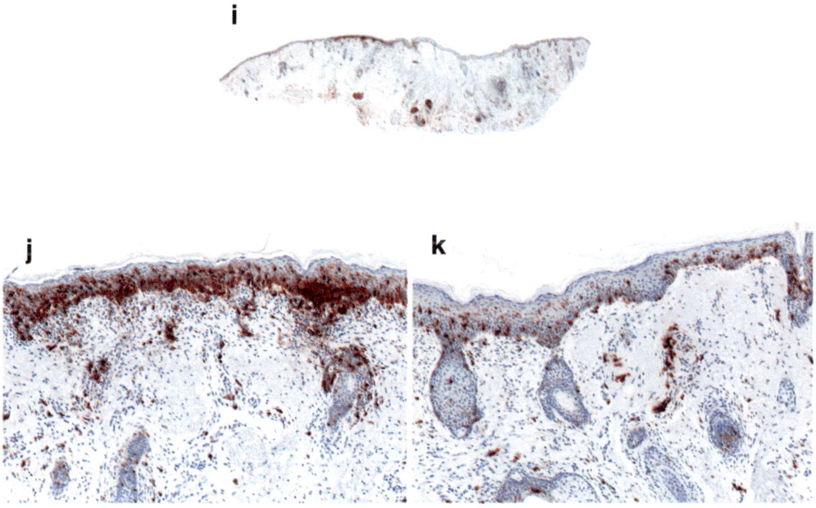

Overall Pattern: Asymmetric, Not Well Defined, Single Cells with Irregular Nesting

Detailed Description

Silhouette

- Not well circumscribed
- Asymmetric
- In epidermis

Patterns

Epidermis

- Right: small, basal, regularly distributed melanocytes
- Left: Increased single cells, focal nesting with horizontal confluence

Cytology

- Right of the scar: Small single cells
- Left of the scar: Medium-sized, partly spindled

Other Changes

- Striking solar elastosis

Immunohistochemistry

- MelanA: Increased melanocytes confluent nesting on the left, and sparsely increased single melanocytes in the basal layer on the right (Fig. 7.36f–h).
- S100: Increased melanocytes confluent nesting on the left, and sparsely increased single melanocytes in the basal layer on the right. Positive staining of dendritic cells in upper layers of the epidermis and dermis (Fig. 7.36i–k).

Integration

Increased melanocytes around re-excision scars are a common source of discussion within centers reporting such specimens. Significantly increased cells can be present in re-excision scars, especially next to the primary surgical site and the site of (previous) suture. This is, in our experience, more marked the less time has passed from the initial excision. Whenever the cells are mostly, but not as a rule, confined to basal layers, and small, this is in line with reactive hyperplasia of melanocytes (Fig. 7.36c, e, h, k). Whenever there are larger cells, varying in size and shape, and formation of nests, especially with confluence, this should usually be regarded as true remnants of a melanoma (Fig. 7.36b, d, g, j). Changes are usually well discernible with H&E staining alone, but immunohistochemistry allows for an easier evaluation of architecture, where in our experience any one of the common melanocytic markers suffices.

Often, primary excisions are dissected macroscopically with "bread loafing," where naturally many parts of the lateral margins are not covered in histological sections. It should therefore be of no surprise to a histopathologist, but also clinician and patient, that even in a primarily "completely excised" melanoma, there can be remnants of melanoma in a re-excision.

Diagnosis: Scar with reactive melanocytic hyperplasia and residual melanoma in situ.

7.1.5.5 Example 5: Epidermal Nests of Melanocytes with a Lichenoid Infiltrate (Fig. 7.37)

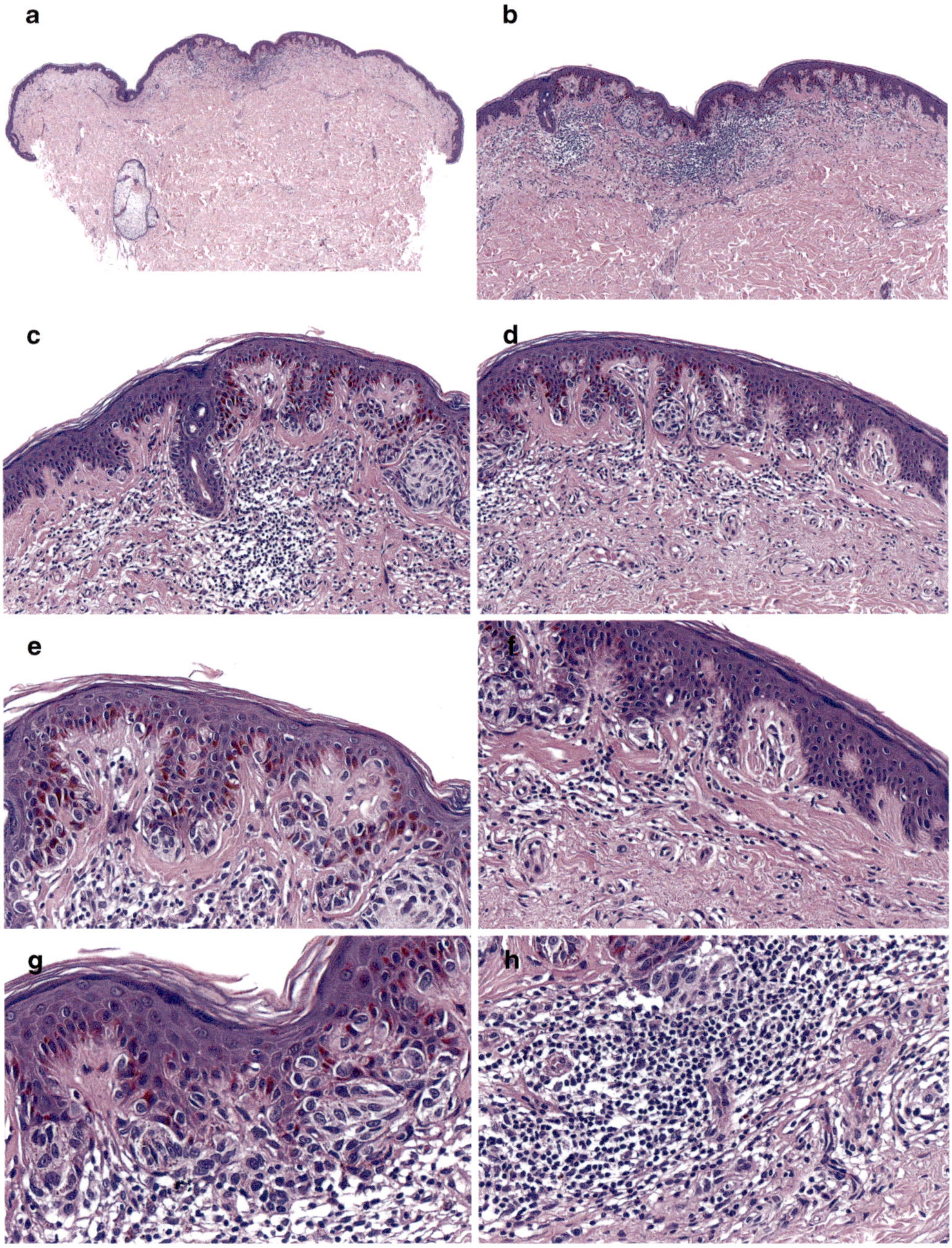

Fig. 7.37 (**a–j**) Regression, sclerosis, recurrence, and inflammation, Example 5. (Courtesy of the Dermatologikum Hamburg)

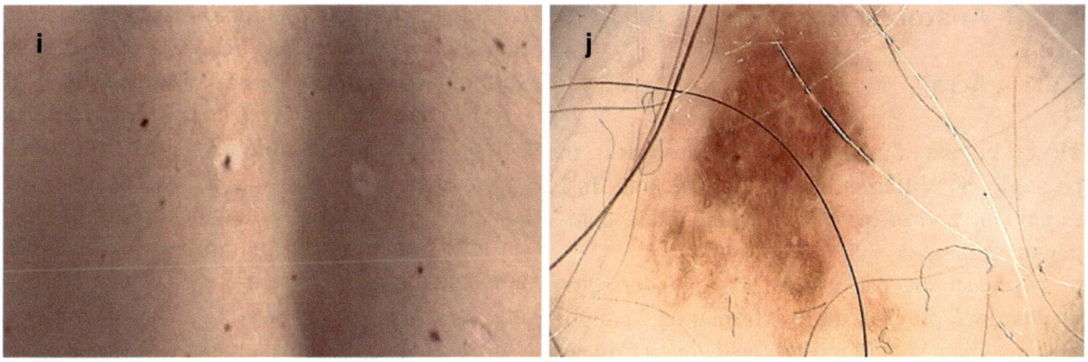

Fig. 7.37 (continued)

Overall Pattern: Symmetric, Poorly Circumscribed

Detailed Description

Silhouette

- Poorly circumscribed
- Epidermal only

Patterns

Epidermis

- Nests at the base of rete ridges.
- Nests vary in size.
- Single melanocytes in the basal layer, regularly distributed.

Dermis

- Few single melanocytes

Cytology

- Epithelioid with enlarged nuclei
- Some nuclei with prominent nucleoli

Other Changes

- Band-like subepidermal lymphocytic infiltrate.
- Infiltrate focally obscures the dermoepidermal junction.
- Fibrosis in the papillary dermis with flattening of the rete ridges on both sides of the lesion.
- So-called lamellar and concentric fibroplasia around rete ridges within the lesion.

Integration

This lesion is obscured by a dense lymphocytic infiltrate (Fig. 7.37a–d) but apart from that has a regular and roughly symmetric architecture. Nests are positioned at the base of rete ridges (Fig. 7.37c–f). At the periphery of the lesion single melanocytes predominate, but they are regularly distributed. The alteration of the papillary dermis on both sides and the slightly epithelioid cytology of the melanocytes can be attributed to the effects of the lymphocytic infiltrate (Fig. 7.37g, h), which is known as the "Halo phenomenon." In this patient, the clinical appearance fits well with the histomorphologic features because a depigmented Halo is also present around the nevus, which therefore is called a Halo nevus (Fig. 7.37i, j). This patient with multiple Halo nevi also had Vitiligo. It seems that this is a junctional nevus, but on closer view, some single melanocytes can be identified in the dermis (Fig. 7.37h). Most likely, this lesion had nests in the dermis, which already have largely regressed due to the effects of the lymphocytic infiltrate.

Diagnosis: Halo nevus.

7.2 Anatomic Sites

7.2.1 Acral

The evaluation of acral melanocytic lesions is, in principle, not different to any anatomic site. Just as anywhere else, nevi can be junctional, compound, or dermal.

The anatomic background of acral dermatoglyphs does provide some information, though. Melanocytic nevi will mostly reside in rete ridges lying below the furrows of the surface, giving rise to the "parallel furrow pattern" in dermatoscopy (Fig. 7.38). Contrastingly, melanomas will (also) be present in epidermal parts below the more broad ridges containing the sweat gland ducts, dermatoscopically visible as structureless or "parallel ridge pattern." Because especially soles are commonly subject to chronic pressure and frictional trauma, one often finds melanin pigment within the stratum corneum above the lesion.

The diagnosis of acral melanoma, from our personal experience, is often delayed due to often inconspicuous pigment clinically. Also, in situ melanoma on acral sites may be almost invisible on H/E stainings alone, similar to in situ melanoma on the face. Therefore, we have the following two rules when evaluating a specimen with a clinical suspicion of melanoma:

- If H/E stainings don't show a clear-cut melanocytic lesion, we perform immunostainings.
- If H/E and immunostainings are both negative, and the specimen size is small—like with a punch biopsy—we recommend a rebiopsy or close clinical follow-up nevertheless.

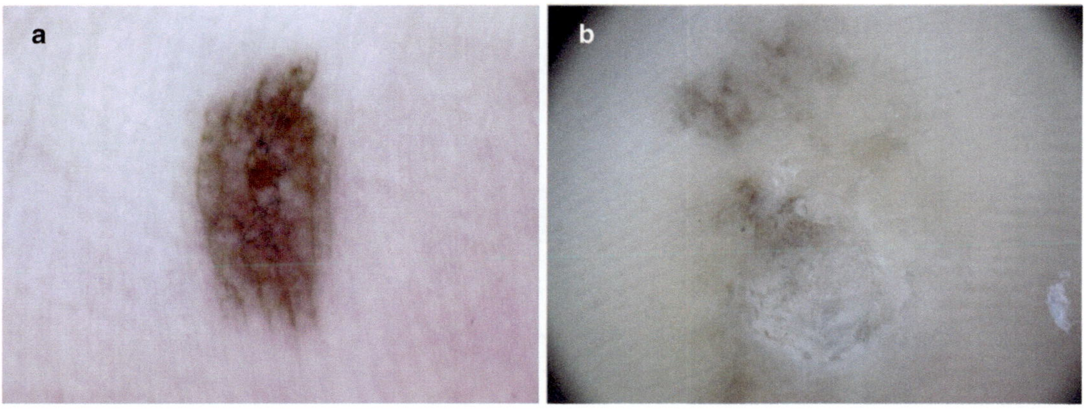

Fig. 7.38 (**a**) Dermatoscopic image of an acral nevus. Notice the pigment is primarily present within the furrows, but not fully restricted to them. One can also see some strands of pigment crossing the furrows. Due to some asymmetry, the clinicians decided to biopsy this lesion, which verified the presence of an acral compound nevus. (**b**) Dermatoscopic image of an acral melanoma. Notice the pigment is often faint, but where present it spans the ridges of dermatoglyphs. (Courtesy of the Department of Dermatology, Medical University of Vienna)

7.2.1.1 Example 1: Large Pigmented Nests (Fig. 7.39)

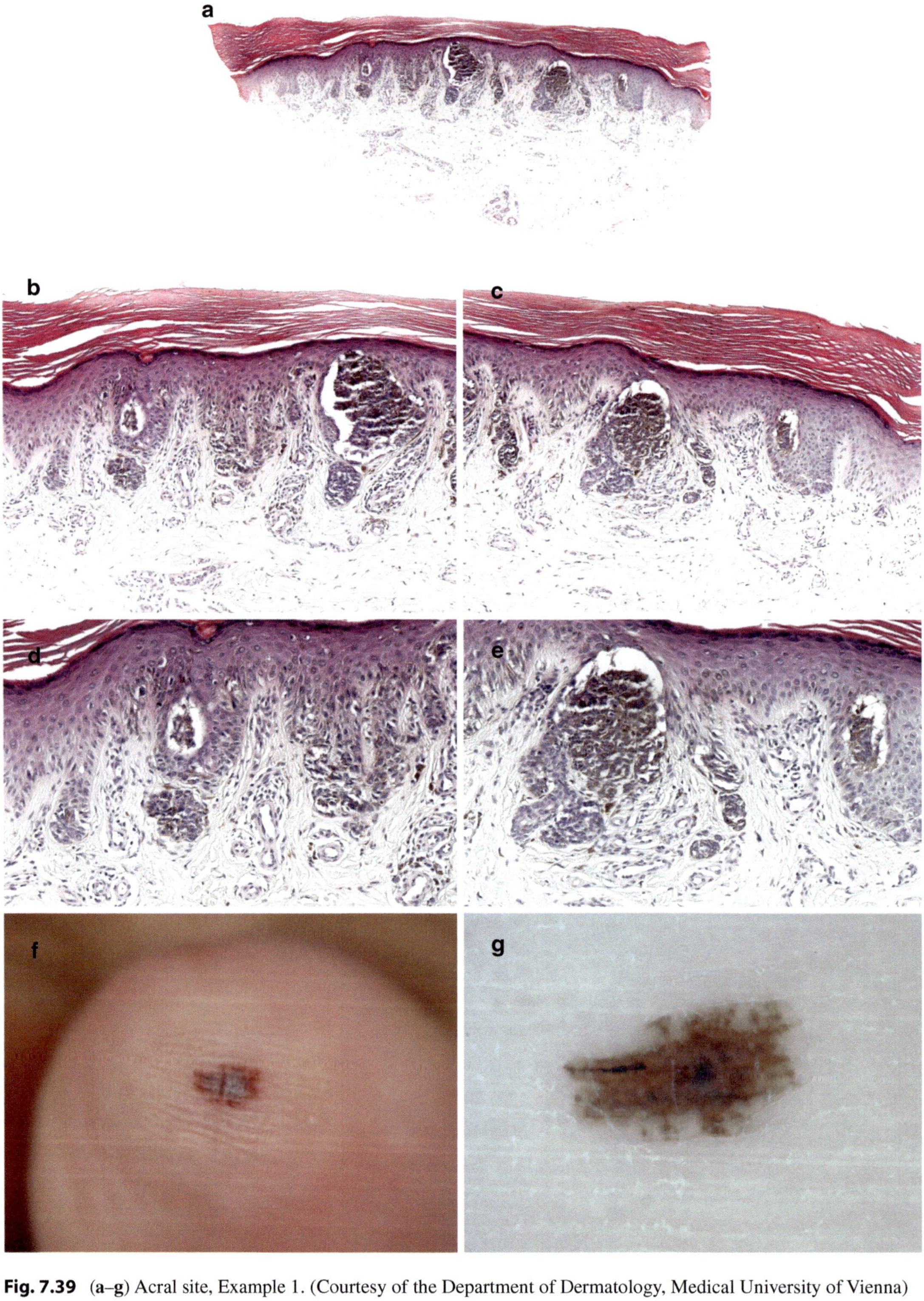

Fig. 7.39 (**a–g**) Acral site, Example 1. (Courtesy of the Department of Dermatology, Medical University of Vienna)

Overall Pattern: Epidermal, Regular, Mainly Large Nests

Detailed Description

Silhouette

- Well circumscribed
- Symmetric
- Epidermal only

Patterns

Epidermis

- Mainly nested
- Varying somewhat in size and shape
- Confined to basal layers

Cytology

- Small, round, monomorphic
- Heavily pigmented

Other Changes

- Minimal pigment in stratum corneum

Integration

The lesion is a small, symmetric and well-circumscribed lesion, with mainly nests in the basal layer of the epidermis (Fig. 7.39a–c). Just as in any other location, this can be interpreted as a junctional nevus. Dermatoscopically, one sees the pigment mainly within the furrows, and brown clods corresponding to the large nests as seen histologically (Fig. 7.39g). This pattern is benign and in accordance with a nevus. The dark line on the left is hemorrhage.

Diagnosis: Acral junctional nevus.

7.2.1.2 Example 2: Small Nests in Epidermis and Papillary Dermis (Fig. 7.40)

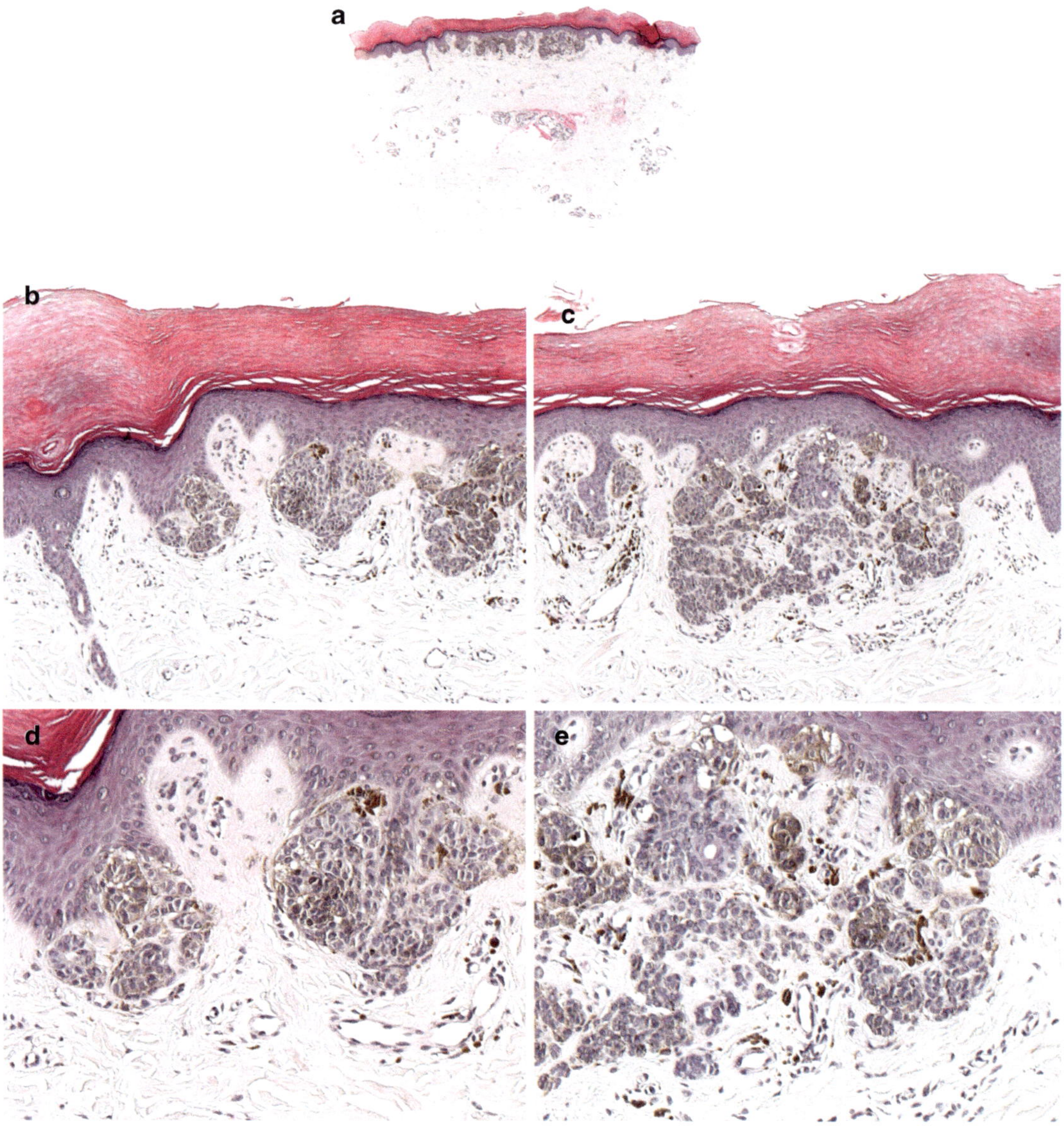

Fig. 7.40 (a–g) Acral site, Example 2. (Courtesy of the Department of Dermatology, Medical University of Vienna)

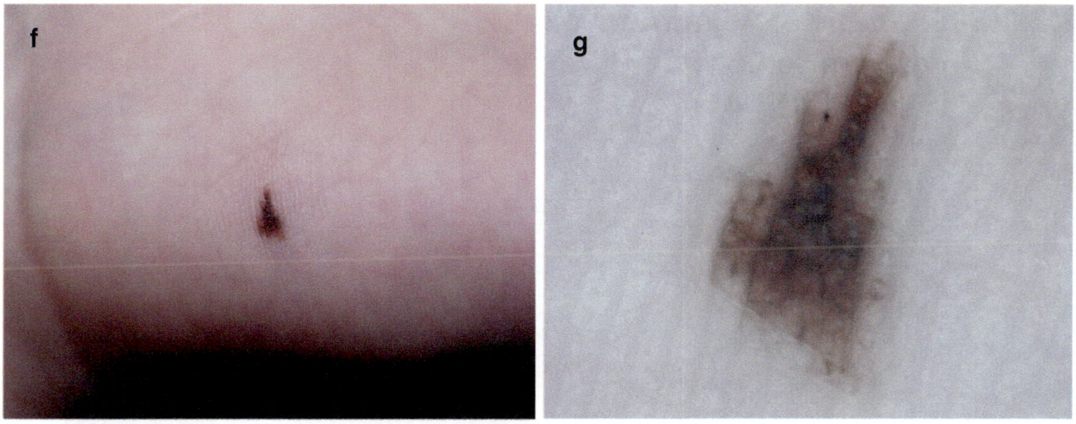

Fig. 7.40 (continued)

Overall Pattern: Epidermal and Superficially Dermal, Symmetric, Nested

Detailed Description

Silhouette

- Well circumscribed
- Symmetric
- In epidermis and papillary dermis

Patterns

Epidermis

- Small- and medium-sized nests, equidistant, mostly situated in the crista profunda limitans

Dermis

- Small round nests

Cytology

- Small, round, monomorphic
- Slightly pigmented

Other Changes

- Sparse melanophages in papillary dermis

Integration

The lesion is a small, symmetric and well-circumscribed lesion, with mainly nests in the basal layer of the epidermis and upper dermis (Fig. 7.40a–c). Just as in any other location, this can be interpreted as a compound nevus based on symmetry, architecture, and good circumscription. The dermatoscopic pattern is entirely benign, as it shows parallel brown pigmentation within the furrows, correlating to nests in the crista profunda limitans (Fig. 7.40g) [159]. The central pigmentation should not be interpreted as "parallel ridge pattern," but as a structureless area corresponding to dermal melanocytes of a compound nevus. Be aware that Saida et al. also found melanocytic nests underlying the ridges in acral nevi [160].

Diagnosis: Acral compound nevus.

7.2.1.3 Example 3: Asymmetric with Large Confluent Nests (Fig. 7.41)

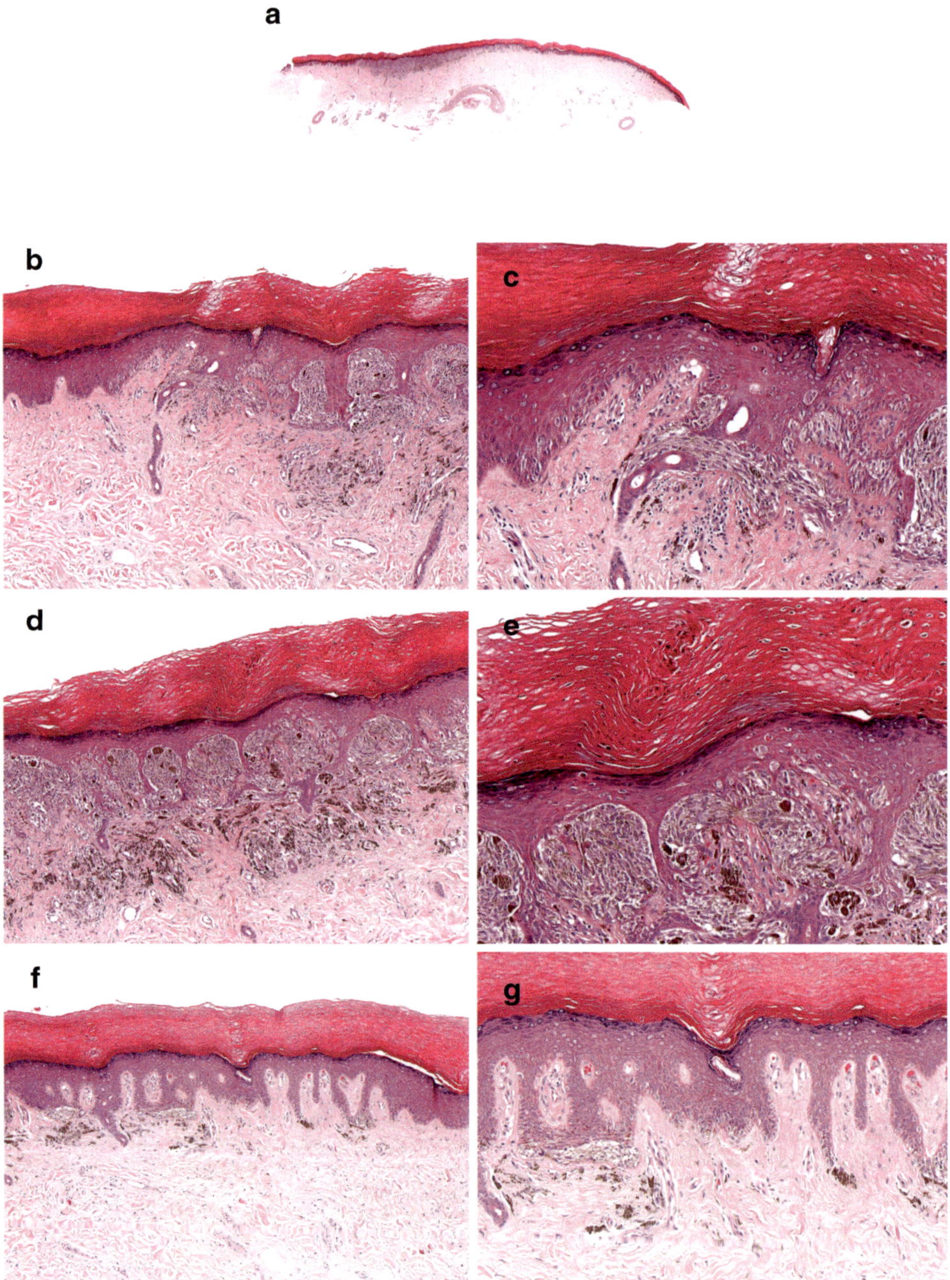

Fig. 7.41 (**a**–**i**) Acral site, Example 3. (Courtesy of the Department of Dermatology, Medical University of Vienna)

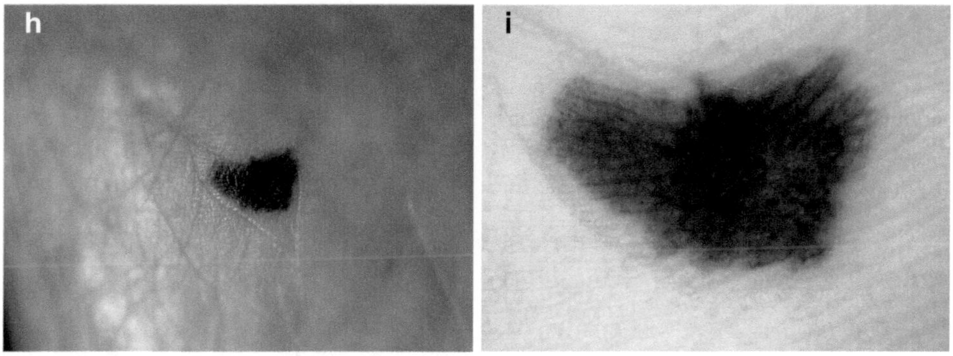

Fig. 7.41 (continued)

Overall Pattern: Asymmetric, Epidermal and Dermal, Nested

Detailed Description

Silhouette

- Not well circumscribed
- Asymmetric
- Epidermis and superficial dermis

Patterns

Epidermis

- Very large nests of unequal size and shape, confluent

Dermis

- Nests and single cells of melanocytes

Cytology

- Large single cells
- Spindled melanocytes in nests
- Fine melanin pigment within the cytoplasm

Other Changes

- Numerous melanophages in the upper dermis

Integration

This lesion fulfills "classic" histologic criteria of melanoma: Asymmetry, pagetoid melanocytes within the epidermis, nests varying in size and shape, confluence, and asymmetric growth into the dermis (Fig. 7.41a-g). A feature more specific, but not exclusive, to acral sites is that nests of melanocytes prominently involve an eccrine duct at the left edge of the lesion (Fig. 7.41c). Dermatoscopically there is pigment as parallel lines within the furrows peripherally, where one can guess there was a pre-existing acral nevus not visible on the histologic slides (Fig. 7.41i). In the middle and to the right, there is an asymmetric eccentric structureless area with dark brown to black color, and white structures. These are dermatoscopic criteria for a melanoma on any body part, and thus in line with the histologic assessment.

Diagnosis: Acral melanoma, invasive.

7.2.2 Face

On the face, the clinical differential diagnosis to melanoma rarely is a nevus for flat lesions. Instead, the more common clinical question is to distinguish melanoma from pigmented actinic keratosis or solar lentigo and lichen planus-like keratosis (LPLK; a seborrheic keratosis in regression), that are difficult to differentiate even with dermatoscopy (Fig. 7.42) [161, 162]. While this differential diagnosis is usually straightforward histopathologically, knowledge of the clinical

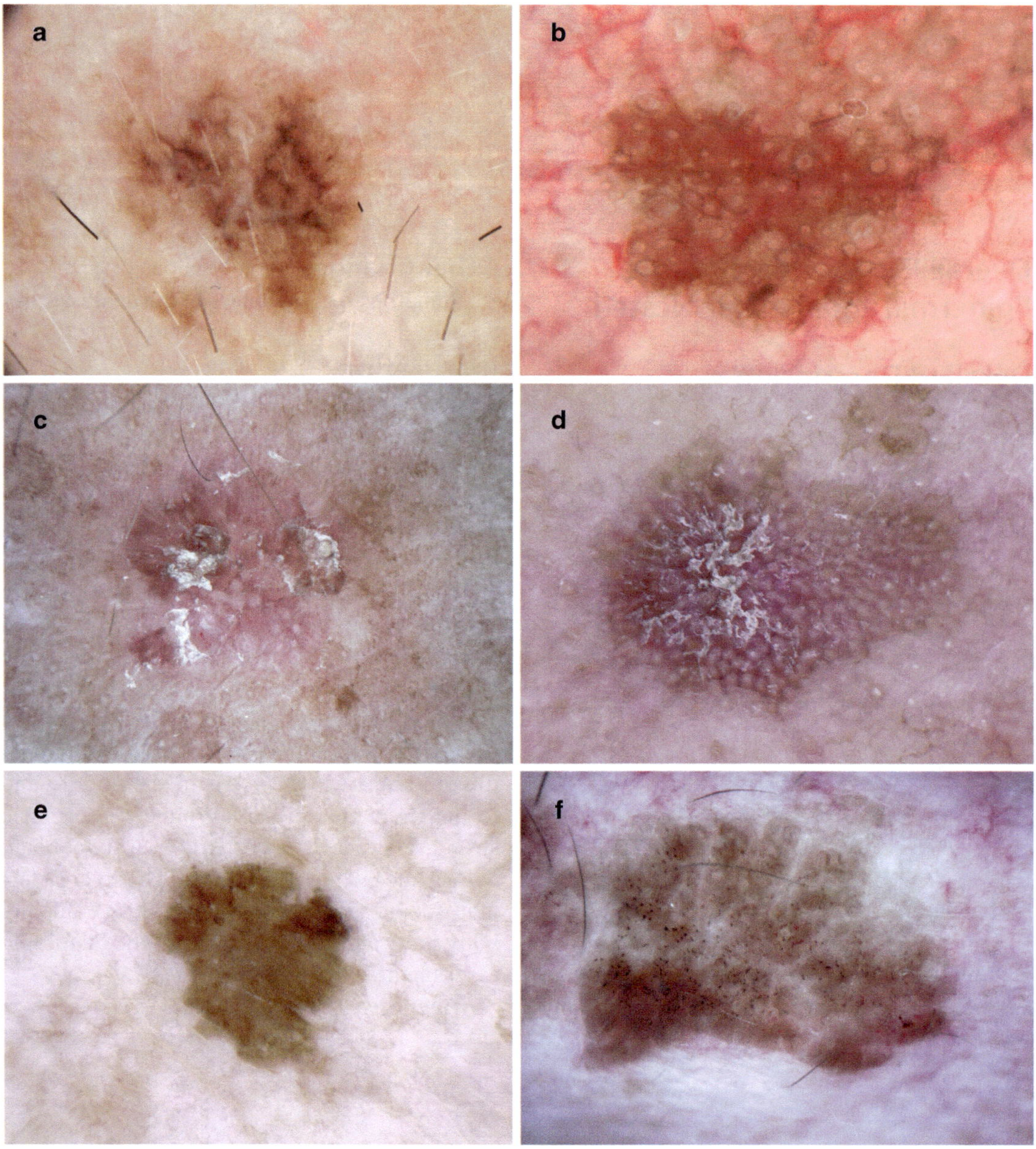

Fig. 7.42 Dermatoscopic images of facial pigmented skin lesions. (**a**) Melanoma in situ with angulated hyperpigmentation. (**b**) Melanoma in situ with structureless brown pigment and gray circles around hair follicles. (**c, d**) Pigmented actinic keratosis with hyperkeratosis corresponding to parakeratosis, prominent follicular openings, and background erythema. (**e**) Solar lentigo with structureless brown pigmentation, and a sharply demarcated border. (**f**) A seborrheic keratosis in regression with structureless brown pigmentation and gray dots corresponding to melanophages. (Courtesy of the Department of Dermatology, Medical University of Vienna)

context can aid to strengthen one's confidence in an equivocal lesion. The utility of MelanA is limited to distinguish pigmented actinic keratosis from melanoma in situ, and in case used should only be interpreted in context with other immunohistochemistry markers [163]. Even then one should be cautious, as sun-damaged skin in general, but also pigmented actinic keratosis can harbor an increased amount of melanocytes. As a more rare occasion, the phenomenon of "pseudomelanocytic nests" should be known and is shown in Example 5.

Melanoma on the face, in contrast to many other anatomic areas, is one usually associated with chronic sun damage, often referred to as lentigo maligna in its in situ stage. This type of melanoma is characterized by a proliferation of single melanocytes, with little nesting especially in early lesions. In small punch biopsies of larger lesions relevant diagnostic criteria can be missed, and we therefore in general prefer a wide and shallow rather than a narrow and deep specimen, that is, a shave biopsy rather than a punch biopsy. This, of course, is not the case for lesions with a clinical suspicion of an invasive part.

Due to the often inconspicuous growth as single cells, the lateral margin of a melanoma on the face is often difficult to ascertain, as melanocytes can also be increased in sun-damaged skin in general. Here, we commonly rely on immunohistochemical stainings to delineate the lesion. Immunohistochemistry is not only needed for margin assessment, but also primary diagnosis. As is the case on acral sites, melanoma in situ can be entirely invisible on hematoxylin & eosin staining alone. We therefore, as a rule, apply immunohistochemistry on a specimen sent with a clinical suspicion of melanoma but no visible melanocytic lesion, in case there is no other unambiguous explanation for the clinical assessment.

Due to problematic anatomic structures, much effort has gone into the more accurate clinical assessment of facial lesions beyond dermatoscopy. In vivo reflectance confocal microscopy, enabling a grayscale en-face view of the epidermis, is actively used for primary diagnosis [164], but also for improving margin control [165, 166], and monitoring non-surgical therapy [167] of melanoma (Fig. 7.43).

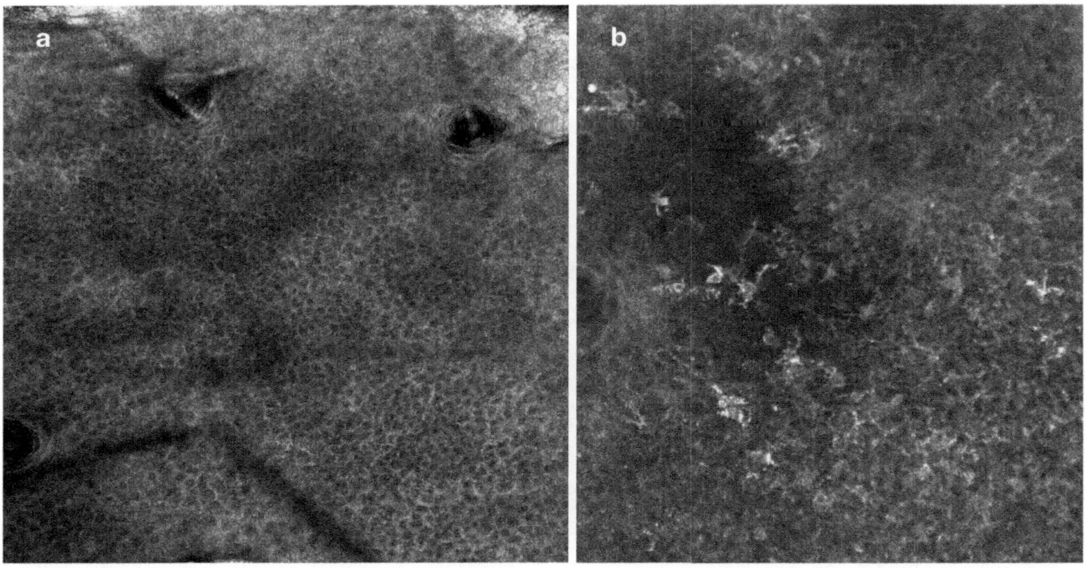

Fig. 7.43 In vivo confocal microscopy of an in situ melanoma on the face. **(a)** En-face view of epidermis with prominent hyperreflective (white) cells with visible dendrites, corresponding to melanocytes in basal and suprabasal layers of a melanoma in situ. **(b)** The same region as shown in **(a)** 24 weeks after therapy with imiquimod, showing a regular epidermis with monomorphous keratinocytes and no visible melanocytes. Interspersed are some hair follicle openings (black circles). (Courtesy of the Department of Dermatology, Medical University of Vienna)

7.2.2.1 Example 1: Single Cells in Flat Epidermis (Fig. 7.44)

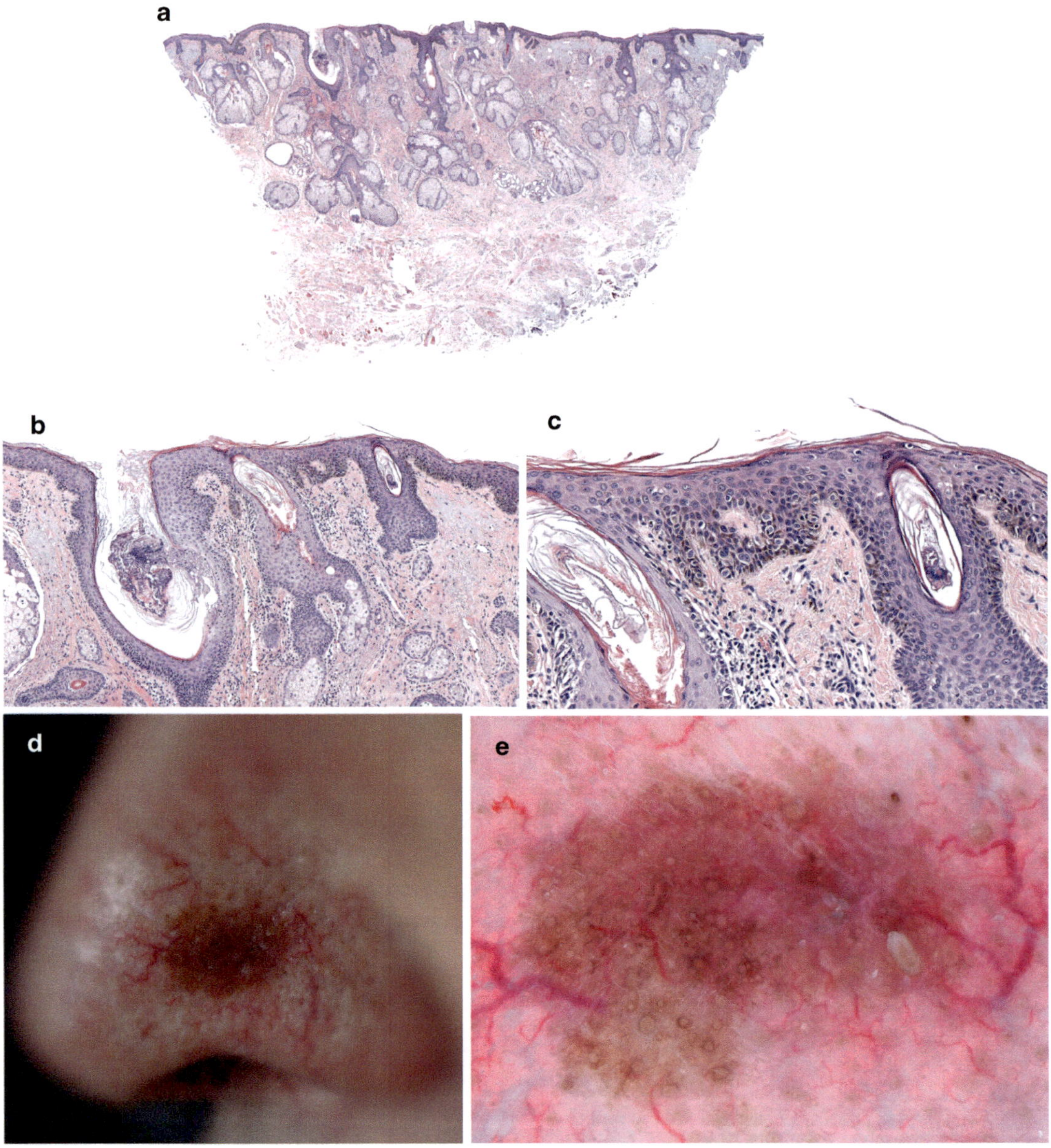

Fig. 7.44 (a–e) Facial site, Example 1. (Courtesy of the Department of Dermatology, Medical University of Vienna)

Overall Pattern: Epidermal, Single Cells, Asymmetric

Detailed Description

Silhouette

- Not well circumscribed
- In epidermis

Patterns

Epidermis

- Only single cells
- In basal, partly also suprabasal, layers
- Growing within basal layers of hair follicles

Cytology

- Large nucleoli and abundant cytoplasm

Other Changes

- Lamellar stratum corneum
- Dilated follicles with Demodex

Integration

This melanocytic proliferation is almost invisible at scanning magnification, but becomes evident on higher magnification (Fig. 7.44a–c). While not necessary in this case, biopsies on the face with the suspicion of melanoma in situ need immunohistochemical stains to reveal the relevant proliferation. Without discernible nests, the differential diagnosis is melanocytic hyperplasia on sun-damaged skin and melanoma in situ. The epithelioid cytology as well as the growth pattern within the hair follicles clearly favor the latter (Fig. 7.44c).

Clinically, one sees a flat macule on the left nasal ala, fitting both a melanoma in situ and a solar lentigo (Fig. 7.44d). Dermatoscopically, there is homogeneous brown pigmentation, correlating to the pigmentation in a flat epidermis devoid of rete ridges (Fig. 7.44e). The combination with a pattern of gray circles, corresponding to melanocytes within the hair follicle, allows for a specific diagnosis dermatoscopically, fitting the histologic assessment.

Diagnosis: Melanoma in situ.

7.2.2.2 Example 2: Asymmetric Horizontal Confluence and Sun Damage (Fig. 7.45)

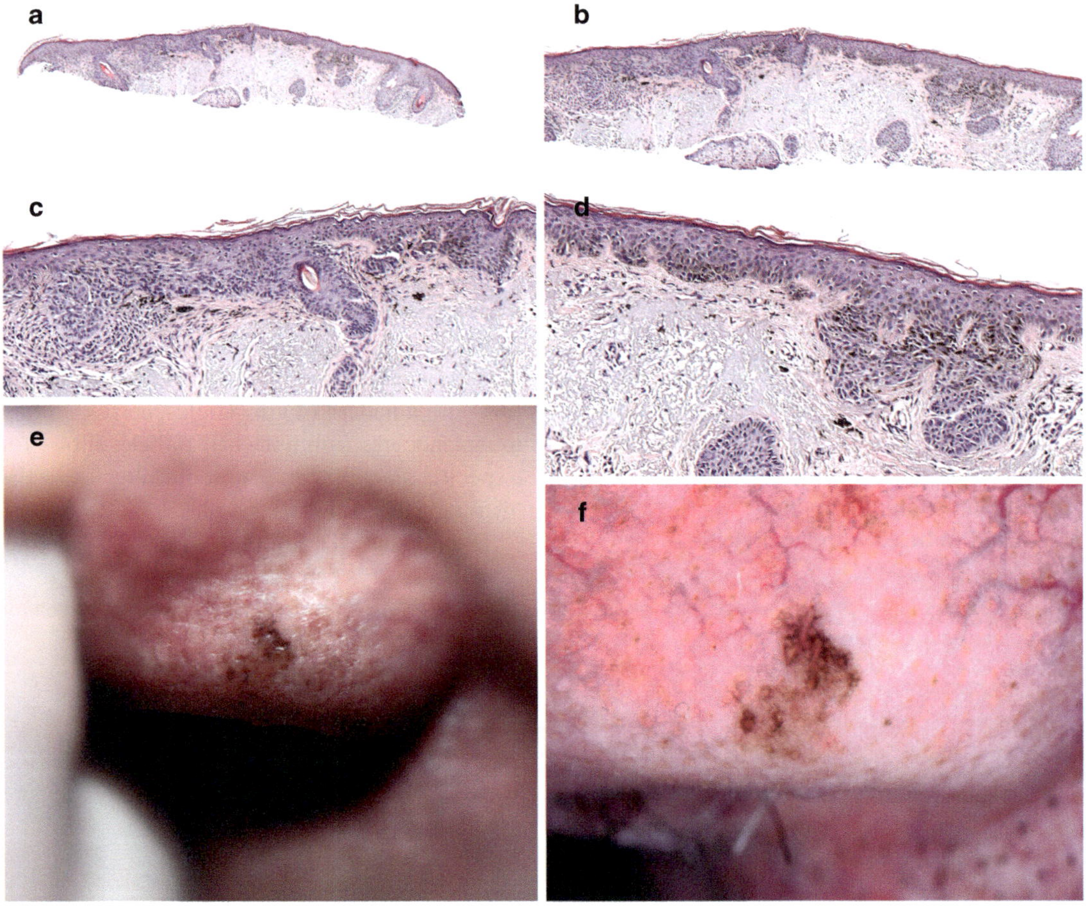

Fig. 7.45 (a–f) Facial site, Example 2. (Courtesy of the Department of Dermatology, Medical University of Vienna)

Overall Pattern: Epidermis Confluent Nests, Asymmetric

Detailed Description

Silhouette

- Not well circumscribed
- Asymmetric
- In epidermis

Patterns

Epidermis

- Nests, varying in size and shape, with horizontal confluence

Cytology

- Round but also spindled

Other Changes

- Lamellar stratum corneum
- Solar elastosis
- Single melanophages within the papillary dermis

Integration

On the basis of sun-damaged skin, such an asymmetric melanocytic proliferation is a melanoma in situ (Fig. 7.45a–d). Dermatoscopically, the lesion is asymmetric as well, with a pattern of structureless brown color, and asymmetrically distributed pigmented circles (Fig. 7.45f). The latter are also termed "asymmetrically pigmented follicular openings" after the early descriptions of this pattern of early melanoma by Schniffner and Stolz [168].

As performed in this case, we prefer a shave biopsy in these types of lesions over a partial punch biopsy, as the clinical probability of an invasive proliferation is low, but the added value of interpretability of horizontal growth histologically is high.

Diagnosis: Melanoma in situ.

7.2.2.3 Example 3: Parakeratosis, Clinical Suspicion of Melanoma (Fig. 7.46)

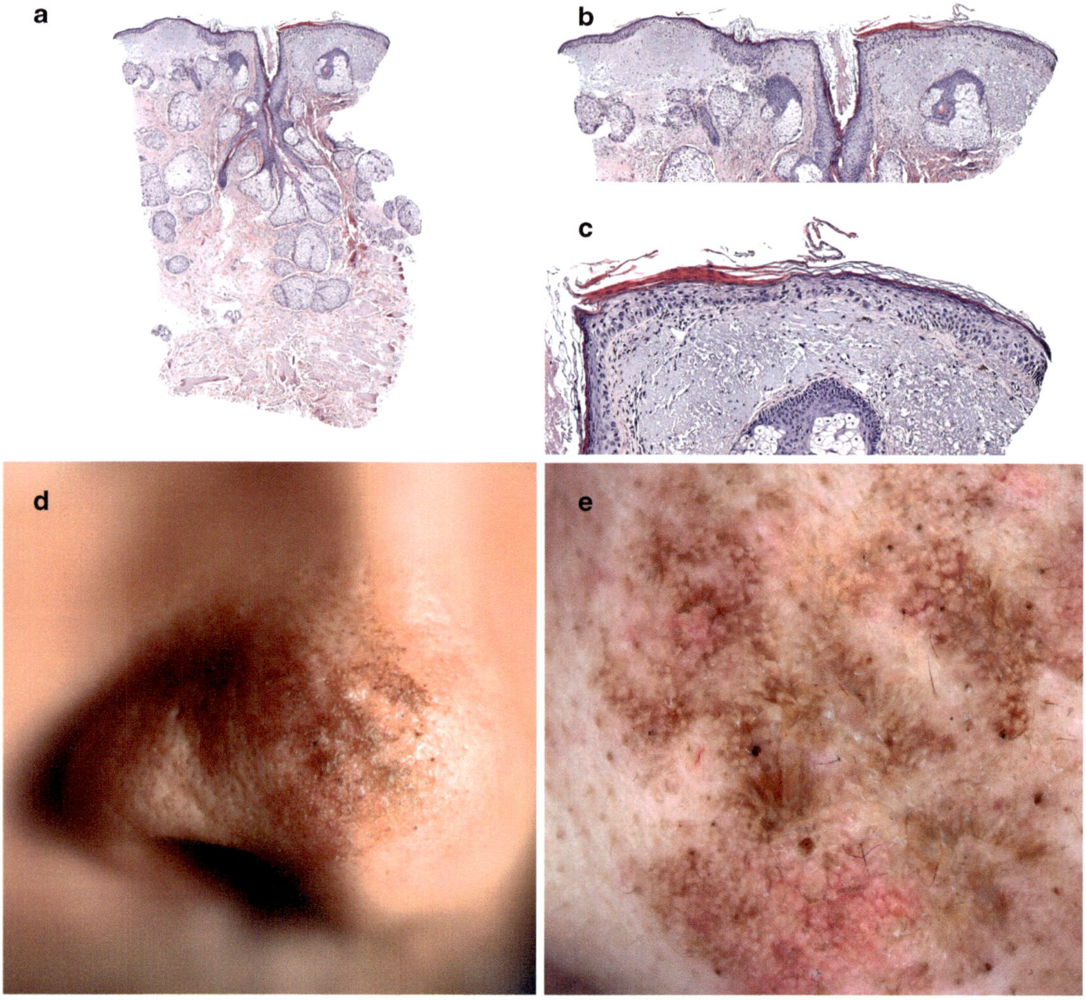

Fig. 7.46 (a–e) Facial site, Example 3. (Courtesy of the Department of Dermatology, Medical University of Vienna)

Overall Pattern: Atypical Keratinocytes, Intraepidermal

Detailed Description

Silhouette

- Not well circumscribed
- Intraepidermal

Patterns

Epidermis

- Atypical crowded keratinocytes
- No melanocytic proliferation

Other Changes

- Parakeratosis
- Solar elastosis
- Widened follicle infundibulum

Integration

Clinically, one sees a pigmented macule on the nose, with asymmetric pigmentation (Fig. 7.46d). Dermatoscopically there is structureless brown pigmentation, which is unspecific in this setting. But one can also make out prominent bright follicles throughout the lesion and background erythema, both features of pigmented actinic keratosis (Fig. 7.46e). So even without immunohistochemical stains one can be confident of the diagnosis when taking into account the clinical and dermatoscopic image—even if the clinician asked to rule out a melanoma. Without such a plausible clinical presentation fitting the histologic patterns, we would almost certainly resort to deeper cuts and immunohistochemical stainings.

Diagnosis: Pigmented actinic keratosis.

7.2.2.4 Example 4: Sun Damage, Morphologically Few Visible Melanocytes (Fig. 7.47)

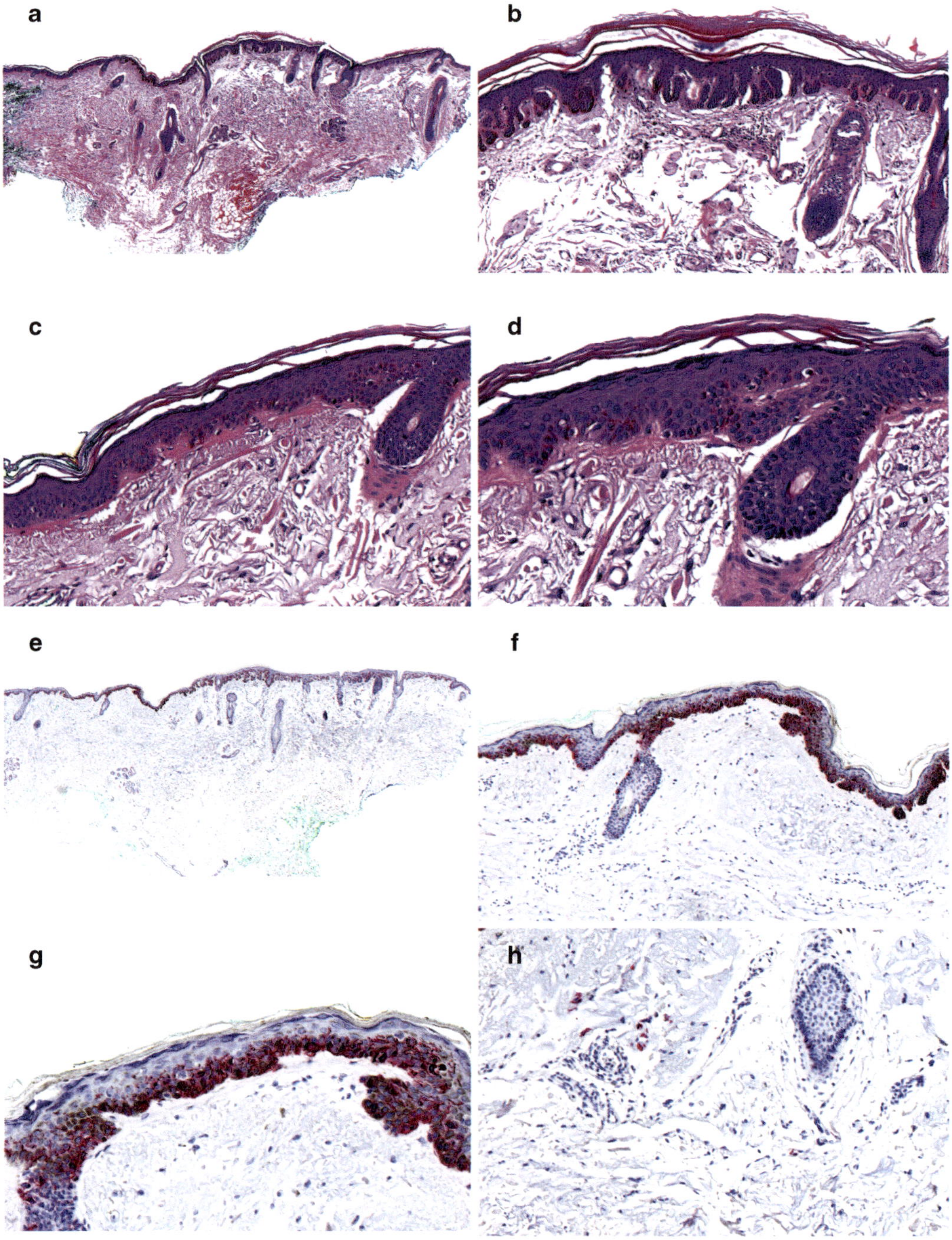

Fig. 7.47 (**a**–**h**) Facial site, Example 4. (Courtesy of the Dermatologikum Hamburg)

Overall Pattern: Epidermal Only, Single Melanocytes, Poorly Circumscribed

Detailed Description

Silhouette

- Epidermal only
- Poorly circumscribed

Patterns

Epidermis

- Single melanocytes only, irregularly distributed
- Some melanocytes in the mid-spinous zone
- Some back-to-back melanocytes

Adnexal Epithelium

- Increased single melanocytes in infundibular epithelium

Dermis

- None

Cytology

- Small melanocytes with dendritic morphology and elongated, high-reaching dendrites

Other Changes

- Solar elastosis
- Elongated rete ridges on the right side, flattened rete ridges on the left
- Hyperpigmentation of basal keratinocytes

Immunohistochemistry

- On MelanA staining (Fig. 7.47a–c) regularly distributed melanocytes in the zone with elongated rete ridges, irregularly distributed, increased numbers of melanocytes in the area with flattened rete ridges
- Few positive dendritic cells in the dermis (Fig. 7.47d)

Integration

A broad lesion has been excised from severely sun-damaged skin. The epidermal configuration on the right side is that of a solar lentigo (Fig. 7.47a, b) and MelanA staining shows only regular distribution of single melanocytes in the basal layer in this area. On the left side, however, the rete ridges are flattened and the number of melanocytes is increased with irregular distribution and some melanocytes in suprabasal layers (Fig. 7.47c, d). The melanocytes are small so that they are not so obvious on conventional H&E staining, but on MelanA they are seen to have very prominent dendrites, a cytologic feature seen commonly in melanoma in situ on sun-damaged skin (Fig. 7.47e–g). The collision of solar lentigo with melanoma in situ is not uncommon as both lesions develop on sun-damaged skin. The meaning of few MelanA-positive cells in the dermis of sun-damaged skin is not known (Fig. 7.47h). They usually do not express other melanocytic markers so that they are not considered to be melanocytes. They are also commonly seen in excisions of epithelial tumors on sun-damaged skin and to date they are interpreted as dendritic cells with aberrant expression of MelanA that have no specific meaning.

Diagnosis: Melanoma in situ on sun-damaged skin (so-called Lentigo maligna) in collision with solar lentigo.

7.2.2.5 Example 5: Nests and Inflammation (Fig. 7.48)

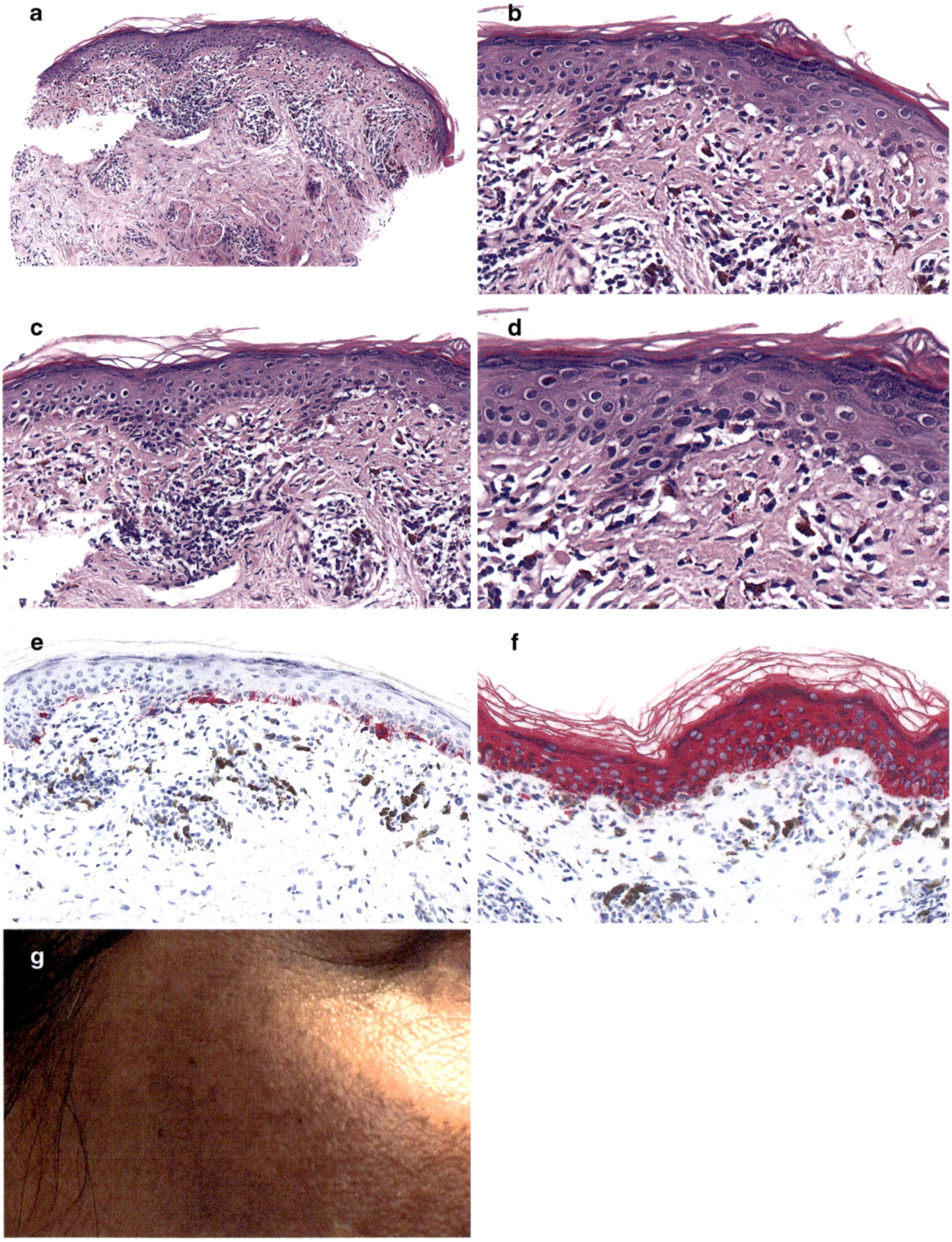

Fig. 7.48 (**a**–**g**) Facial site, Example 5. (Courtesy of the Dermatologikum Hamburg)

Overall Pattern: Single Melanocytes and Small Nests, Irregularly Distributed

Detailed Description

Silhouette

- Subtle proliferation in the basal layer
- Biopsy

Patterns

Epidermis

- Single melanocytes and small nests, irregularly distributed

Dermis

- None

Cytology

- Heavily pigmented, epithelioid, and dendritic

Other Changes

- Numerous melanophages
- Band-like lymphocytic infiltrate
- Necrotic keratinocytes
- Solar elastosis

Immunohistochemistry

- MelanA stains single melanocytes and some larger aggregations that look like nests of melanocytes (Fig. 7.48e).
- Pan-cytokeratin (Fig. 7.48f) shows that the nest-like aggregations contain necrotic keratinocytes together with melanocytes and some lymphocytes.

Integration

In this small biopsy taken from sun-damaged skin of the face, the first impression is that of a subtle melanocytic lesion consisting mainly of single melanocytes and few nests which is obscured to some extent by a lymphocytic infiltrate (Fig. 7.48a–d). The differential diagnosis is an inflammatory condition that imitates a melanocytic lesion so that immunohistochemical stainings for melanocytic markers should be ordered. Confusingly, MelanA seems to confirm a melanocytic lesion with irregularly distributed single melanocytes and nests (Fig. 7.48e). However, some necrotic keratinocytes are also present within the nested structures and in the papillary dermis. Pan-cytokeratin staining confirms necrotic keratinocytes between melanocytes in the nest-like structures and in the papillary dermis (Fig. 7.48f). The biopsy comes from a patient with actinic lichen planus who had developed reticulated hyperpigmentation on both cheeks. The interface dermatitis with some flattening of the rete ridges, hypergranulosis and hyperkeratosis and prominent melanophages fits well with the diagnosis of actinic lichen planus which is confirmed also by the clinical picture (Fig. 7.48g). The imitation of nests on H&E and MelanA in interface dermatitis has been designated MelanA-positive pseudo-nests.

Diagnosis: Actinic lichen planus with MelanA-positive pseudo-nests.

7.2.3 Nail

Melanocytic lesions of the nail unit can be located in the nail bed or in the nail matrix. When situated in the nail matrix, they usually present as longitudinal melanonychia (melanonychia striata), a brown-black band of pigment in the nail plate. Clinically, a longitudinal melanonychia with increasing width towards the matrix region is suspicious of melanoma [169]. When melanoma extends from the nail matrix to the proximal and/or lateral nail fold, it presents clinically as "Hutchinson sign," i.e., pigmentation of the skin of the nail fold. These clinical signs are very helpful to decide for biopsy of a pigmented lesion of the nail unit, but they are not entirely pathognomonic. Periungual hyperpigmentation may occur for example in pigmented Bowen's disease of the nail unit or hyperpigmentation of the nail bed and matrix may shine through the thin skin of nail folds, which has been termed the "Pseudo-Hutchinson's sign" [170]. Multiple pigmented bands are generally a benign finding as seen in racial pigmentation in darker-skinned patients or in Laugier-Hunziker-Baran syndrome. Narrow and solitary bands are produced by melanocytic nevi or simple lentigo of the nail matrix. Ulceration, total melanonychia, nail plate destruction, and polychromia are clinical and dermatoscopic features of advanced melanomas of the nail unit. It has to be kept in mind that, just like in any other site, melanoma of the nail unit may at times be amelanotic and may not produce pigmentation at all.

When a melanocytic proliferation of the nail matrix is suspected, biopsy with histopathologic examination is the gold standard for diagnosis. However, biopsy of the nail unit is not an easy undertaking. The nail fold and nail plate need to be removed to access the nail matrix, which usually requires an experienced nail surgeon. The biopsy material from the matrix is often soft and tiny, so that proper orientation is challenging for the technician [171]. From the histopathologist's perspective, a complete excision sampling nail matrix, nail bed, nail plate, and proximal nailfold would be much more desirable, but as long as melanocytic nature and malignancy of a lesion is in doubt, clinicians will attempt to keep trauma to the nail matrix minimal in the hope that the nail regrows without defect. For the same reason, some clinicians practice nail clippings rather than nail matrix biopsies under the assumption that a melanocytic lesion and especially a melanoma will be typified by suprabasal melanocytes that will, at one point, also pepper the nail plate. While a nail plate with scattered melanocytes can be considered as evidence for a melanocytic lesion in the nail matrix, it cannot be taken as a sure sign of melanoma, especially in a young person. In contrast, lack of melanocytes in the nail plate does not exclude the possibility of a melanocytic lesion, not even of melanoma. In early melanoma in situ of the nail unit, suprabasal melanocytes may not be a prominent feature.

In general, most criteria for melanocytic nevi and melanoma that apply on other sites of the body can also be used in the nail unit. Nevi will show a regular nested arrangement, simple lentigo should have regularly distributed melanocytes, and melanoma should have variation in size and shape of nests with focal predominance of single melanocytes. Likewise, the uncertainty arising from incomplete sampling in which symmetry and circumscription cannot be assessed is the same as on any other site of the body. Usually, it is not so problematic to histologically diagnose a fully developed melanoma of the nail unit, because features of melanoma in situ will be present in the nail matrix as well as in the nail fold (Hutchinson sign), where criteria used in acral skin apply accordingly. Invasive melanomas of the nail unit will show pleomorphism, lack of maturation, and eventually ulceration. It is important to note that, if a biopsy of the nail matrix reveals an invasive melanoma, the depth of invasion at this site may not be representative for the whole specimen. In a study on 14 cases, dermal invasion involved the nail matrix area as well as other areas of the nail unit. Except for one case, the nail matrix area showed thinner dermal invasion compared with dermal invasion in other areas of the nail unit [172].

In contrast to a straightforward diagnosis of invasive melanoma of the nail unit, it can be exceedingly difficult to diagnose early melanoma in situ in a small biopsy and to differentiate it from simple lentigo or junctional nevus of that site. In recent years, criteria for diagnosis have been refined and the following features have been emphasized for melanoma in situ of the nail unit: Sparse irregular junctional melanocytic proliferation with focal confluent melanocytes ("back-to-back"), poorly circumscribed proliferation with predominance of single cells over nests, variable pagetoid spread [173], small to medium nuclear enlargement, mild to moderate nuclear atypia such as hyperchromasia and irregular contours of nuclei are often seen. Multinucleated melanocytes, inflammatory infiltrate, and cutaneous adnexal extension were seen to be associated with early invasion [174]. Melanocytes with prominently dendritic shape and heavy pigmentation as well as high-reaching dendrites have also been described [56], features that may also be observed in mucosal melanomas including those on the conjunctiva. Especially when the lesion is subtle in H&E stainings, the architecture of the melanocytic proliferation can effectively be emphasized with immunohistochemical stainings such as MelanA, HMB45, and SOX10 [174]. PRAME has been recently suggested as a relatively sensitive and highly specific marker in differentiating benign from malignant melanocytic lesions of the nail unit, but the degree of PRAME expression correlated also with patients' age and clinical size of the lesion [175], and some PRAME expression was also observed in entirely benign lesions.

7.2.3.1 Example 1: Asymmetric Longitudinal Nail Pigmentation (Fig. 7.49)

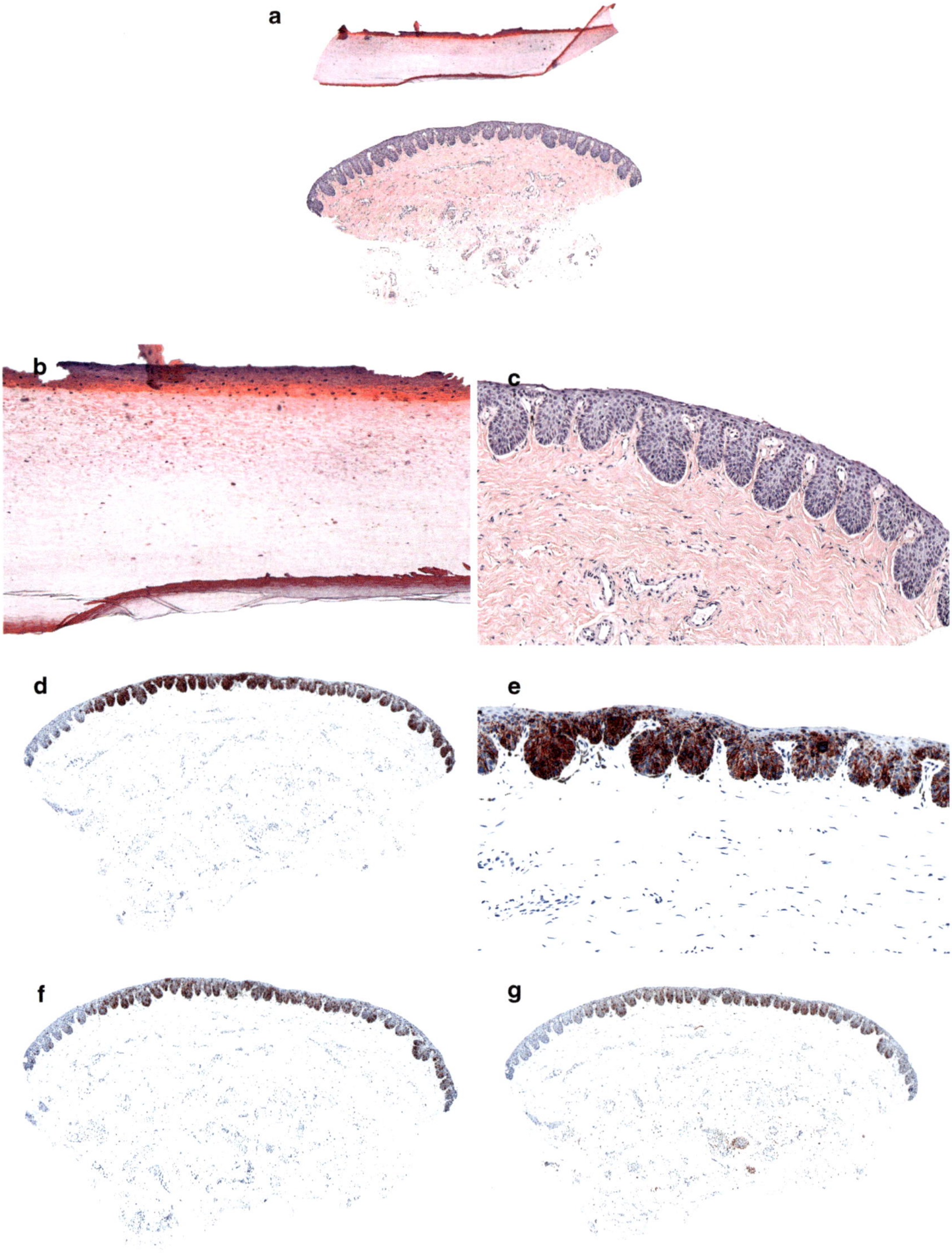

Fig. 7.49 (**a–i**) Nails, Example 1. (Courtesy of the Department of Dermatology, Medical University of Vienna)

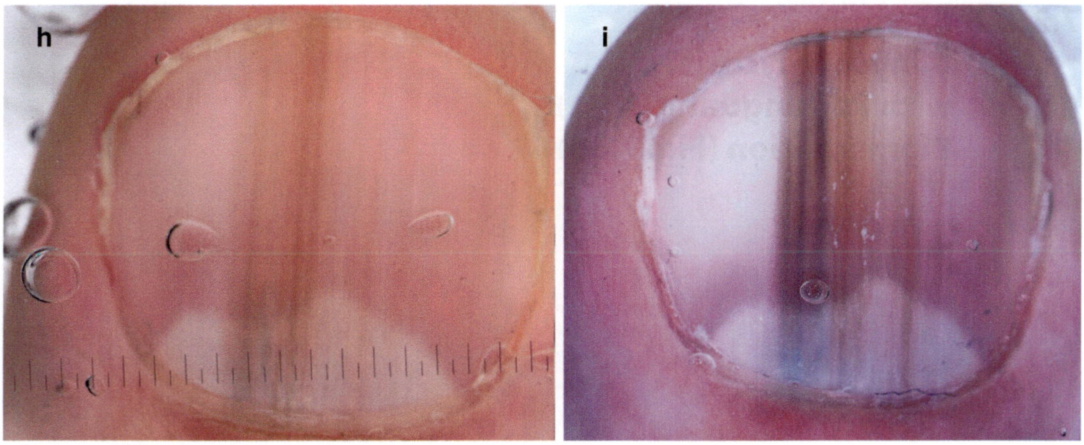

Fig. 7.49 (continued)

Overall Pattern: Broad, Not Well Circumscribed, Intraepithelial

Detailed Description

Silhouette

- Not well circumscribed
- Fairly asymmetric
- In epithelium/matrix

Patterns

Nail matrix epithelium

- Single cells of varying size and shape

Cytology

- Single melanocytes hard to discern on hematoxylin/eosin stainings

Other Changes

- Melanin pigment and single melanocytes within the nail plate

Immunohistochemistry

- HMB45 (Fig. 7.49d, e), MelanA (Fig. 7.49e), and S100 (Fig. 7.49f) reveal a melanocytic proliferation that is essentially invisible with H&E staining alone.

Integration

Whenever we are confronted with a pigmented lesion in question from nail matrix, face, or acral sites, where little is visible on H&E staining, we apply immunohistochemical stainings as a rule (Fig. 7.49d–f). As exemplified here, quite often it will reveal a significant, and otherwise invisible, melanocytic neoplasm (Fig. 7.49a–c). Albeit only intraepithelial, the lesion is asymmetric, and also spans almost the whole specimen in width, both not expected in a benign lesion. Retained melanocytes within the nail plate are a soft clue to nail matrix melanoma.

The consecutive dermatoscopic images underline the diagnosis of melanoma, with bands of pigmentation asymmetric in size and shape, almost a third of the nail involved, and increasing pigment over time (Fig. 7.49h, i).

Diagnosis: Melanoma in situ.

7.2.3.2 Example 2: "Onychomycosis" with Periungual Pigmentation (Fig. 7.50)

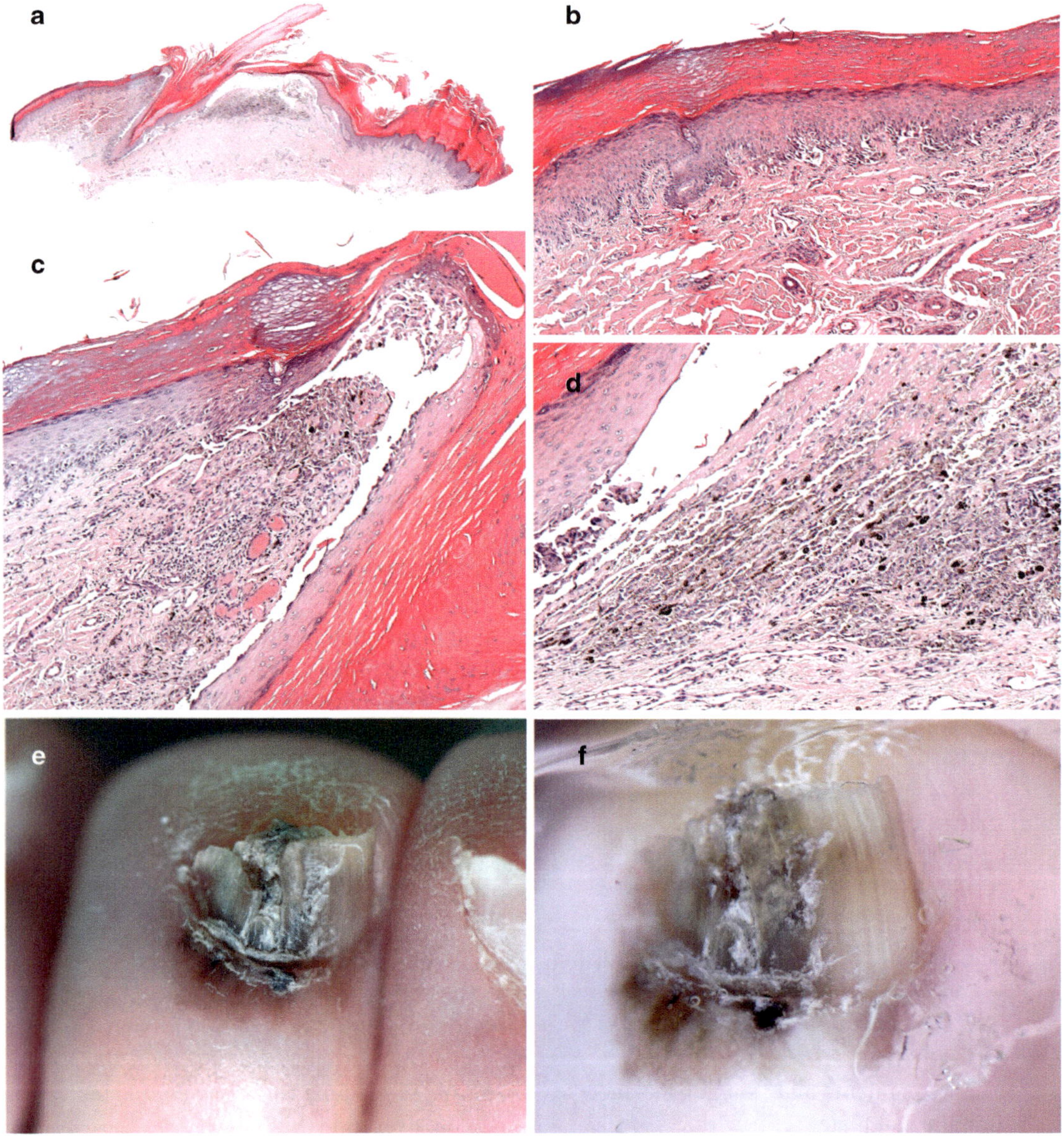

Fig. 7.50 (a–f) Nails, Example 2. (Courtesy of the Department of Dermatology, Medical University of Vienna)

Overall Pattern: Asymmetric, Nested, Epidermal and Dermal

Detailed Description

Silhouette
- (Not) well circumscribed
- In epidermis and dermis

Patterns

Epidermis
- Single cells and nests varying in size and shape
- Broad: Reaching from the epidermis of the proximal nail fold, over the nail matrix, into the proximal nail bed
- Clefting

Dermis
- Nests and sheets of melanocytes with fine melanin pigment
- Interspersed melanophages

Cytology
- Small, round

Other Changes
- Dystrophic nail

Integration
This case is from a female patient in her mid 40s, with the third toenail being treated for onychomycosis for multiple months now. The dermatoscopic images show asymmetric pigmentation of more than half of the nail, nail dystrophy, and a "Hutchinson sign" on the proximal nail fold (Fig. 7.50e, f), all underlining the histologic. As evident from the histologic specimen (Fig. 7.50a), the clinical certainty was high enough to warrant an excision of the complete nail unit already initially.

Diagnosis: Melanoma, invasive.

7.2.3.3 Example 3: Slightly Changing Melanonychia Striata (Fig. 7.51)

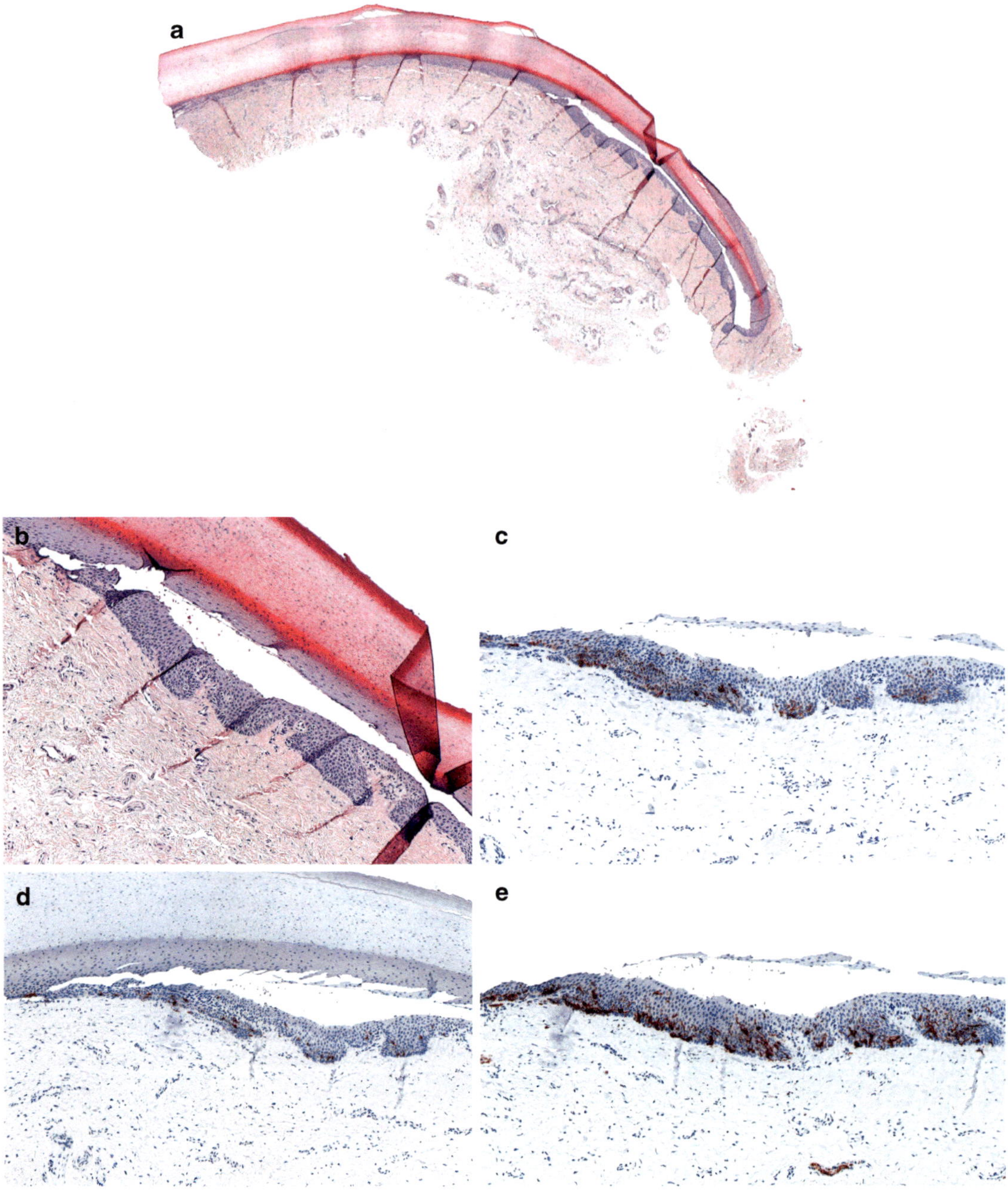

Fig. 7.51 (**a**–**g**) Nails, Example 3. (Courtesy of the Department of Dermatology, Medical University of Vienna)

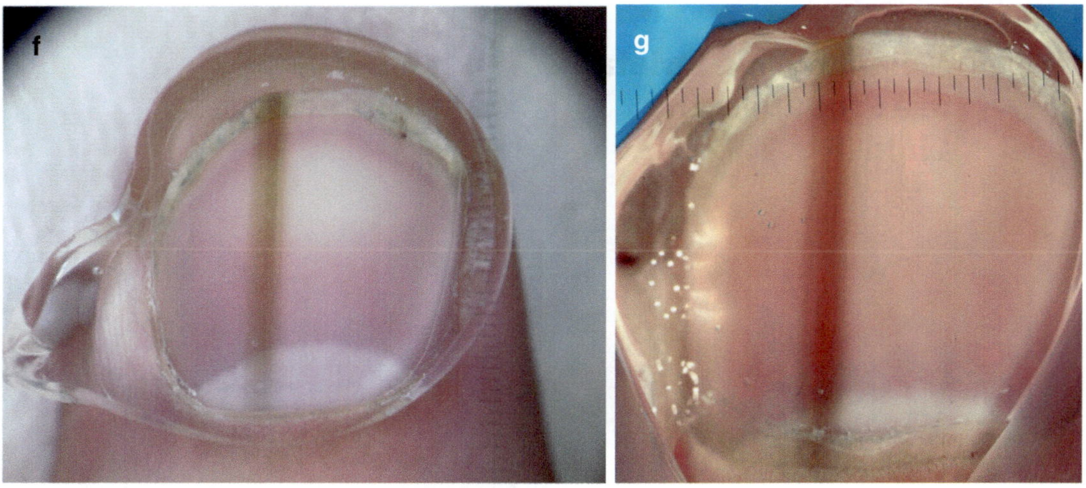

Fig. 7.51 (continued)

Overall Pattern: Small, Increased Single Cells, Some Suprabasal

Detailed Description

Silhouette

- Not well circumscribed
- Symmetric
- In nail matrix

Patterns

Nail matrix epithelium

- Single cells, only visible with immunohistochemistry, mostly basal, some suprabasal

Cytology

- Large, evenly sized, some with long dendrites

Immunohistochemistry

- Positive staining with HMB45 (Fig. 7.51c), S100 (Fig. 7.51e), and less with MelanA (Fig. 7.51d)

Other Changes

- Focal parakeratosis in covering nail plate

Integration

This kind of situation is always challenging. Clinically and dermatoscopically one sees a longitudinal pigmentation, only faintly increasing in size and pigmentation (Fig. 7.51f, g). The changes are only somewhat concerning, but also not bland enough to be reassuring. Histopathology, in our view, adds to the confusion. On the one hand the changes are small, on the other hand the number of melanocytes certainly increased, within suprabasal layers, and with prominent and long dendrites (Fig. 7.51a–e). In our experience, histopathologic reports for such lesions will span from certain melanoma in situ to benign (atypical) melanocytic hyperplasia. We mostly accept that such lesions will fall into a diagnostic gray zone, and talk to clinicians and patients to at least ensure the changes are completely excised.

Diagnosis: Difficult to interpret, we cannot exclude early melanoma in situ.

7.2.3.4 Example 4: Melanonychia Striata in a Prepubescent Child (Fig. 7.52)

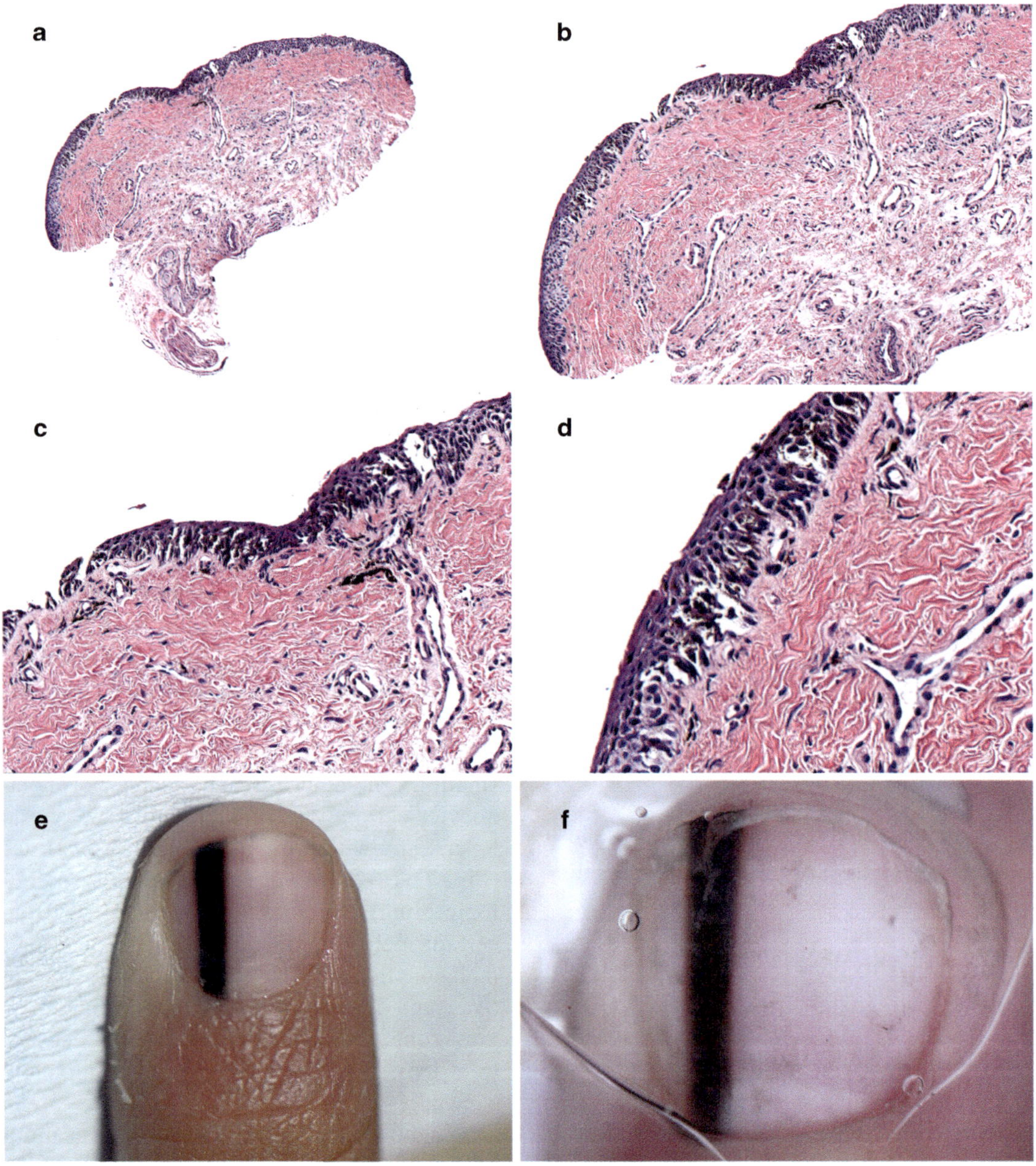

Fig. 7.52 (**a–f**) Nails, Example 4. (Courtesy of the Department of Dermatology, Medical University of Vienna)

Overall Pattern: Small, Junctional, Nested

Detailed Description

Silhouette

- Well circumscribed
- Symmetric
- In nail matrix

Patterns

Nail matrix epithelium

- Nests of heavily pigmented melanocytes

Cytology

- Large, evenly sized, some with long dendrites

Other Changes

- Melanophages in the upper dermis

Integration

This is a heavily pigmented melanonychia striata in a prepubescent child. The pigmentation at the distal end of the nail plate is thicker than at the proximal part (Fig. 7.52e, f). This indicates that the lesion was growing but growth has stopped. The lesion will get smaller and the pigmentation will fade, which is a common finding in nail matrix nevi of prepubescent children. The biopsy of the nail matrix shows nests of heavily pigmented melanocytes but also some dendritic single melanocytes (Fig. 7.52c, d). The lesion is small, symmetric, and well circumscribed (Fig. 7.52a, b). Given the clinical context this can only be a nevus.

Diagnosis: Junctional nevus of the nail matrix.

7.2.3.5 Example 5: Slightly Changing Melanonychia Striata (Fig. 7.53)

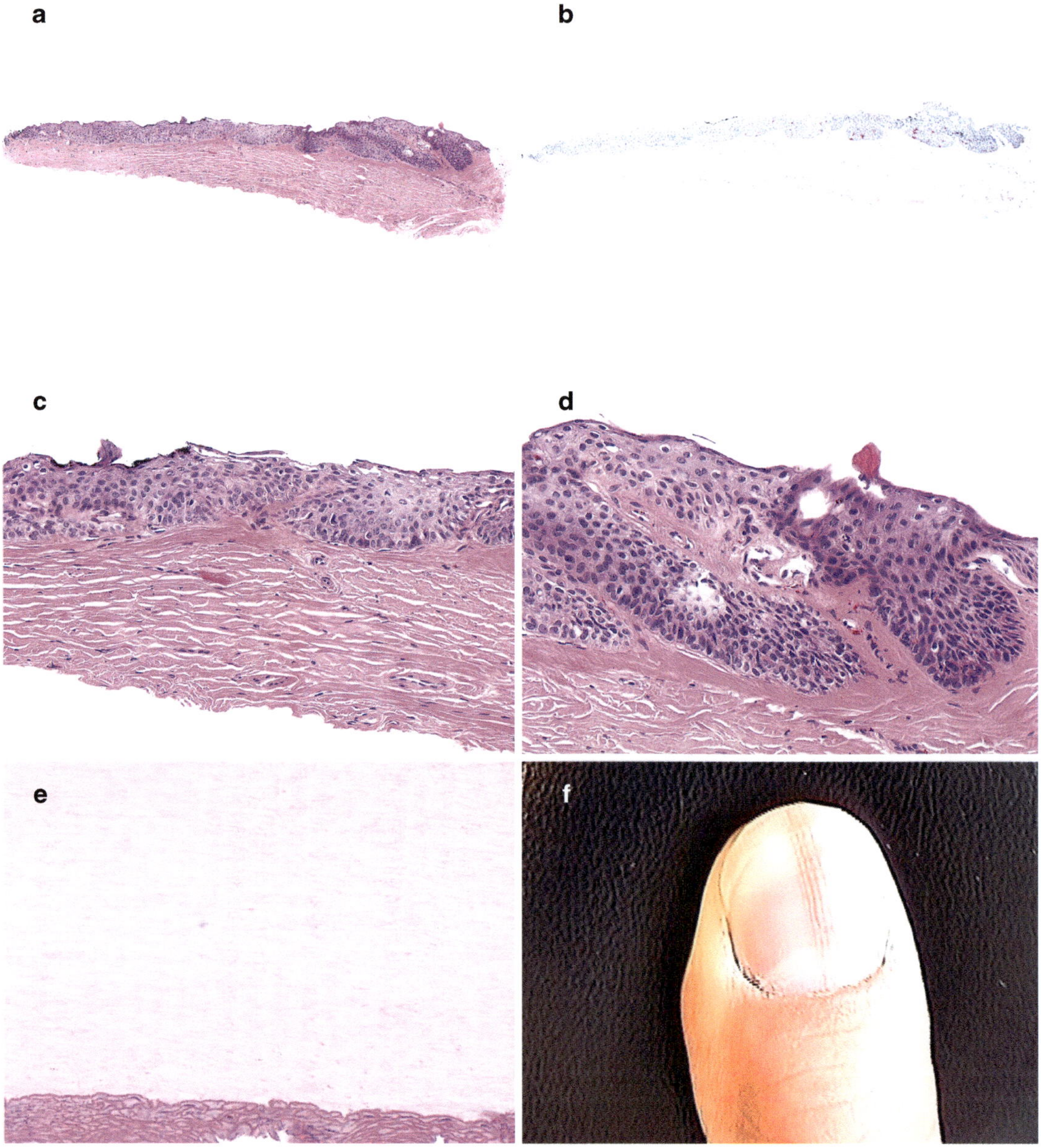

Fig. 7.53 (**a**–**f**) Nails, Example 5. (Courtesy of the Dermatologikum Hamburg)

Overall Pattern: Subtle Pigmentation the Nail Matrix, Biopsy

Detailed Description

Silhouette

- Ill-defined subtle pigmentation of the nail matrix
- Biopsy

Patterns

Nail matrix epithelium

- Pigmented basal keratinocytes, melanocytes not increased
- Pigmentation most prominent at the base of rete ridges

Dermis

- None

Cytology

- Monomorphic

Other Changes

- Elongated rete ridges
- Melanophages in the superficial dermis

Integration

This biopsy taken from the nail matrix of a melanonychia striata does not show obvious changes at scanning magnification (Fig. 7.53a). On close-up view, a subtle pigmentation at the base of rete ridges is seen, but it consists only of pigmented keratinocytes (Fig. 7.53c, d). The number of melanocytes is not increased, which is seen better in the MelanA stain (Fig. 7.53b). A second specimen showing the nail plate also has no melanocytes but only a subtle deposition of finely granular pigment in the nail keratin (Fig. 7.53e). Clinically, the patient presented with a melanonychia striata that showed slight variation in pigmentation during follow-up and an associated benign melanosis of the vulva, a typical presentation of Laugier-Hunziker-Baran syndrome, a hereditary pigmentary disorder. Essentially the changes in the nail unit are identical to those seen on the genitalia in this condition, namely, pigmentation of keratinocytes in the basal layer, accentuated at the base of rete ridges.

Diagnosis: Melanonychia striata of Laugier-Hunziker-Baran Syndrome (idiopathic lenticular mucocutaneous pigmentation).

7.2.4 "Special" Sites (Navel, Mamilla, Genital, Axilla)

In some regions of the body, melanocytic nevi more commonly show unusual histopathological features such as asymmetry, irregularly shaped nests, melanocytes in suprabasal layers, cytologic atypia, and occasional mitosis. These regions have been termed "Special site" and include genitalia, flexural areas, mamilla and milk line, umbilicus and, already addressed in a separate paragraph, acral skin [176, 177]. Nevi of special sites illustrate convincingly that histopathologic features in melanocytic lesions always have to be integrated with clinical information, especially the site of the lesion.

Since nevi of special sites share features with traumatized and recurrent nevi, reasons for histopathologic variation in the aforementioned areas may include chronic irritation, friction, previous trauma, and scarring. Moreover, especially on the genitalia, it has to be taken into account that melanocytic lesions on mucosal surface or in close proximity to mucosa have a different architecture with less prominent rete ridges. Last, melanocytic lesions may appear differently in collision with a second skin condition. As an example, nevi on the vulva appear highly irregular both clinically and histopathologically when colliding with Lichen sclerosus [178, 179].

7.2.4.1 Example 1: Flat Lesion on the Mamilla (Fig. 7.54)

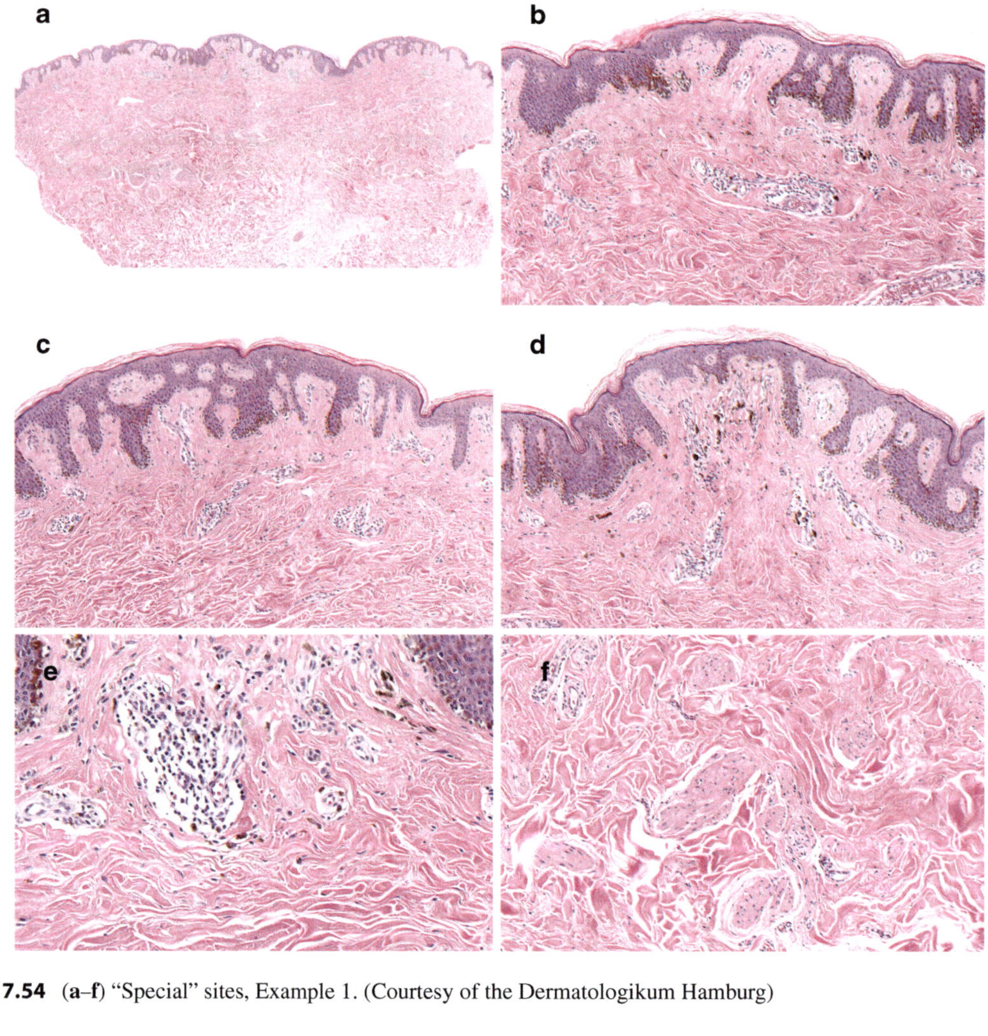

Fig. 7.54 (**a**–**f**) "Special" sites, Example 1. (Courtesy of the Dermatologikum Hamburg)

Overall Pattern: Single Melanocytes, Poorly Circumscribed, Symmetric

Detailed Description

Silhouette
- Poorly circumscribed
- Symmetric
- Largely epidermal

Patterns

Epidermis
- Single melanocytes at the junction predominate.
- Few small nests at the base of rete ridges.
- Some confluence of nests.

Dermis
- Few nests in the dermis in the center of the lesion
- Some maturation

Cytology
- Small, monomorphic

Other Changes
- Hyperpigmentation of the basal layer
- Flattened rete ridges in the center
- Irregular elongation of rete ridges at the sides
- Fibrosis in the subepidermal dermis in the center
- Prominent melanophages
- Numerous muscle fascicles in the deeper dermis

Integration
A predominance of single melanocytes and poor circumscription together with irregular epidermal hyperplasia and some flattening of rete ridges (Fig. 7.54a, b, d) may raise the suspicion of a melanoma in situ in this lesion. However, a small dermal nested part is positioned in the very center of the lesion giving it an overall symmetric appearance (Fig. 7.54e). The suprapapillary epidermis is spared from single melanocytes (Fig. 7.54b–d). Moreover, no scatter of melanocytes is seen and the dermal part shows some maturation. The muscle fascicles in the dermis identify the special site of this lesion, which is the mamilla (Fig. 7.54f).

Diagnosis: Lentiginous compound nevus on the mamilla.

7.2.4.2 Example 2: Lesion on the Mamilla (Fig. 7.55)

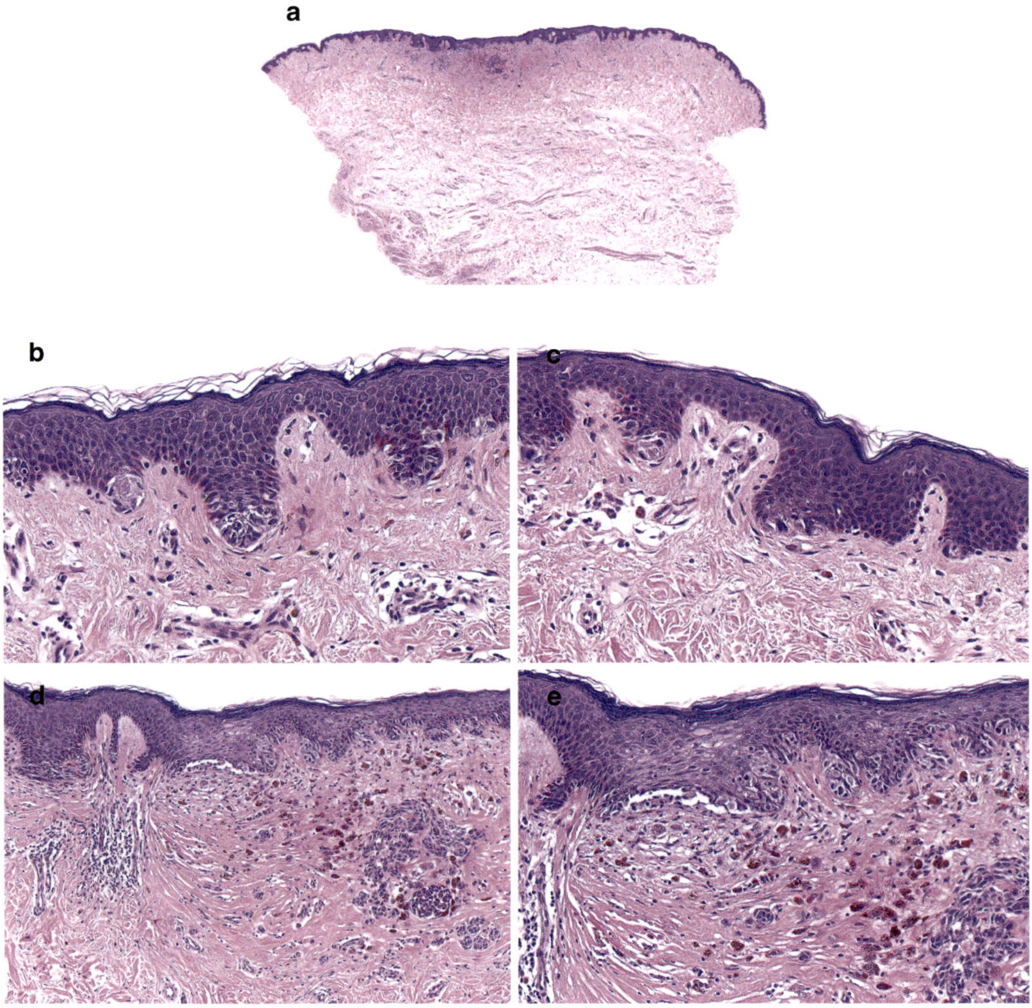

Fig. 7.55 (**a**–**i**) "Special" sites, Example 2. (Courtesy of the Dermatologikum Hamburg)

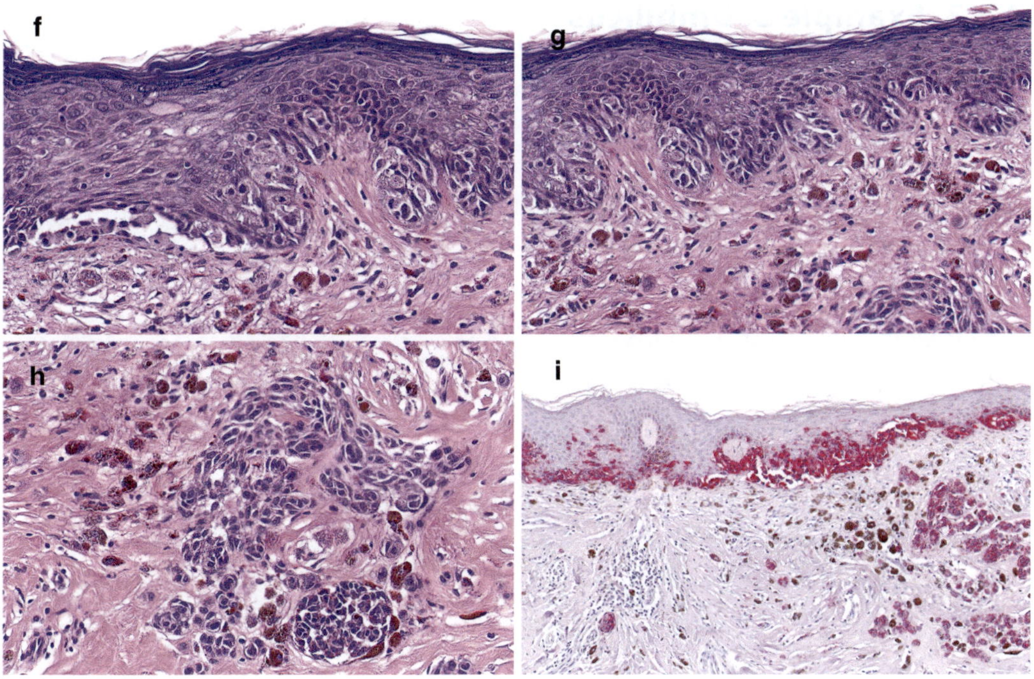

Fig. 7.55 (continued)

Overall Pattern: Nested, Epidermal and Dermal, Symmetric

Detailed Description

Silhouette

- Symmetric
- Well circumscribed
- Epidermal and dermal

Patterns

Epidermis

- Nested at the junction
- Some horizontal confluence of nests
- Single melanocytes between nests
- Some melanocytes in suprabasal layers

Dermis

- Nested
- Maturation

Cytology

- Enlarged, richly pigmented in the epidermis
- Smaller with less pigment in the dermis

Other Changes

- Fibrosis in the dermis in the center of the lesion
- Numerous melanophages
- Muscle fascicles in the deeper dermis

Immunohistochemistry

- MelanA shows confluence of nests, single melanocytes between nests, and some melanocytes in suprabasal layers of the epidermis (Fig. 7.55i).

Integration

The lesion is symmetric, well circumscribed, predominantly nested and shows maturation in the dermis, which all indicate the diagnosis of a nevus (Fig. 7.55a, d, e). Unusual features include the cytology with enlarged hyperpigmented melanocytes (Fig. 7.55h), the irregular arrangement of single melanocytes and nests in the epidermis and some suprabasal melanocytes (Fig. 7.55f, g, i). In the context of the fibrosis in the superficial dermis, the intraepidermal features can be interpreted as signs of previous trauma (Fig. 7.55d, e). They are very similar to what is seen in recurrent or persistent nevi. The muscle fibers in the dermis signal the site, namely, the mamilla (Fig. 7.55a).

Diagnosis: Melanocytic compound nevus on the mamilla.

7.2.4.3 Example 3: Umbilicus (Fig. 7.56)

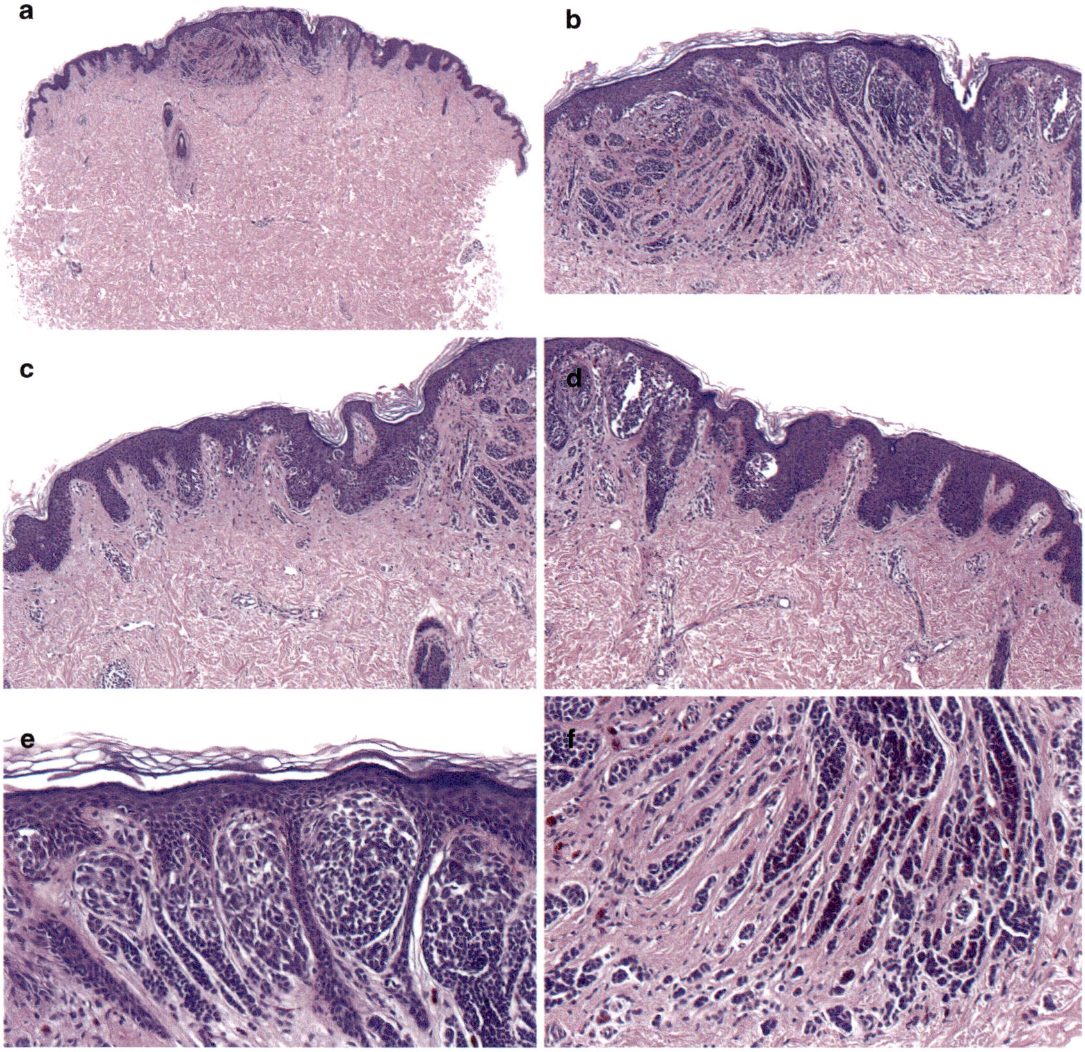

Fig. 7.56 (**a**–**f**) "Special" sites, Example 3. (Courtesy of the Dermatologikum Hamburg)

Overall Pattern: Somewhat Asymmetric, Poorly Circumscribed, Epidermal and Dermal

Detailed Description

Silhouette

- Poorly circumscribed
- Epidermal and dermal
- Asymmetric

Patterns

Epidermis

- Nests at the base of rete ridges.
- Some confluence of nests.
- Single cells between nests.
- Few melanocytes and nests of melanocytes in suprabasal layers.
- Single melanocytes predominate at the periphery of the lesion on both sides.

Dermis

- Nests of melanocytes
- Maturation

Cytology

- Slightly epithelioid and pigmented in the epidermis
- Small with very little cytoplasm in the dermis

Other Changes

- Focal flattening of rete ridges
- Irregular elongation of rete ridges
- Focal subepidermal fibrosis

Integration

The first impression in this lesion is that of a congenital nevus given the prominent dermal maturation and the nested arrangement in the epidermis (Fig. 7.56a). At closer view, however, the circumscription in the epidermis is not so good and single melanocytes can be identified between nests with some nests and single melanocytes in suprabasal layers (Fig. 7.56b–d), so that either a melanoma in situ arising in a nevus or a nevoid melanoma can be considered in the differential diagnosis. In this constellation of findings, it is important to know that the lesion comes from the umbilicus, a so-called special site. Conceptually the umbilicus can be regarded as a site of previous trauma (after section and involution of the umbilical cord) and all features seen in nevi recurring in a scar can also be seen in a nevus in this area. Suprabasal melanocytes and some confluence of nests as well as focal flattening of rete ridges and subepidermal fibrosis can be expected in a nevus from that site (Fig. 7.56e, f).

Diagnosis: Congenital nevus from the umbilicus.

7.2.4.4 Example 4: Vulvar Pigmentation with Sclerosis (Fig. 7.57)

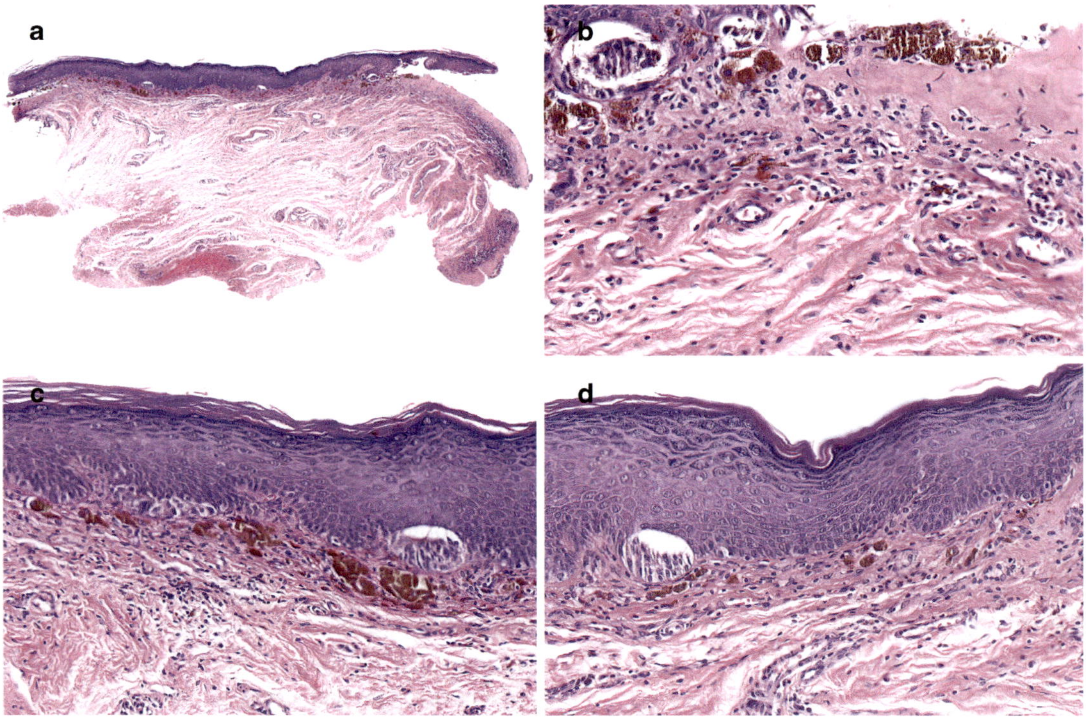

Fig. 7.57 (**a**–**d**) "Special" sites, Example 4. (Courtesy of the Dermatologikum Hamburg)

Overall Pattern: Epidermal, Irregular, Single Melanocytes Predominate, Reaching the Margins

Detailed Description

Silhouette

- Epidermal only
- Irregular
- Reaching the margins

Patterns

Epidermis

- Single melanocytes predominate.
- Few nests of even size at the junction.

Cytology

- Epithelioid, pigmented
- Monomorphic

Other Changes

- Acanthosis and hypergranulosis
- Clefting around nests
- Subepidermal clefting at one side
- Subepidermal eosinophilic sclerosis at one side
- Band-like subepidermal lymphocytic infiltrate
- Band of melanophages
- Richly vascular loose connective tissue in the dermis

Integration

This lesion comes from the skin of the vulva which can be concluded from the structure and composition of the connective tissue (Fig. 7.57a). A melanocytic lesion is present at the junction and it is reaching both margins so that circumscription and symmetry cannot be assessed. Even though the lesion is irregularly distributed, it is positioned solely at the junction and the size of nests is quite even (Fig. 7.57b–d). The lesion is accompanied by a band-like lymphocytic infiltrate and a distinctive subepidermal sclerosis typical of lichen sclerosus, which is a relatively common disease of the vulva (Fig. 7.57b). In the context of an interface dermatitis, the architecture of melanocytic nevi is altered and can also produce an irregular, asymmetric clinical appearance, which is partly due to the prominent infiltrate of melanophages.

Diagnosis: Junctional melanocytic nevus on the vulva in collision with lichen sclerosus.

7.2.5 Conjunctiva

Melanocytic lesions on the conjunctiva are difficult to interpret because most of us do not have much experience with this particular anatomic site. In general, the criteria for diagnosis are the same as on any other site, but the accompanying epithelial changes are different [180, 181]. Conjunctiva is a thin mucous membrane that covers the bulbus and the inner side of the eyelid. It is a nonkeratinized stratified squamous epithelium that consists of 2–5 layers of columnar or cuboidal cells and variable numbers of mucin-producing goblet cells. It also contains regularly distributed melanocytes and Langerhans cells. Especially in palpebral conjunctiva invaginations of surface epithelium form tubular and cystic structures (so-called pseudo glands of Henle). Below the epithelium, there is a loose fibrovascular connective tissue (substantia propria), which regularly shows quite a number of inflammatory cells, mostly lymphocytes and plasma cells. Since conjunctiva is a soft and thin epithelium, orientation and cutting of specimens from the conjunctiva is more challenging compared with skin. Misorientation and cutting artifacts like disruption of the epithelium are common and complicate histologic assessment.

Most conjunctival nevi are noticed in childhood and adolescence and therefore a pigmented lesion that develops on the conjunctiva of an adult is always suspicious. Conjunctival nevi almost always involve the bulbar conjunctiva and caruncle. Most are compound lesions with melanocytes in epithelium and lamina propria. Within the epithelium, a nested pattern predominates. In the dermis, nests and interstitial strands with maturation are seen. Solid and cystic inclusions of conjunctival epithelium are a common finding and we designate the arrangement of melanocytes around those cysts as pericystic. Inflammatory infiltrates are frequent in melanocytic lesions on the conjunctiva. In children, lesions are still growing and may show mitotic figures. Junctional conjunctival nevi are seen only in very young children and they also show a nested pattern of melanocytes in the basal part of the epithelium. Purely subepithelial nevi also not so common, they are less pigmented with bland cytology but may show balloon cell differentiation.

Conjunctival melanoma is a rare disease, with approximately 20 cases per year being diagnosed in large countries such as Germany [182–184]. It may develop de novo or, less commonly, arise in a nevus as a pigmented or nonpigmented lesion, commonly in the limbal area. Involvement of the cornea is extremely rare. In general, any pigmented lesion presenting in an adult in the palpebral conjunctiva or fornix should be considered suspicious for melanoma. A confusing terminology has been used to designate intraepithelial acquired pigmented lesions of the conjunctiva in adults, that is "Primary acquired melanosis with/without atypia" [185]. Doubtlessly there are also benign acquired pigmented patches in the adult conjunctiva such as a conjunctival analogue of solar lentigo or benign melanosis, but both are pigmented epithelial lesions with no increase in number of melanocytes. In contrast, any acquired intraepithelial proliferation of melanocytes in an adult should be considered a melanoma in situ, no matter how much cytologic atypia is discernible, because junctional melanocytic nevi of the conjunctiva practically do not exist in the adult. Conjunctival melanoma in situ develops most commonly at the limbus and epibulbar interpalpebral region; the eyelid epidermis may also be involved. Invasive melanomas of the conjunctiva almost always show intraepithelial involvement in the form of melanoma in situ. Genetic alterations of conjunctival melanoma include mutations in the *BRAF*, *NRAS,* and *TERT* promoter genes, which are also found in cutaneous melanomas.

7.2.5.1 Example 1: Conjunctiva (Fig. 7.58)

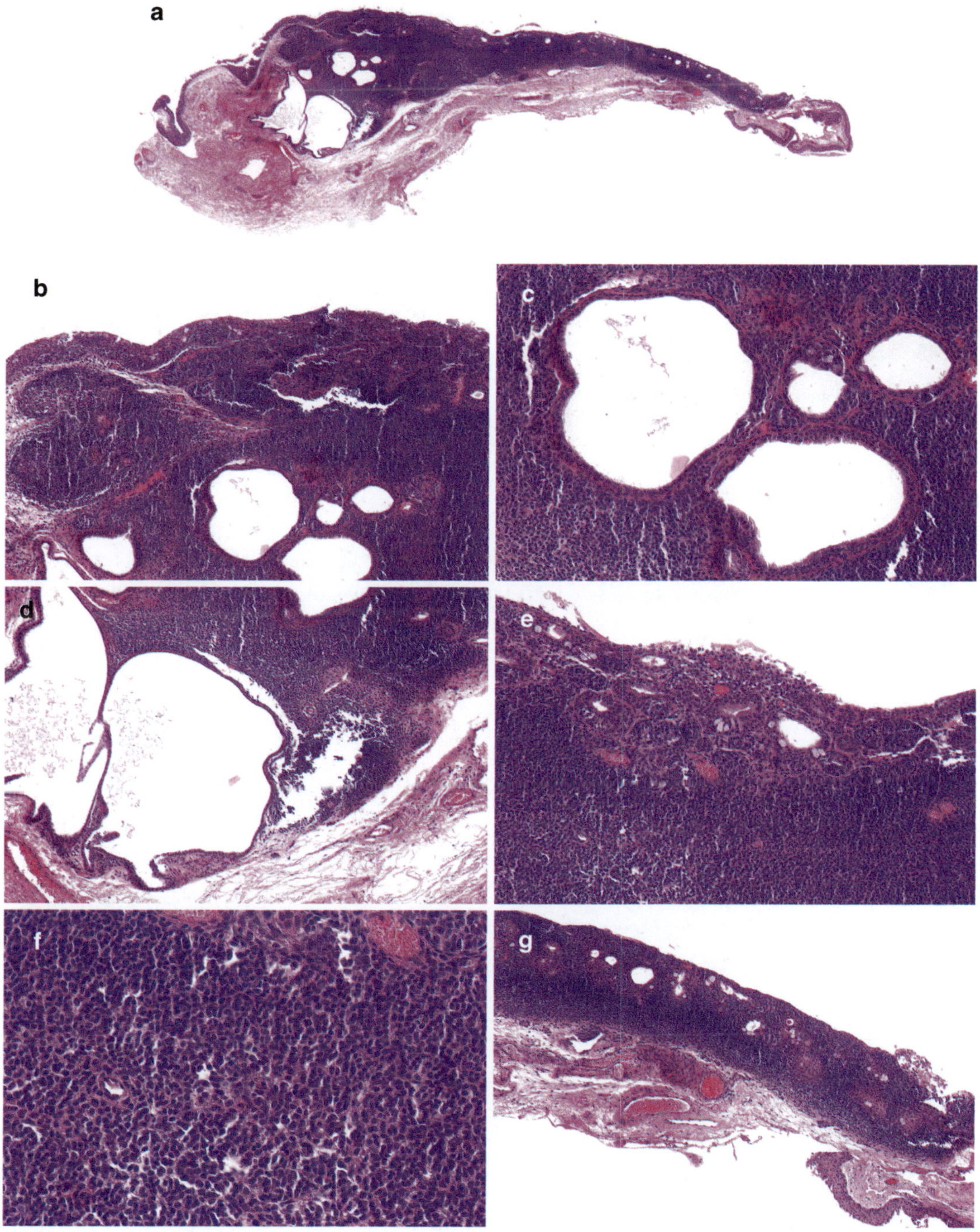

Fig. 7.58 (a–j) Conjunctiva, Example 1. (Courtesy of the Dermatologikum Hamburg)

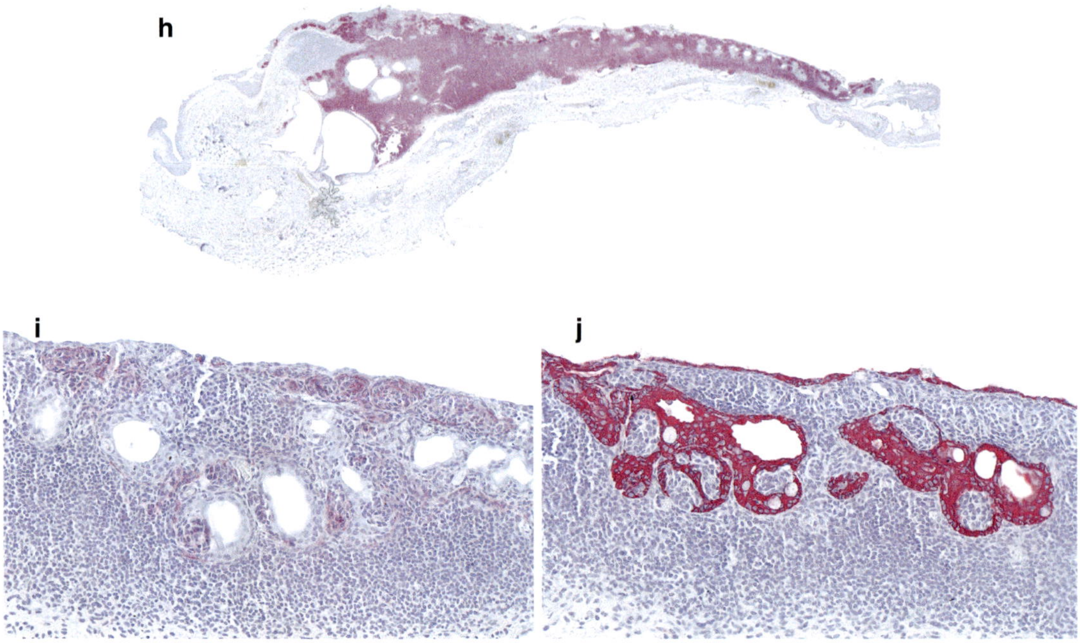

Fig. 7.58 (continued)

Overall Pattern: Epithelial and Lamina Propria, Nested, Pericystic

Detailed Description

Silhouette

- Well circumscribed
- In epithelium and lamina propria

Patterns

Epithelium

- Nested, some confluence
- Single melanocytes between nests, evenly distributed
- No suprabasal melanocytes

Lamina Propria

- Small nests, closely arranged
- Interstitial strands
- Pericystic arrangement
- Some maturation

Cytology

- Round to oval
- Monomorphic
- No crowding, no mitoses, no necrotic cells

Other Changes

- Prominent cystic change
- Lymphoplasmacytic infiltrate

Immunohistochemistry

- MelanA shows the silhouette with good circumscription (Fig. 7.58h).
- HMB45 is not expressed in the proliferation in the lamina propria (Fig. 7.58i).
- Pan-cytokeratin can highlight the epithelial cystic proliferations (Fig. 7.58j).

Integration

This lesion is well circumscribed and mostly nested in the intraepithelial part (Fig. 7.58a, h). In the lamina propria, melanocytes are monomorphic with maturation (Fig. 7.58e, f) and arrangement around prominent epithelial cystic change (Fig. 7.58b–d). The good circumscription can better be appreciated in the MelanA immunostain, pan-cytokeratin helps to identify the epithelial cystic proliferations. Within these proliferations, a nested pattern of intraepithelial melanocytes appears as a negative-image (Fig. 7.58j). This lesion came from the conjunctiva of an 8-year-old African child.

Diagnosis: Congenital melanocytic nevus of the conjunctiva.

7.2.5.2 Example 2: Conjunctiva (Fig. 7.59)

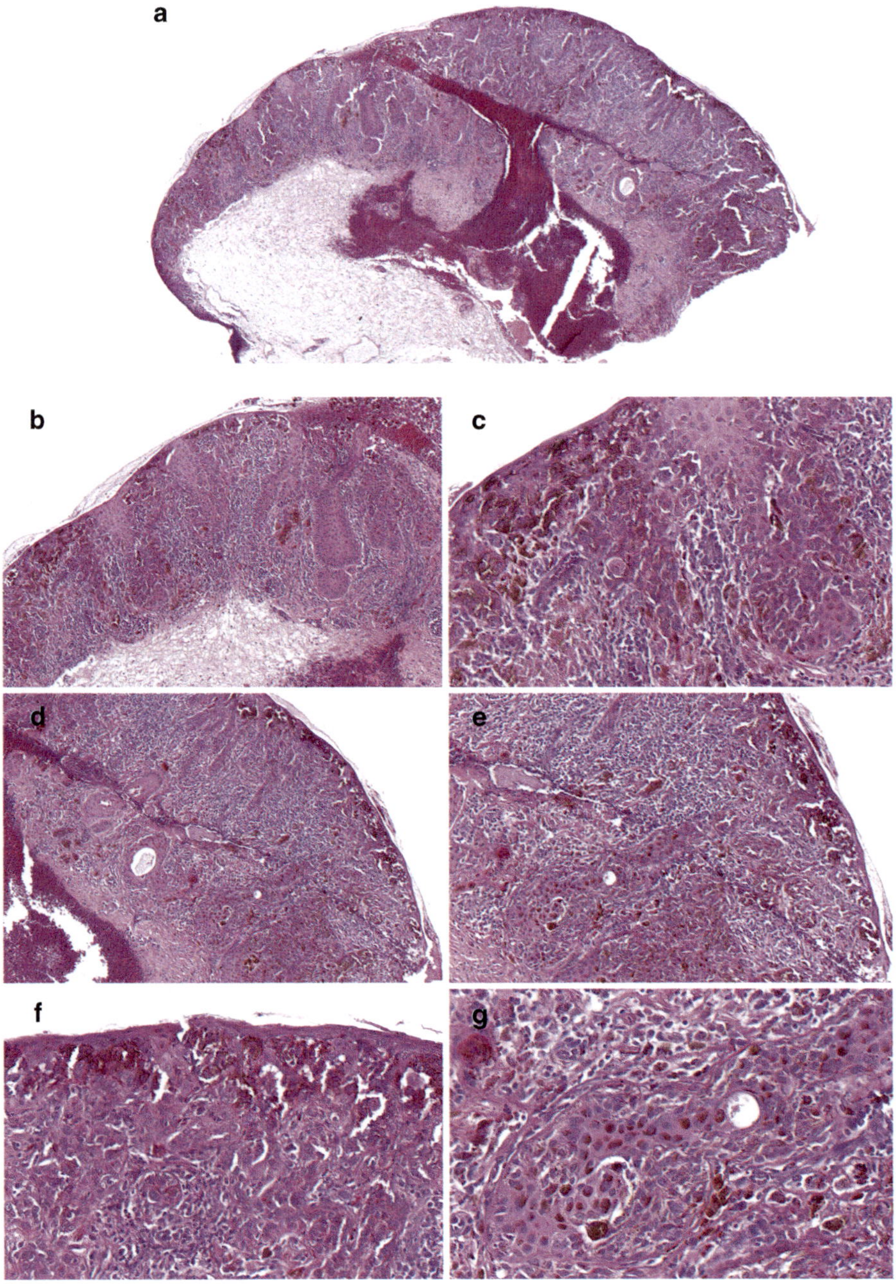

Fig. 7.59 (**a**–**j**) Conjunctiva, Example 2. (Courtesy of the Dermatologikum Hamburg)

Fig. 7.59 (continued)

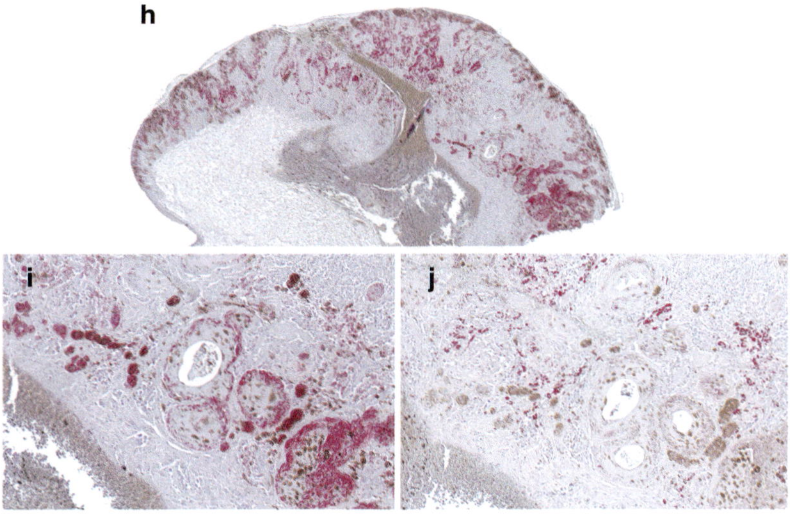

Overall Pattern: Nested, Epithelium and Lamina Propria

Detailed Description

Silhouette

- Well circumscribed
- Epithelium and lamina propria

Patterns

Epithelium

- Nested, some confluence
- Nests also prominent in epithelial hyperplasia
- Single melanocytes between nests, regularly distributed
- No suprabasal melanocytes, but heavy pigmentation in epithelial cells

Lamina propria

- Nested
- Pericystic arrangement
- Maturation

Cytology

- Round to oval, heavily pigmented
- Monomorphic
- No crowding, no mitoses, no necrotic cells

Other Changes

- Prominent epithelial hyperplasia with some cystic change
- Heavy pigmentation of epithelial cells
- Numerous melanophages
- Prominent lymphoplasmacytic infiltrate

Immunohistochemistry

- MelanA shows the silhouette with good circumscription (Fig. 7.59h, i).
- HMB45 is not expressed in the nests in the lamina propria (Fig. 7.59j).

Integration

This lesion is well circumscribed and mostly nested in the intraepithelial part (Fig. 7.59a, h). Even though this lesion seems to involve the lamina propria extensively, most of the nests of melanocytes are actually located within the hyperplastic epithelium (Fig. 7.59b–g). Only few small nests are seen in the connective tissue and there is also an inflammatory cell infiltrate and numerous melanophages. In the lamina propria, melanocytes are monomorphic with maturation. The good circumscription can better be appreciated in the MelanA immunostain. Nests in the lamina propria do not express HMB45, which only stains some melanophages in this case. This lesion came from the conjunctiva of an 11-year-old African child and had been present since birth.

Diagnosis: Congenital melanocytic nevus of the conjunctiva.

7.2.5.3 Example 3: Conjunctiva (Fig. 7.60)

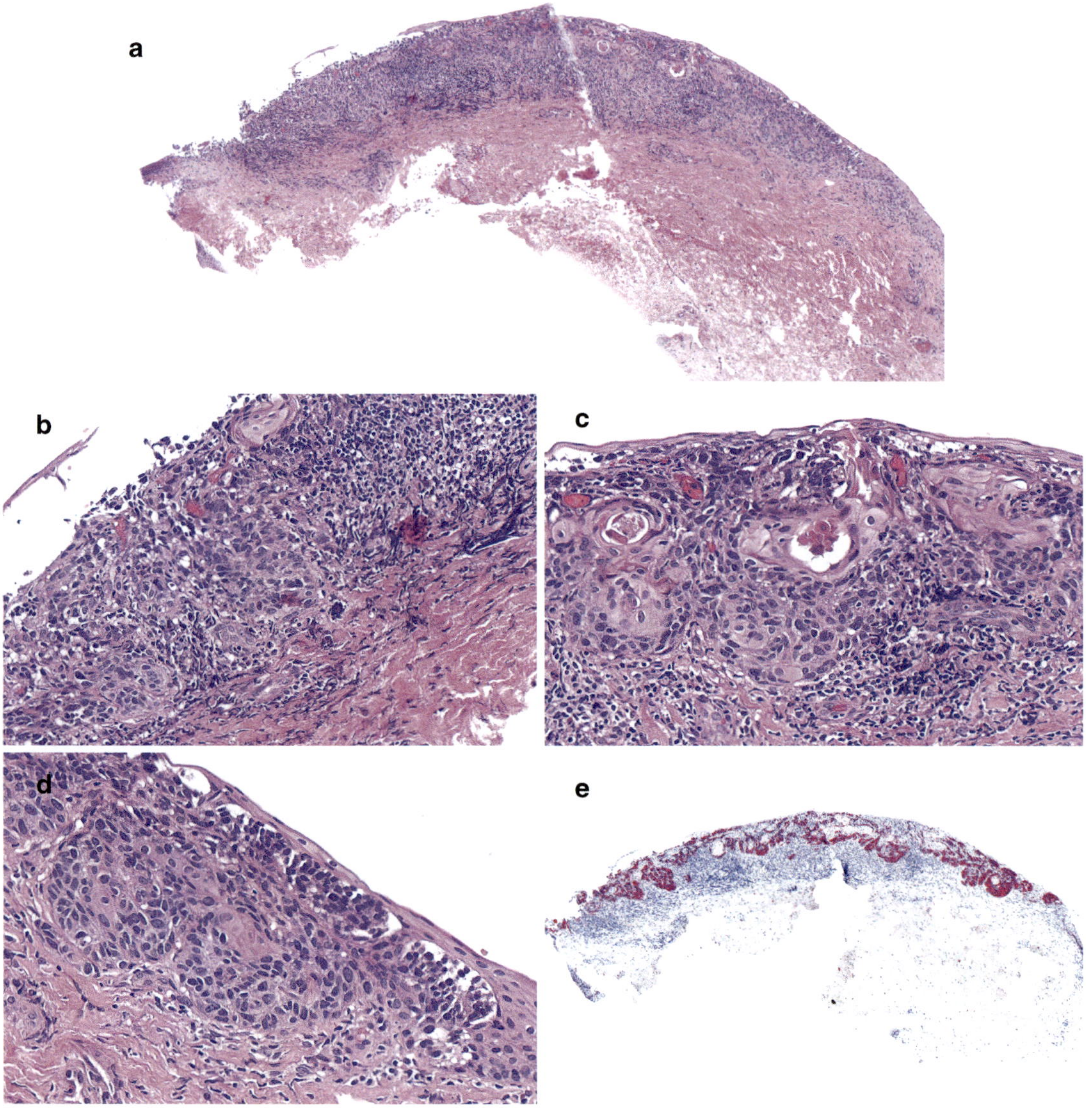

Fig. 7.60 (**a**–**e**) Conjunctiva, Example 3. (Courtesy of the Dermatologikum Hamburg)

Overall Pattern: Well Circumscribed, in Epithelium and Lamina Propria

Detailed Description

Silhouette

- Well circumscribed
- In epithelium and lamina propria

Patterns

Epithelium

- Nested, some confluence
- Nests also in epithelial hyperplasia
- No suprabasal melanocytes

Lamina propria

- Small nests in the center of the lesion

Cytology

- Epithelioid
- Monomorphic
- No crowding, no mitoses, no necrotic cells

Other Changes

- Some epithelial hyperplasia with some cystic change
- Focal clefting
- Lymphoplasmacytic infiltrate

Immunohistochemistry

- MelanA shows the silhouette with good circumscription (Fig. 7.60e).

Integration

This lesion is well circumscribed and mostly nested in the intraepithelial part including the epithelial hyperplasia (Fig. 7.60a, e). Few small nests are present in the lamina propria in the center of the lesion. Melanocytes are epithelioid but monomorphic (Fig. 7.60b–d). The good circumscription and involvement of the lamina propria can better be appreciated in the MelanA immunostain (Fig. 7.60e). This is a congenital lesion from the conjunctiva of a 6-year-old African child.

Diagnosis: Congenital melanocytic nevus of the conjunctiva.

7.2.5.4 Example 4: Conjunctiva (Fig. 7.61)

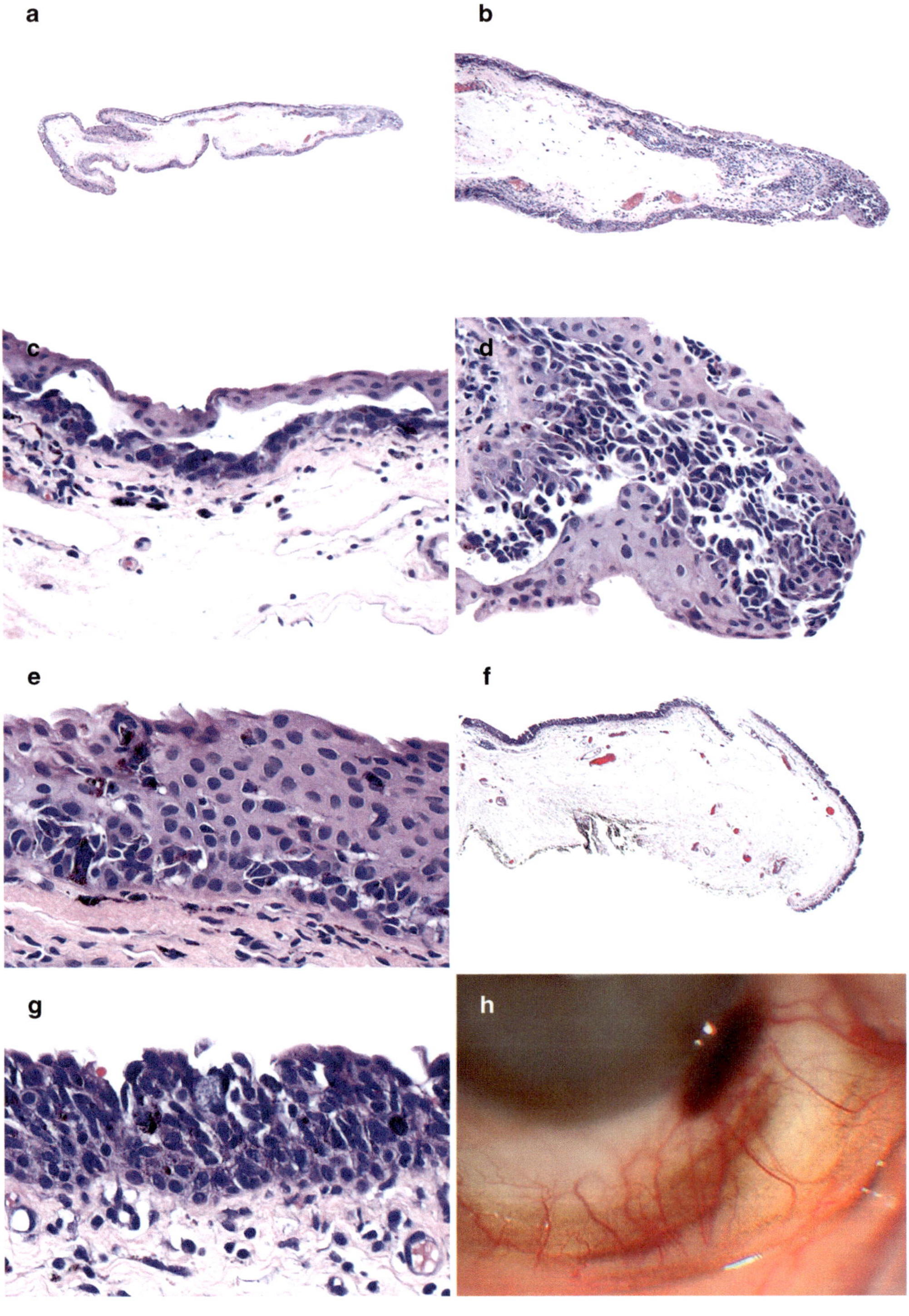

Fig. 7.61 (**a–h**) Conjunctiva, Example 4. (Courtesy of Almut Böer-Auer)

Overall Pattern: Broad Lesion, Confluence of Nests, Only Epithelial

Detailed Description

Silhouette

- Asymmetric
- Poorly circumscribed
- Only epithelial

Patterns

Epithelium

- Single melanocytes, irregularly distributed.
- Nests of melanocytes, confluent to large and irregular aggregations.
- Single cells predominate over nests.
- Melanocytes in suprabasal layers of the epithelium.

Lamina propria

- None

Cytology

- Pleomorphic with prominent dendrites
- Enlarged and irregular nuclei, some hyperchromatic
- Crowding of nuclei
- No mitoses, no necrotic cells

Other Changes

- Elongated clefts
- Some lymphocytic infiltrate and melanophages

Integration

An un-sharply demarcated and irregularly pigmented large macule is seen on the lower bulbar conjunctiva of a Caucasian adult (Fig. 7.61h). Two biopsies were performed (Fig. 7.61a, f). An irregular and broad proliferation of melanocytes is present in the conjunctival epithelium (Fig. 7.61a, b). It consists of nests and single melanocytes. Nests are confluent to form large and bizarre-shaped aggregations (Fig. 7.61c, d). In foci, single melanocytes predominate. Some melanocytes are present in suprabasal layers of the epithelium (Fig. 7.61e). In other foci, proliferations of melanocytes have replaced almost the entire epithelium. The findings shown here are diagnostic of melanoma in situ of the conjunctiva. Changes in the second biopsy specimen taken from the same lesion are more subtle. A proliferation of single melanocytes is present in basal and suprabasal layers of the conjunctiva (Fig. 7.61g). Melanocytes are pleomorphic and have prominent dendrites.

Diagnosis: Melanoma in situ of the conjunctiva.

7.2.5.5 Example 5: Caruncula (Fig. 7.62)

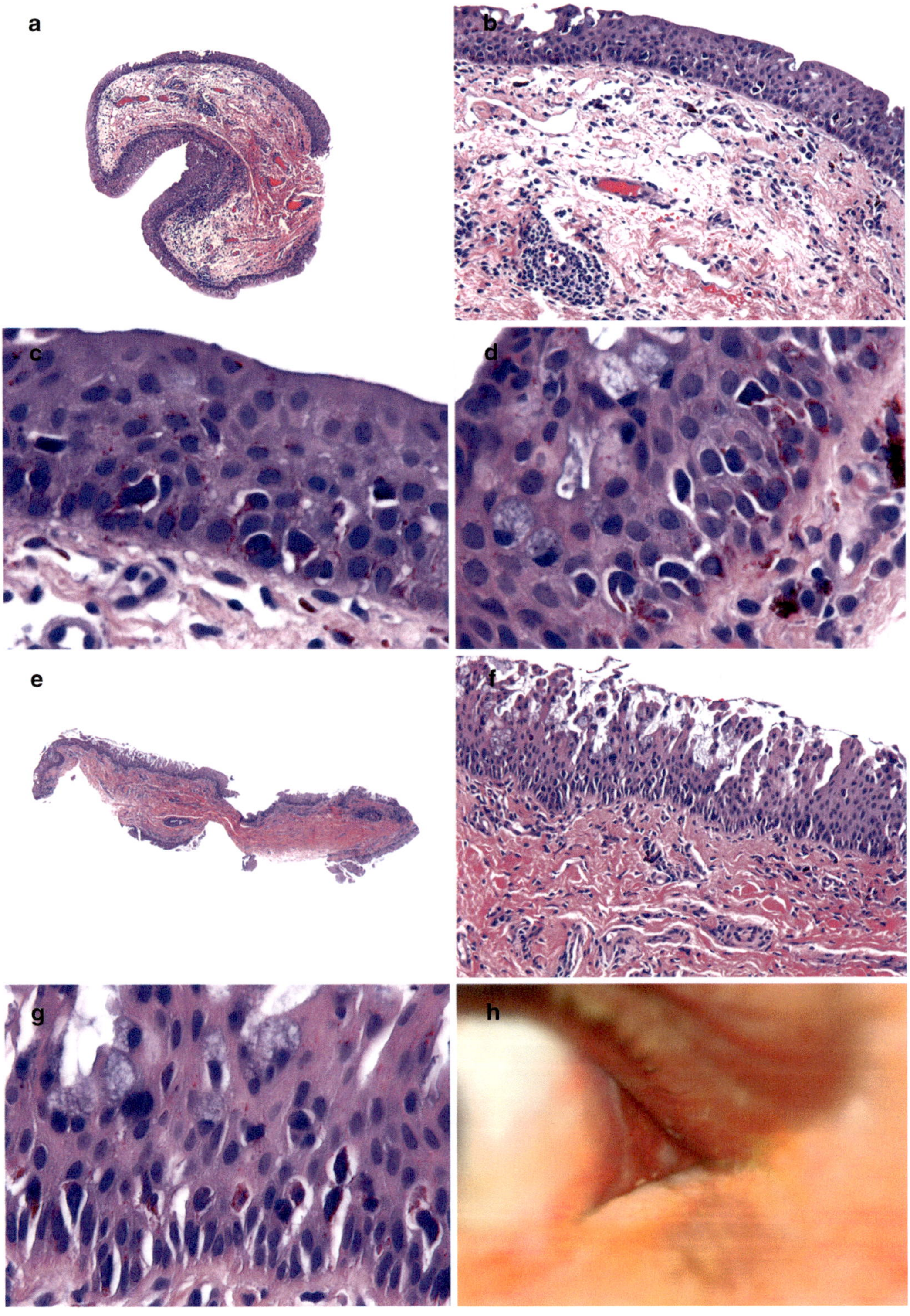

Fig. 7.62 (**a**–**h**) Conjunctiva, Example 5. (Courtesy of Almut Böer-Auer)

Overall Pattern: Only Epithelial, Single Melanocytes Predominate

Detailed Description

Silhouette
- Asymmetric
- Poorly circumscribed
- Only epithelial

Patterns

Epithelium
- Single melanocytes, irregularly distributed
- Back-to-back melanocytes
- Melanocytes in upper layers
- No obvious nesting

Lamina propria
- None

Cytology
- Enlarged with hyperchromatic nuclei
- Prominent and high-reaching dendrites
- Crowding of nuclei

Other Changes
- Melanophages
- Some lymphocytic infiltrate

Integration
A subtle pigmented lesion of the caruncle was biopsied (Fig. 7.62h). Two specimens of this lesion are shown (Fig. 7.62a, e). A proliferation of single melanocytes is present in the basal layer (Fig. 7.62b–d). Some melanocytes are present above the junction (Fig. 7.62c). Melanocytes are heavily pigmented and show prominent dendrites (Fig. 7.62d). Even though no nests of melanocytes are present in this biopsy specimen, the changes are diagnostic of melanoma in situ of the conjunctiva. In the second specimen, single melanocytes are present in the basal layer and in suprabasal layers (Fig. 7.62e–g).

Diagnosis: Melanoma in situ of the conjunctiva.

7.2.5.6 Example 6: Conjunctiva, Nonpigmented Lesion (Fig. 7.63)

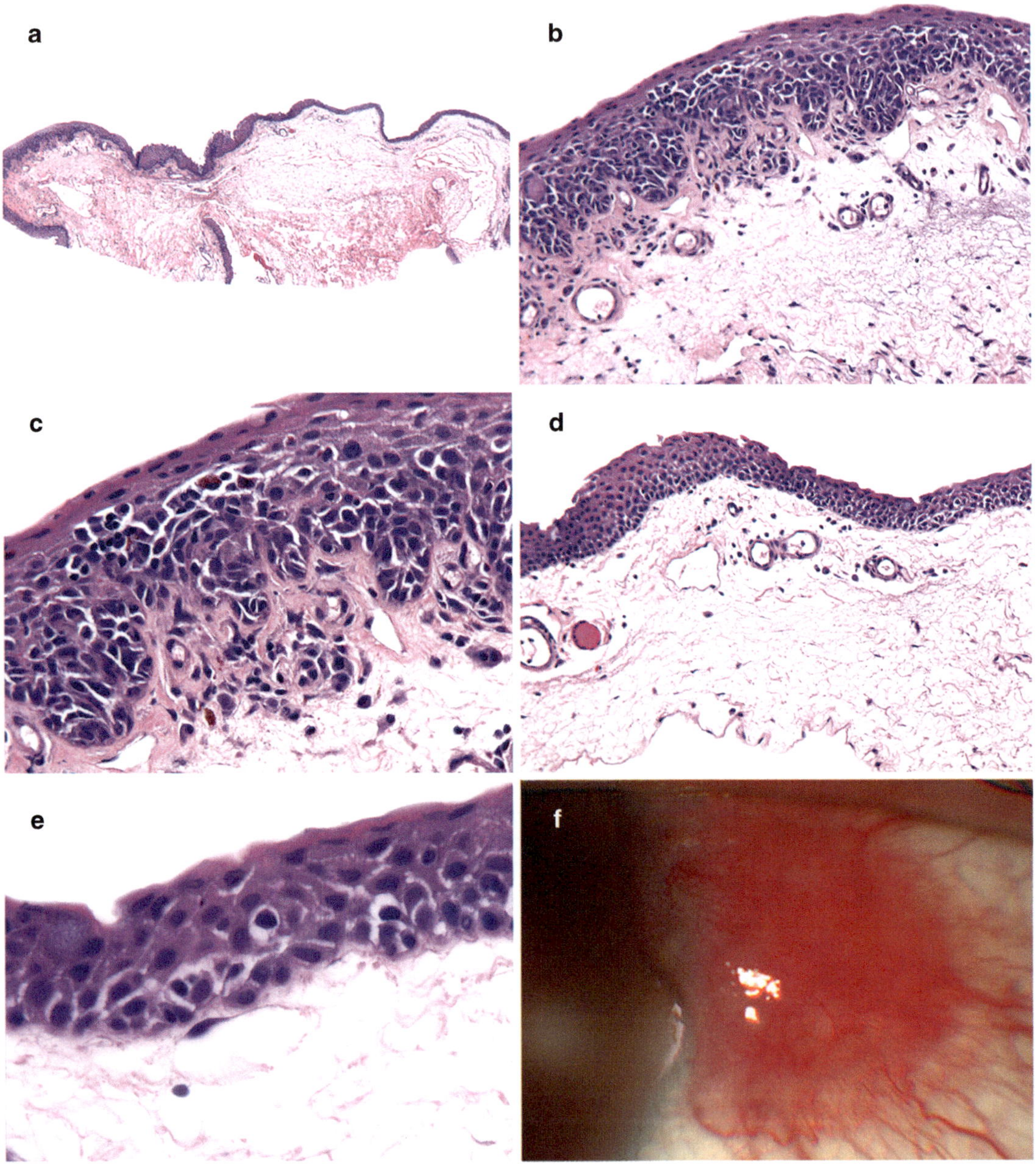

Fig. 7.63 (a–f) Conjunctiva, Example 6. (Courtesy of Almut Böer-Auer)

Overall Pattern: Epithelium and Lamina Propria, Single Melanocytes, Irregularly Distributed

Detailed Description

Silhouette

- Asymmetric
- Poorly circumscribed
- In epithelium and focally in the lamina propria

Patterns

Epithelium

- Single melanocytes, irregularly distributed
- Back-to-back melanocytes
- Melanocytes in upper layers
- Nests confluent to irregular aggregations

Lamina propria

- Focal nests and single melanocytes

Cytology

- Enlarged with hyperchromatic nuclei
- Crowding of nuclei

Integration

A red papule surrounded by telangiectasia is seen on the bulbar conjunctiva (Fig. 7.63f). A proliferation of melanocytes is present in the conjunctival epithelium (Fig. 7.63a). Melanocytes are confluent to form bizarre aggregations (Fig. 7.63b, c). Single melanocytes and small aggregations are also seen in suprabasal layers of the epithelium. Few melanocytes are also present in the superficial lamina propria (Fig. 7.63c). In adjacent areas of the conjunctiva, the proliferation consists only of single melanocytes, which are slightly pleomorphic and partly located in suprabasal layers (Fig. 7.63d, e).

Diagnosis: Amelanotic melanoma of the conjunctiva, focally invasive in the lamina propria.

7.3 Clinical Setting

7.3.1 Partial Biopsies

In the daily routine of dermatopathology, partial biopsies of melanocytic lesions are not uncommon. For a conventional dermal nevus, removal by shave technique is a frequent practice. Such specimens, even though incomplete, are not so problematic for the dermatopathologist because the specimen still can be oriented well by the technician and in most cases the lesion is largely dermal without epidermal involvement so that there is no suspicion of malignancy. However, melanocytic lesions may also arrive in the laboratory in the form of curettings, as multiple fragmented pieces, especially when the clinician did not suspect a melanocytic lesion but a seborrheic keratosis, an actinic keratosis, or a superficial pigmented basal cell carcinoma. Such material is always challenging under the microscope, mainly for three reasons: (1) symmetry and circumscription of the lesion cannot be assessed, (2) the material cannot be oriented well in the paraffin block and sections of the specimen will show epidermis and dermis cut in various angles or even in transverse cut, and (3) because it is upon the histopathologist to consider a melanocytic lesion at all—even though the clinician is not specifically asking for it. Especially in the setting of chronically sun-damaged skin, it is worthwhile for the dermatopathologist to always think of a melanoma in situ, and, because they can be quite subtle on H&E, request help from immunostainings if there is any suspicion.

Sometimes, large melanocytic lesions are biopsied with a punch because a suspicious area in a large congenital nevus is sampled or because in a large lesion the clinical diagnosis between melanoma and a simulator of it is not solvable. A typical clinical setting is so-called lentigo maligna (melanoma in situ on sun-damaged skin) versus solar lentigo, in which punch biopsy is a common practice. If the punch reveals melanoma not restricted to the epidermis, assessment of thickness can only be given preliminary, because the biopsy may not have sampled the thickest area of the lesion. Final assessment of the thickness can only be provided together with the complete excision of the lesion.

If a diagnosis cannot be made with certainty in a partial biopsy, this should be stated in the report straightforwardly and complete removal of the lesion with reassessment of the diagnosis in the excisional specimen has to be performed. Ideally, partial biopsy and complete excision should be assessed by the same diagnostician and the slides of the partial biopsy should be reviewed when the excision arrives for sign-out.

The following examples should serve to illustrate how to handle uncertainty in partial biopsies.

7.3.1.1 Example 1: Curetting (Fig. 7.64)

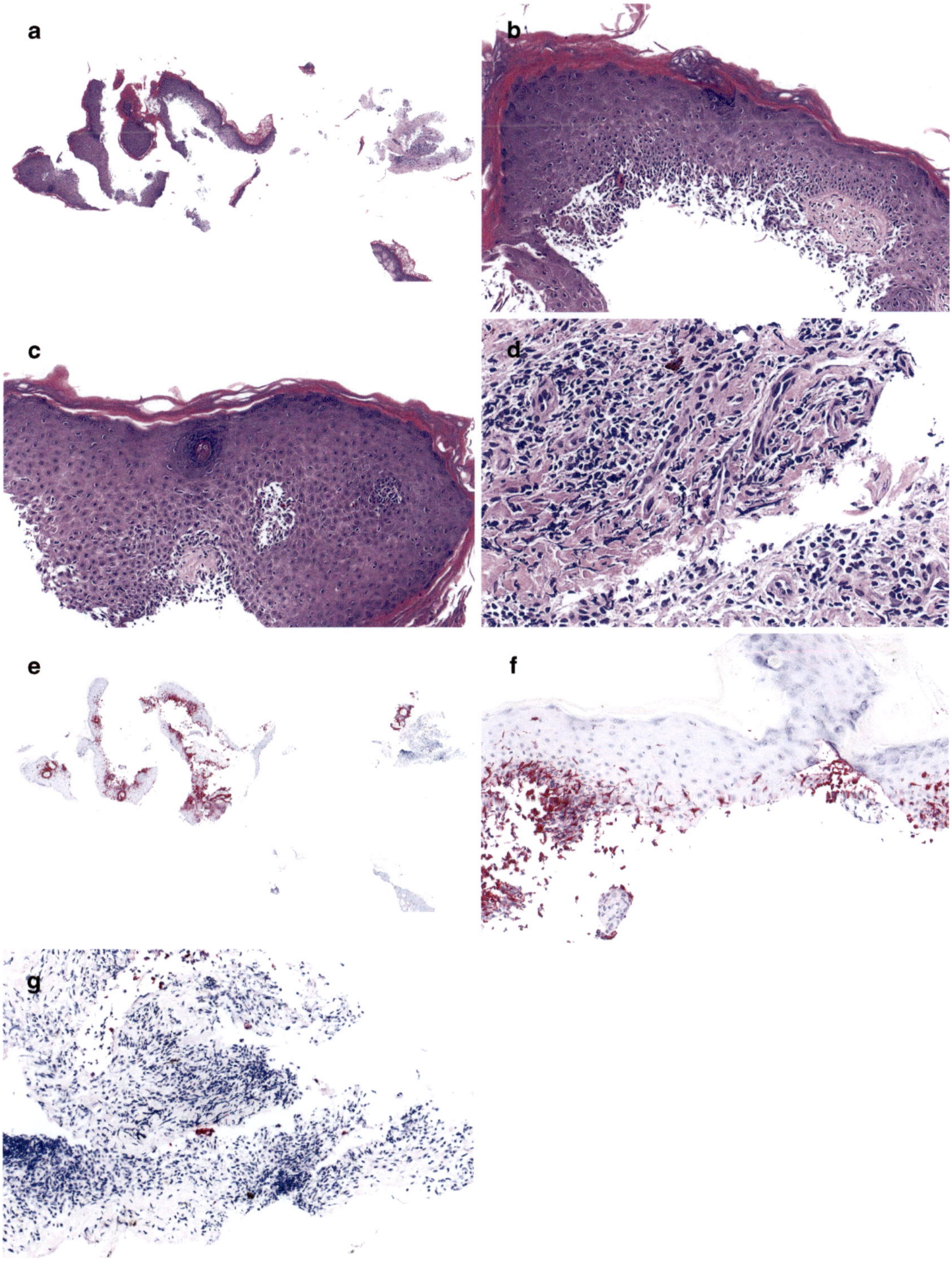

Fig. 7.64 (**a–g**) Partial biopsies, Example 1. (Courtesy of the Dermatologikum Hamburg)

Overall Pattern: Fragmented Shave Specimen, Single Melanocytes, Poorly Circumscribed

Detailed Description

Silhouette
- Poorly circumscribed
- Epidermal only

Patterns

Epidermis
- Single melanocytes, irregularly distributed
- Some suprabasal melanocytes
- Focal irregularly shaped nests

Dermis
- None

Cytology
- Small with prominent pigmentation and hyperchromatic nuclei
- Prominent dendrites

Other Changes
- Dense lymphocytic infiltrate
- Some acanthosis

Integration

The first diagnosis that comes to mind in this fragmented shave specimen is lichen planus-like keratosis given the epidermal acanthosis, the dense subepidermal infiltrate, and the impression of some alteration at the dermoepidermal junction (Fig. 7.64a, b). At closer view, however, an irregular proliferation of melanocytes is seen at the junction (Fig. 7.64c). The melanocytes are relatively small with hyperchromatic nuclei so that they can be misinterpreted as lymphocytes at lower magnifications. MelanA presents the melanocytic proliferation much more obviously (Fig. 7.64e–g). It consists predominantly of single melanocytes with some confluence to irregularly shaped nests. In shave specimens and curettings often the orientation of the epidermis is not optimal and melanocytes may look suprabasal even though they are positioned in the basal layer, which actually is cut obliquely. In this specimen, however, the melanocytes are clearly present in the mid-spinous zone and in the granular layer, which cannot be explained by tangential cut (Fig. 7.64f). Moreover, the melanocytes have a dendritic morphology, which becomes apparent only in the MelanA stain. No definite dermal involvement of the melanocytic lesion can be identified. Some MelanA-positive cells within the lymphocytic infiltrate have likely been placed there by the microtome from junctional nests (Fig. 7.64g). Since symmetry and circumscription cannot be assessed in this specimen, the diagnosis of a melanoma should be favored with the need of re-excision and reevaluation in the excisional specimen. A possible differential diagnosis is a surface of a recurrent nevus ("pseudomelanoma"), but no obvious scar is sampled in the biopsy and only small parts of the dermis are seen anyhow.

Diagnosis: Melanoma in situ, most probably, re-excision mandatory with reevaluation of the diagnosis in context with the re-excision.

Follow-up: In the re-excision of this lesion, no residual melanocytic lesion was found. There was just a fresh superficial scar from the recent shave operation. The absence of a dermal part of a nevus in the re-excision makes the differential diagnosis of recurrent nevus with pseudomelanoma features much less likely. The final diagnosis therefore remained melanoma in situ.

7.3.1.2 Example 2: Shave Biopsy (Fig. 7.65)

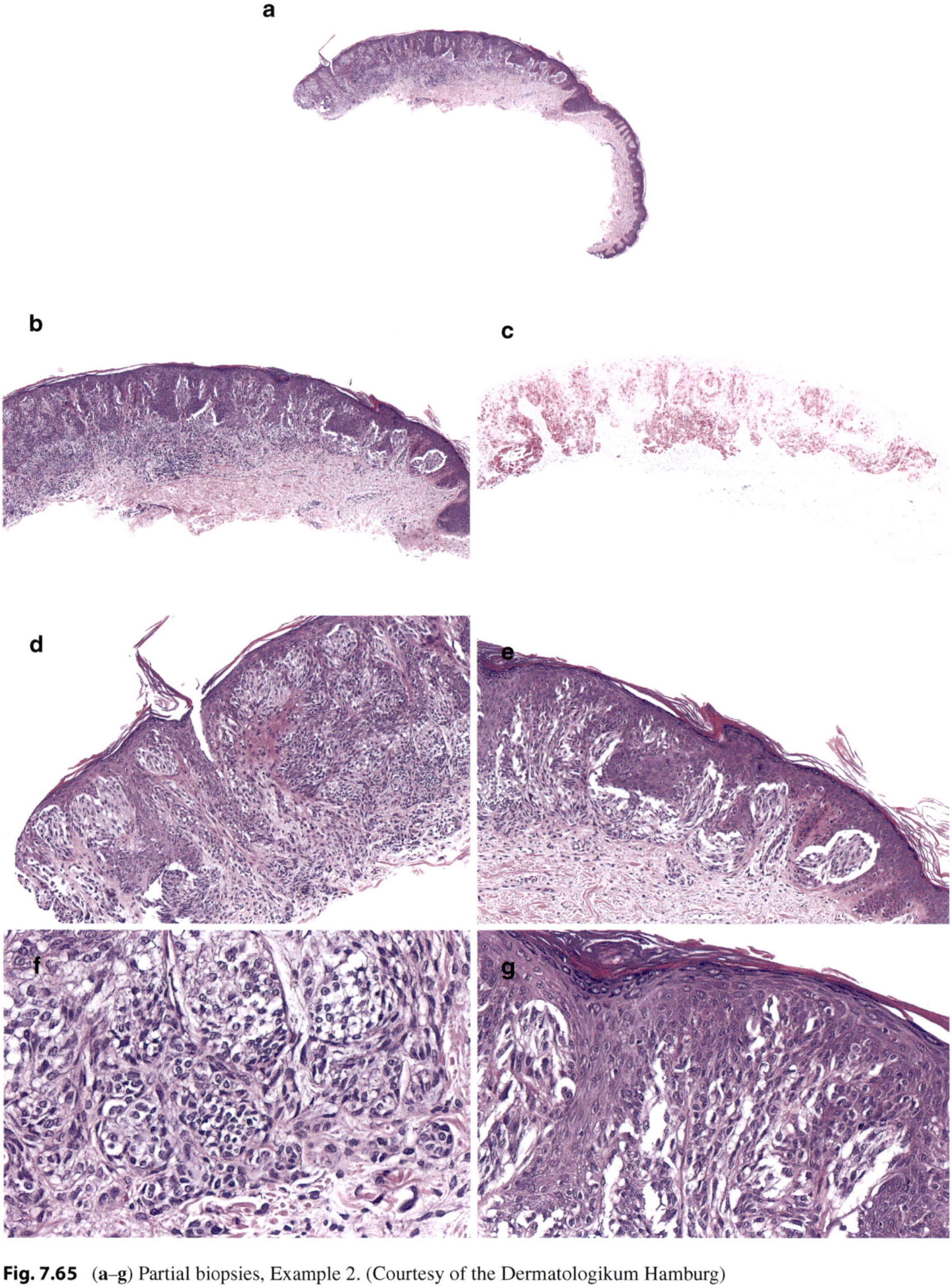

Fig. 7.65 (**a**–**g**) Partial biopsies, Example 2. (Courtesy of the Dermatologikum Hamburg)

Overall Pattern: Nested, Epidermal and Dermal, Well Circumscribed, Incomplete Excision

Detailed Description

Silhouette

- Shave specimen
- Well circumscribed to one side
- Epidermal and dermal

Patterns

Epidermis

- Large nests at the base of rete ridges
- Some confluence of nests
- Single melanocytes between nests
- Some melanocytes and small nests in upper layers of the epidermis

Dermis

- Nests of melanocytes
- Some maturation

Cytology

- Large epithelioid and spindled
- Moderately pleomorphic nuclei
- No mitoses

Immunohistochemistry

- MelanA: Sharp circumscription at one side.
- MelanA: Single melanocytes are more numerous in the epidermis than seen on H&E.
- MelanA: On the left side single cells predominate over nests.

Other Changes

- Clefts between nests and epidermis
- Acanthosis, hypergranulosis, and hyperkeratosis
- Some lymphocytic infiltrate

Integration

This lesion with spitzoid cytology has many features of a Spitz nevus, such as large nests in the epidermis and maturation in the dermal part (Fig. 7.65a–c, f). The epidermis is hyperplastic with elongated rete ridges, but no Kamino bodies are seen (Fig. 7.65d, e, g). The most difficult aspect of this lesion is the fact that it is only a partial biopsy. Symmetry and circumscription cannot be assessed and the sharp circumscription on one side can be misleading. Moreover, the lesion seems to be mostly nested on H&E while single melanocytes are much more prominent on immunostaining with MelanA (Fig. 7.65c). The high number of single melanocytes is unusual for a Spitz nevus but could be interpreted as the result of outside irritation. Because of the uncertainty in this specimen, it is essential to make sure that the lesion is excised completely.

Diagnosis: The differential diagnosis is between a spitzoid melanoma and an irritated Spitz nevus. The lesion extends to one margin so that symmetry and circumscription cannot be assessed. Complete excision is necessary.

Read on to see the follow-up of this lesion.

Excision: Nodular Lesion After Shave Biopsy (Fig. 7.66)

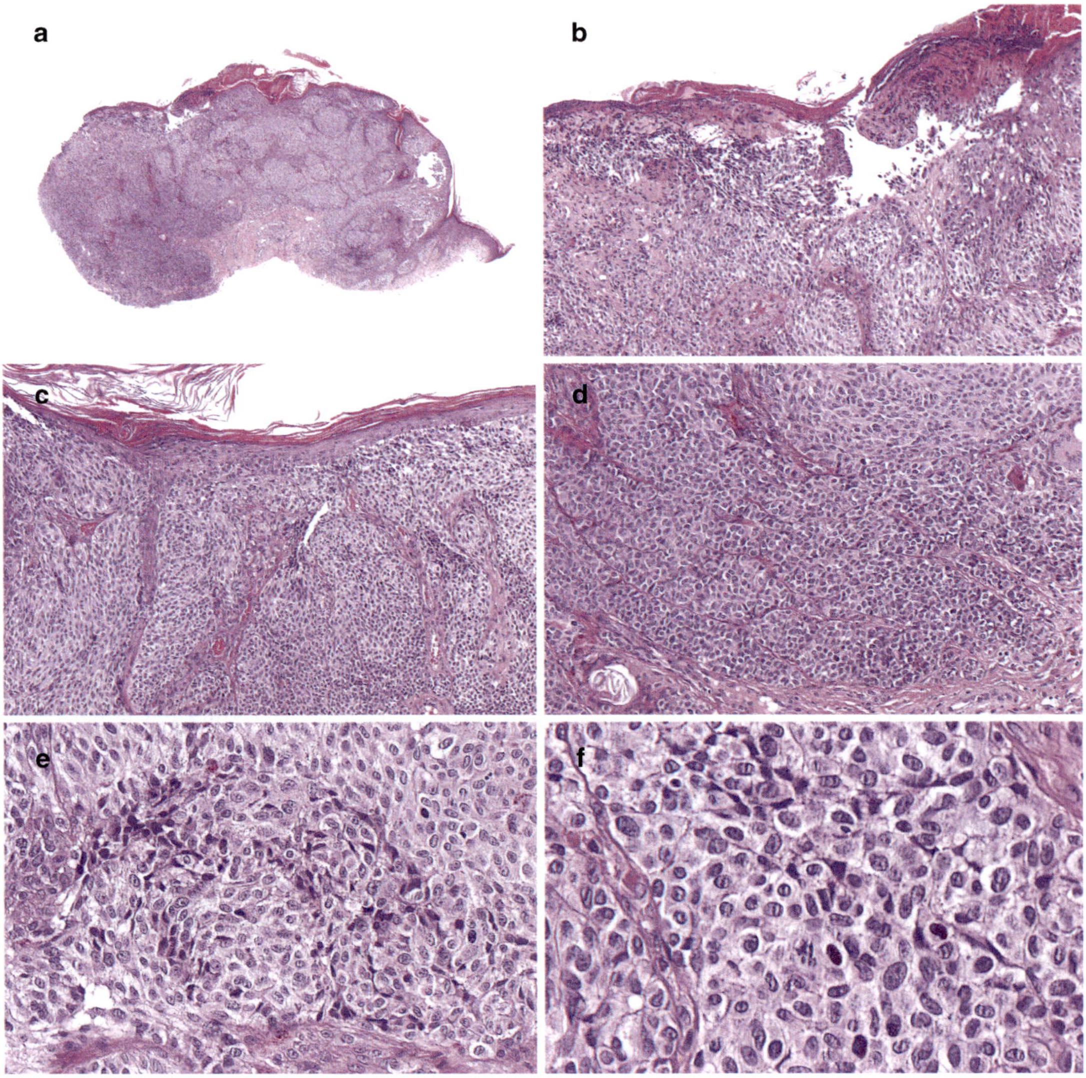

Fig. 7.66 (**a**–**f**) Partial biopsies, Example 2 (follow-up). (Courtesy of the Dermatologikum Hamburg)

Overall Pattern: Nodular, Ulcerated, Epidermal and Dermal

Detailed Description

Silhouette

- Ulceration with crust
- Asymmetric
- Relatively well circumscribed to one side
- Extending to margins
- Epidermal and dermal

Patterns

Epidermis

- Large nests with confluence replacing the epidermis (consumption)
- Single melanocytes between nests in irregular distribution

Dermis

- Large nodules and sheets of melanocytes
- Some maturation

Cytology

- Large epithelioid and spindled melanocytes in the upper part
- Large melanocytes with little cytoplasm in the deeper part
- Large and pleomorphic, heterochromatic nuclei
- Mitoses, including atypical forms
- Zones of necrotic melanocytes

Other Changes

- Thinned epidermis with ulceration
- Some lymphocytic infiltrate

Integration

This lesion is malignant because of an asymmetric silhouette and a replacement of the epidermis by pleomorphic melanocytes with ulceration (Fig. 7.66a–c). In the dermis, large nodules and sheets of pleomorphic cells are irregularly distributed. Even though there is some maturation in the dermal part, the aggregations are large and irregularly shaped (Fig. 7.66c, d). While the cells qualify as spitzoid in the upper part of the lesion, in the lower part, the cells consist mostly of enlarged nuclei with little cytoplasm. Nuclei show crowding and mitoses including atypical forms as well as necrotic melanocytes are seen (Fig. 7.66e, f).

This lesion is the recurrence of the lesion shown in Example 2. The lesion came from the left dorsal thigh of a 56-year-old man. Even though complete excision for Example 2 had been recommended, it was not performed and the lesion regrew in a period of 9 months. In this excision of the recurrence, the diagnosis of melanoma is obvious and it gives the chance to reconsider the weighting of criteria for diagnosis in Example 2. In fact the single melanocytes between nests in Example 2 are really numerous, which is best appreciated in the MelanA stain (Fig. 7.65c). In the setting of a partial biopsy, predominance of single cells over nests, even in foci, is a strong hint to melanoma.

Diagnosis: Spitzoid melanoma, ulcerated.

7.3.1.3 Example 3: Punch Biopsies of a Large Lesion on the Face

Punch Biopsy 1 (Fig. 7.67)

Punch Biopsy 2 (Fig. 7.68)

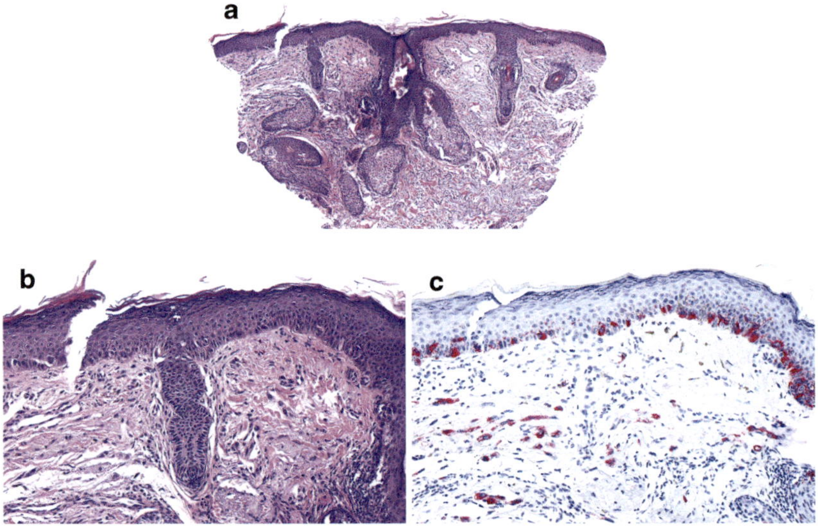

Fig. 7.67 (a–c) Partial biopsies, Example 3 (biopsy 1). (Courtesy of the Dermatologikum Hamburg)

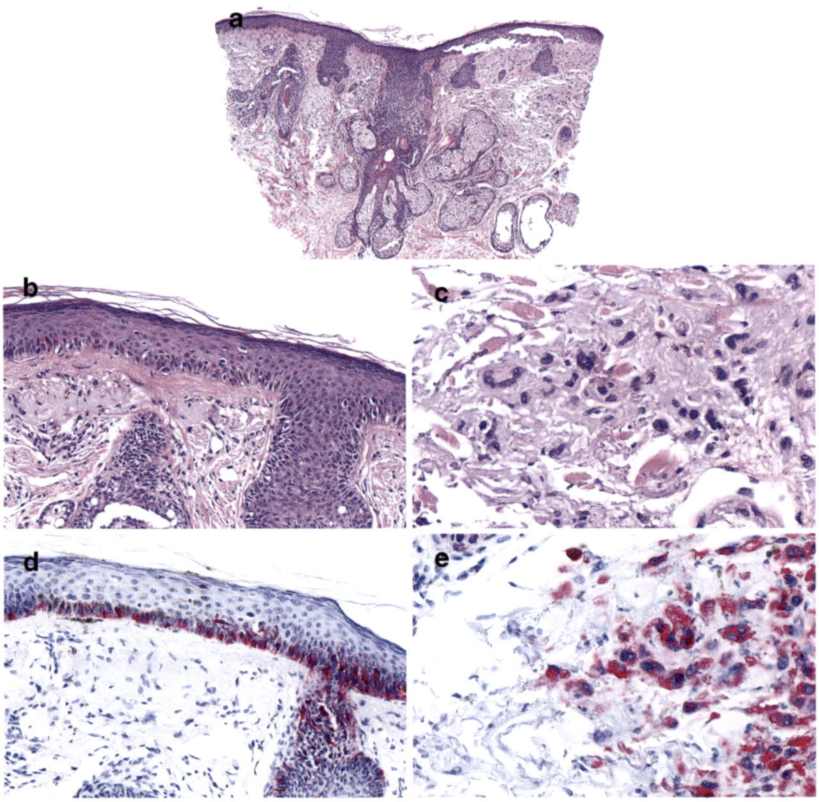

Fig. 7.68 (a–e) Partial biopsies, Example 3 (biopsy 2). (Courtesy of the Dermatologikum Hamburg)

Overall Pattern: Epidermal and Dermal, Irregular Single Melanocytes, Two Biopsies from One Lesion

Detailed Description

Silhouette

- Poorly circumscribed
- Epidermal and dermal

Patterns

Epidermis

- Single cells only
- Irregular distribution, few back-to-back melanocytes
- Few melanocytes in suprabasal layers

Adnexal epithelium

- Single melanocytes, irregularly distributed in the second biopsy

Dermis

- Scattered single melanocytes
- Irregular aggregations at the edge of the second biopsy

Cytology

- Enlarged with prominent dendrites
- Pleomorphic nuclei

Other Changes

- Solar elastosis
- Flattened rete ridges

Immunohistochemistry

- MelanA expression in pleomorphic cells in the epidermis and dermis (Figs. 7.67c and 7.68d, e)

Integration

The findings in these two biopsies taken from a large pigmented patch on the nose of an elderly woman are quite subtle at first sight. The density of melanocytes in the epidermis in the first biopsy is comparable to that seen in melanocytic hyperplasia on sun-damaged skin (Fig. 7.67a–c). Only a few suprabasal melanocytes and prominent and elongated dendrites are suspicious for a melanoma in situ. The dermal cells could be easily misconstrued as fibroblasts, histiocytes, or endothelial cells (Fig. 7.67b), but they express MelanA, so that they can either be melanocytes or dendritic cells with aberrant MelanA expression (Fig. 7.67c). However, these cells in the dermis are pleomorphic and epithelioid rather than dendritic so that they are better interpreted as melanocytes. Together with the second biopsy, the interpretation of the lesion becomes easier. Here the single melanocytes also involve adnexal epithelia in irregular fashion (Fig. 7.68b, d) and the dermal proliferation is denser, at least at one edge of the biopsy (Fig. 7.68c, e). This pattern is not compatible with dendritic cells with aberrant MelanA expression, so that the only possible conclusion is an invasive melanoma.

Diagnosis: Invasive melanoma on sun-damaged skin, biopsies.

Excision (Fig. 7.69)

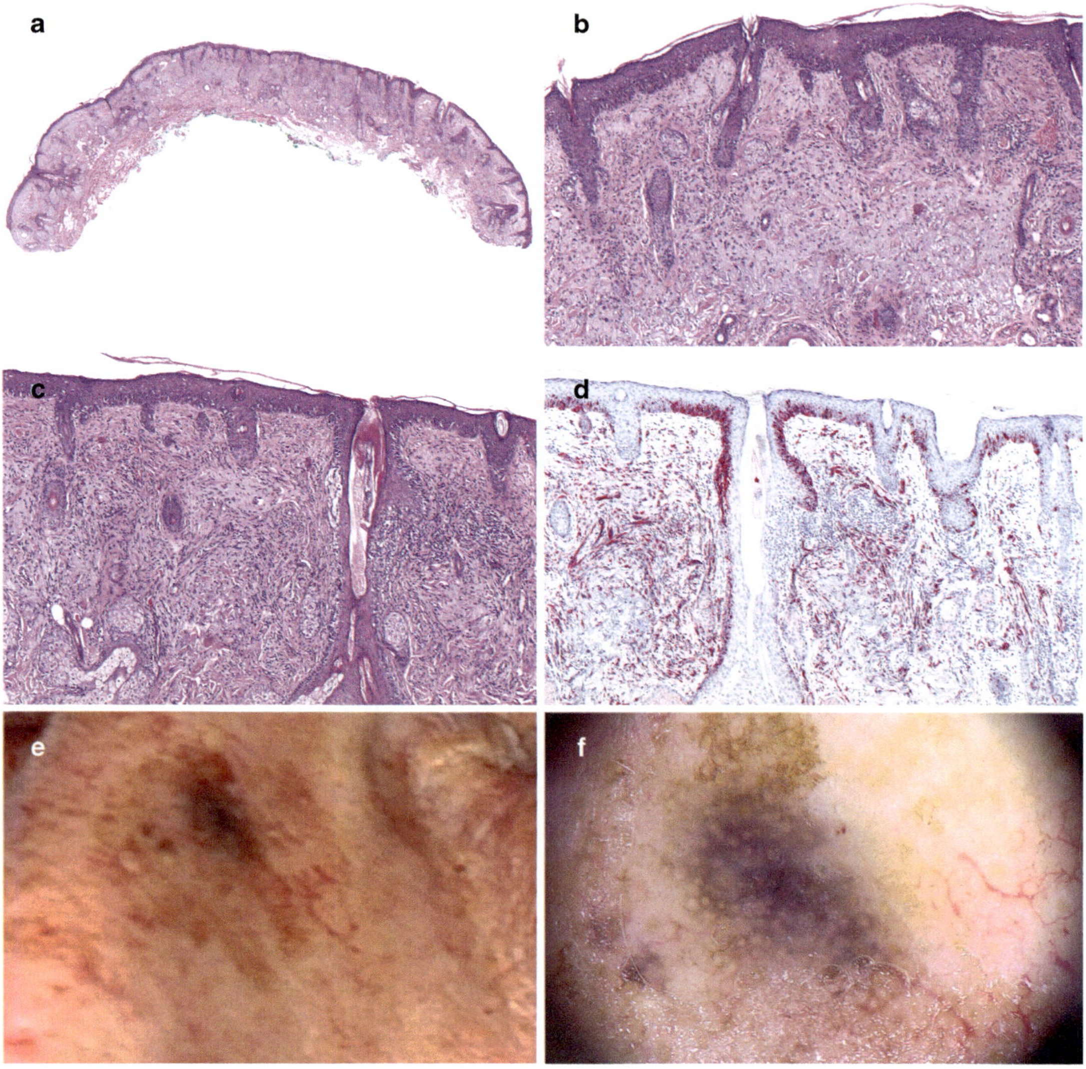

Fig. 7.69 (**a**–**f**) Partial biopsies, Example 3 (follow-up). (Courtesy of the Dermatologikum Hamburg)

Overall Pattern: Epidermal and Dermal, Irregular Single Melanocytes

Detailed Description

Silhouette
- Poorly circumscribed
- Epidermal and dermal

Patterns

Epidermis
- Single cells only
- Irregular distribution, back-to-back melanocytes
- Some melanocytes in suprabasal layers

Adnexal epithelium
- Single melanocytes and nests, irregularly distributed
- Involvement of deeper parts of follicular and sebaceous epithelium

Dermis
- Scattered single melanocytes
- Interstitial strands and fascicles
- Irregular aggregations

Cytology
- Enlarged with prominent dendrites in the epidermis
- Epithelioid and spindled in the dermis
- Pleomorphic nuclei

Other Changes
- Flattened rete ridges
- Fibrosis
- Solar elastosis
- Patchy lymphocytic infiltrate

Immunohistochemistry
On MelanA (Fig. 7.69d) positivity in irregular epidermal melanocytes and prominent expression in adnexal structures in the form of single melanocytes and nests. Extensive interstitial expression in the dermis

Integration
This is the excisional specimen (Fig. 7.69a–c) of the patient whose two biopsies were presented in the preceding pictures (Figs. 7.67, and 7.68). The diagnosis of invasive melanoma is now obvious, here with desmoplastic features in the dermis (Fig. 7.69c, d). The clinical picture shows the difficulty of differentiation between solar lentigo with evolving seborrheic keratosis from melanoma in sun-damaged skin of the face (Fig. 7.69e, f). For this reason, the two biopsies were taken prior to complete excision of the lesion. In direct comparison, this is an instructive example to understand the selectivity of a biopsy procedure, i.e., that findings in a small biopsy can be quite subtle (Fig. 7.67) even though the lesion is an obvious melanoma on excision. Imagine you had only the first biopsy and no MelanA staining at hand, how easy it would be to misread this as sun-damaged skin with some melanocytic hyperplasia. This reinforces the need for full clinical information, size of a lesion, evolution of a lesion, site and age of the patient when interpreting a small biopsy. It also illustrates the tremendous contribution of immunohistochemistry in such instances. In the first biopsy it was the expression of MelanA in the dermal cells (Fig. 7.67c) that attracted the eye to study more closely the cytology of these cells, which is clearly beyond what is acceptable as “dermal dendritic cells with aberrant MelanA expression.”

Diagnosis: Invasive melanoma on sun-damaged skin.

7.3.1.4 Example 4: Small Nests and Single Melanocytes, Biopsy of a Large Lesion (Fig. 7.70)

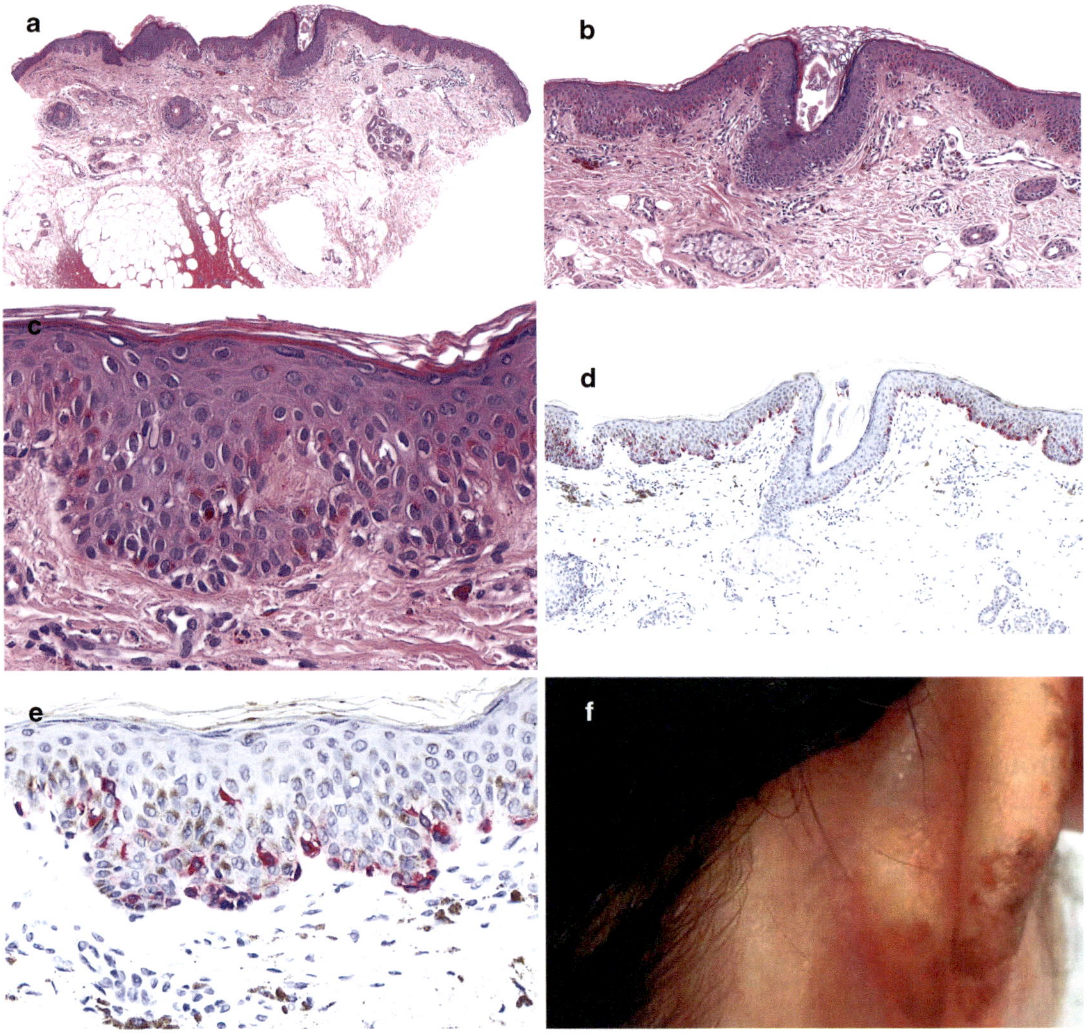

Fig. 7.70 (**a**–**f**) Partial biopsies, Example 4. (Courtesy of the Dermatologikum Hamburg)

Overall Pattern: Epidermal Only, Single Cells Predominate, Biopsy

Detailed Description

Silhouette

- Epidermal only
- Punch biopsy, circumscription cannot be assessed

Patterns

Epidermis

- Single melanocytes increased at the base of rete ridges, evenly distributed
- Few nests at the junction

Dermis

- None

Cytology

- Small, monomorphous

Other Changes

- Epidermal hyperplasia with elongated rete ridges
- Basal hyperpigmentation
- Melanophages

Immunohistochemistry

- MelanA expressed at the junction, at the base of rete ridges in single melanocytes and incipient nests, few melanocytes positive in the middle of the epidermis (Fig. 7.70d, e)

Integration

Epidermal hyperplasia with elongated rete ridges is impressive in this section. At intermediate magnification, a subtle melanocytic lesion is discernible. Intraepidermal melanocytes are seen only in the basal layer and with even distribution (Fig. 7.70b, c). The biopsy comes from the ear as it can be concluded from the number and size of vellus follicles. On MelanA staining, few melanocytes seem to be present in the middle of the epidermis, but they actually represent basal melanocytes at adjacent high-reaching dermal papillae (Fig. 7.70d, e). In general, any proliferation of single melanocytes on facial skin should be treated with suspicion especially when only a small biopsy is available and information on size and evolution of the lesion should be requested if not provided with the specimen. This lesion had been present since birth and clinical presentation is typical of a nevus spilus (Fig. 7.70f). Without the clinical picture, a definite diagnosis is difficult, but in the absence of solar elastosis and with preserved and elongated rete ridges and regular distribution of melanocytes at the base of rete ridges, the diagnosis of a lentiginous junctional nevus should also be favored on histopathology with a comment that correlation with clinical appearance is necessary.

Diagnosis: Lentiginous junctional nevus, biopsy, clinically Nevus spilus.

7.3.2 Newborns, Babies, and Children

It is sometimes assumed that age should have no influence on our decisions. Indeed, it is difficult to understand why the same lesion diagnosed as "Spitz nevus" or "atypical Spitz tumor" in a child should be melanoma in an adult. However, there is a reason for this, and it is the base rate. Melanoma is extremely rare in prepubertal children, and this must be taken into account. All other things being equal, children are much less likely to have melanoma than adults, and it would be a mistake to discount the base rate. Spitzoid lesions are the most common diagnostic problem in children. In addition, deep penetrating nevi and blue nevi can also cause problems, and we refer to the relevant examples in the subchapters. Furthermore, epidermal parts of congenital nevi when biopsied during the first year of life may mimic melanoma with irregular nests and single cells in higher levels of the epidermis. Another differential diagnosis, although less common, is the distinction between proliferative nodules and melanoma developing in a congenital nevus. Historically, the likelihood of melanoma developing in congenital nevus has been slightly overestimated due to selection bias that can be attributed to retrospective study designs. However, the rarity of melanoma diagnosis and the fact that most difficult decisions involve deep dermal lesions make diagnosis of lesions in children particularly challenging.

7.3.2.1 Example 1: Lesion of a 3-Week-Old Infant (Fig. 7.71)

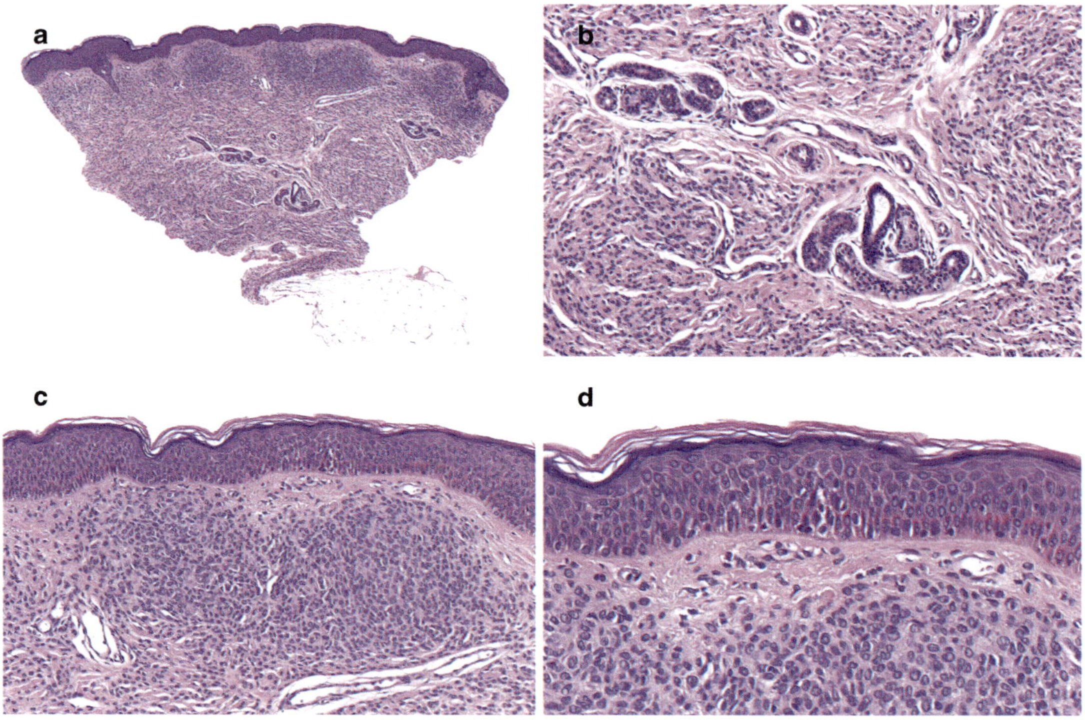

Fig. 7.71 (a–f) Newborns, babies, and children, Example 1. (Courtesy of the Dermatologikum Hamburg)

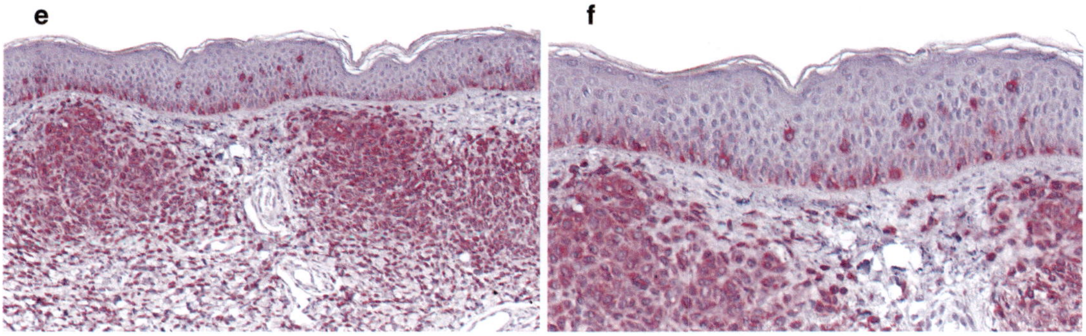

Fig. 7.71 (continued)

Overall Pattern: Large Nests and Interstitial Strands in the Entire Dermis

Detailed Description

Silhouette
- Entire dermis
- Biopsy

Patterns

Epidermis
- Single melanocytes in the basal layer, irregularly distributed, few cells above the junction

Dermis
- Large ill-defined nests in the upper dermis
- Interstitial strands filling the entire dermis
- Maturation

Subcutis
- Interstitial strands extending from the deep dermis into subcutaneous septa

Cytology
- Monomorphic, lymphocytoid with little cytoplasm and small, roundish nuclei
- Smaller nuclei in the deeper dermis/subcutis

Other Changes
- Flattened rete ridges

Integration
Without any clinical information it is not so easy to think of a melanocytic lesion in this biopsy in the first place. The interstitial distribution of cells in the dermis with sparing of a small subepidermal band of uninvolved connective tissue may call to mind leukemic infiltration of the skin, but a vaguely nested arrangement in the upper dermis and maturation of cells in the dermis is suggestive of a congenital nevus (Fig. 7.71a–c). The proliferation involves the superficial subcutis as can be concluded from the position of eccrine coils, which are densely surrounded by the proliferation (Fig. 7.71c). MelanA stain confirms the melanocytic nature of the lesion but also identifies an intraepidermal proliferation of single melanocytes with several melanocytes above the junction (Fig. 7.71d–f). This biopsy comes from a 3-week-old infant with a large congenital nevus. Suprabasal melanocytes are often seen in congenital nevi shortly after birth and they must not be mistaken for evolving melanoma in situ in that age.

Diagnosis: Congenital nevus, deep, shortly after birth, biopsy.

7.3.2.2 Example 2: Lesion of a 9-Week-Old Infant (Fig. 7.72)

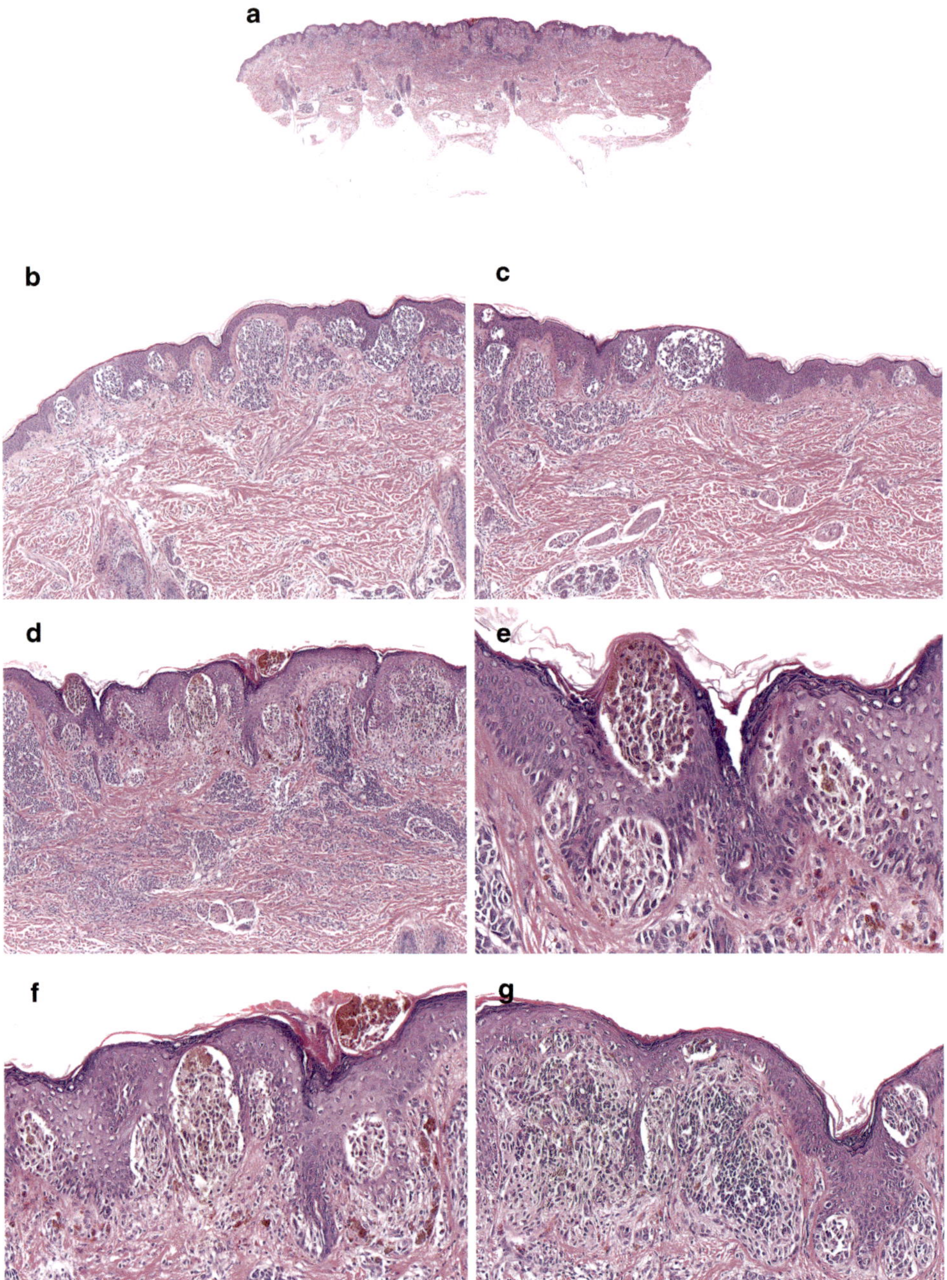

Fig. 7.72 (**a**–**i**) Newborns, babies, and children, Example 2. (Courtesy of the Dermatologikum Hamburg)

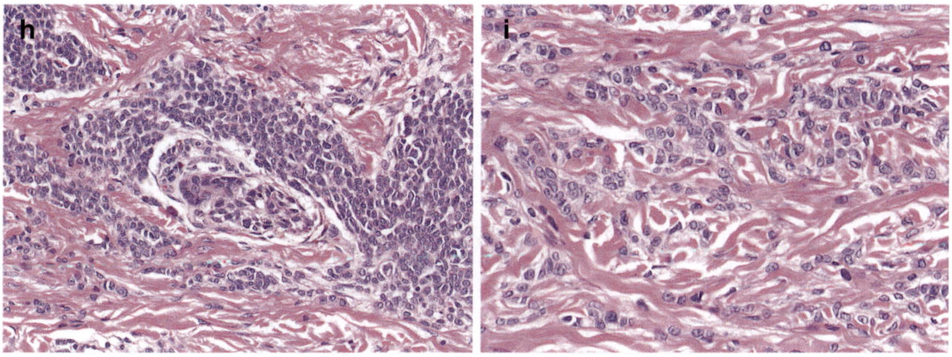

Fig. 7.72 (continued)

Overall Pattern: Asymmetric, Epidermal and Dermal, Nested and Interstitial

Detailed Description

Silhouette

- Asymmetric
- Epidermal and dermal
- Well circumscribed

Patterns

Epidermis

- Nested
- Variable size of nests with some large nests
- Nests in suprabasal layers including the cornified layer
- Heavy pigmentation of some intraepidermal nests

Adnexal epithelium

- Nests in eccrine ductal epithelium

Dermis

- Nests in the upper dermis
- Interstitial and periadnexal strands in the mid and deeper dermis
- Myotropism
- Maturation

Cytology

- Two populations of melanocytes: one slightly epithelioid without pigment, the other larger with strongly pigmented cytoplasm
- Each population monomorphic

Other Changes

- Acanthosis and hypergranulosis
- Irregular distribution of melanophages
- Increased interstitial fibroblasts

Integration

The nested pattern in the epidermis and periadnexal and interstitial pattern in the dermis identify the lesion as a congenital nevus (Fig. 7.72a, c, d, i). There are also melanocytes in eccrine ductal epithelium (Fig. 7.72i). and within arrector pili muscle (Fig. 7.72d). and there is maturation, which also indicates a congenital nevus. However, the lesion is asymmetric, because of a second population of melanocytes, which is heavily pigmented (Fig. 7.72g). Within the epidermis, the pigmented melanocytes form nests, but some are very large and some are present in suprabasal layers (Fig. 7.72d–g). For a melanoma developing in a congenital nevus, a predominantly nested pattern would be unusual, because melanoma in situ almost always shows numerous single melanocytes. Therefore, the lesion is best interpreted as a combined congenital nevus. The unusual epidermal component is explained by the fact that this lesion comes from a very small child, a 9-week-old infant. The increased number of fibroblasts in the dermis is a hint to the skin of a baby.

Diagnosis: Combined congenital nevus in a 9-week-old infant.

7.3.2.3 Example 3: Dermal Lesion with Thin Epidermis in a Child (Fig. 7.73)

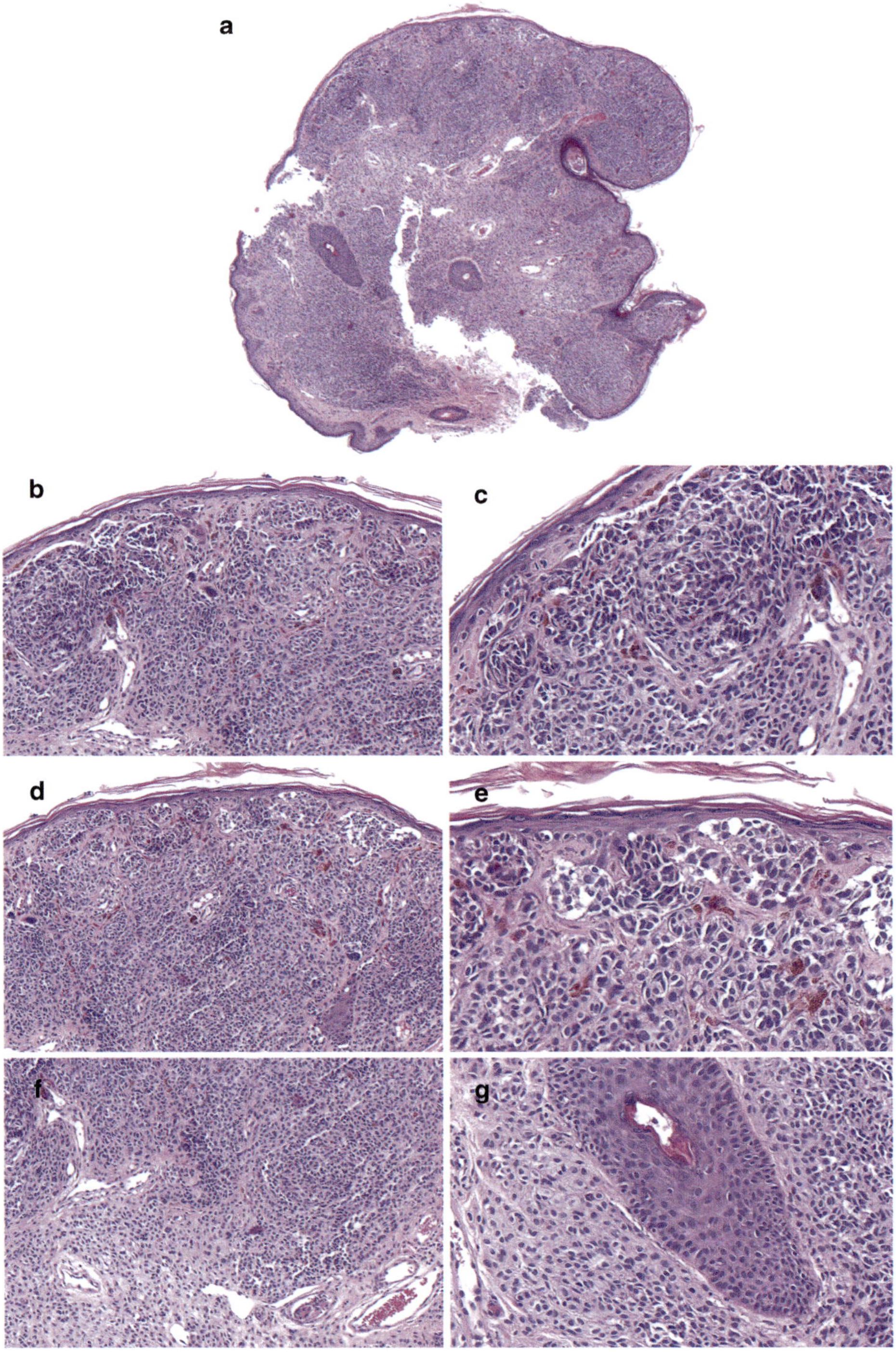

Fig. 7.73 (**a**–**j**) Newborns, babies, and children, Example 3. (Courtesy of the Dermatologikum Hamburg)

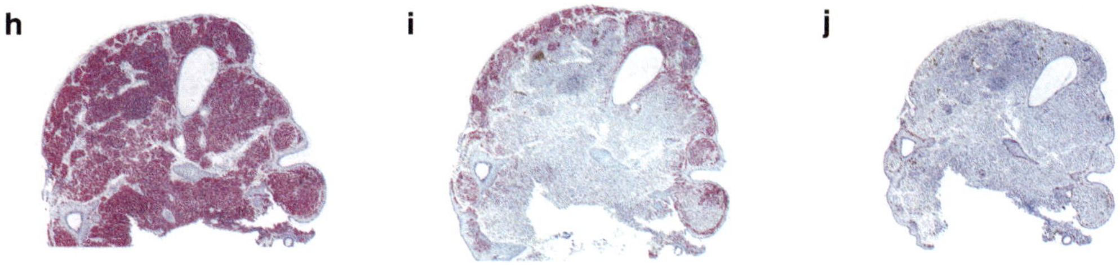

Fig. 7.73 (continued)

Overall Pattern: Polypoid, Largely Dermal, Adnexocentric

Detailed description

Silhouette

- Polypoid, largely dermal

Patterns

Epidermis

- Few nests at the junction
- Single melanocytes in the basal layer of the epidermis, regularly distributed

Dermis

- Nests in the upper dermis
- Periadnexal and interstitial strands in the deeper dermis
- Maturation

Cytology

- Epithelioid in the upper dermis
- Small in the deeper dermis
- Some variation in size and shape of nuclei, but with homogenous chromatin
- Some multinucleated melanocytes

Other Changes

- Thin epidermis
- Adnexal epithelial hyperplasia with cystic dilation of infundibula
- Melanophages
- Dilated vessels

Immunohistochemistry

- MelanA highlights the dermal distribution of melanocytes with nesting in the upper part and interstitial and periadnexal arrangement below (Fig. 7.73h). The epidermal involvement is minimal with few nests and single cells in the basal epidermis.
- HMB 45 demonstrates a loss of immunoreactivity with progressive descent in the dermis (Fig. 7.73i).
- No expression of Ki67 is seen in the dermal proliferation of melanocytes (Fig. 7.73j).

Integration

This largely dermal lesion with a nested and interstitial pattern in the dermis and maturation is typical of a dermal nevus (Fig. 7.73a), but the epidermis is thin, simulating the pattern of "consumption" (Fig. 7.73b–e). Close inspection shows that there is minimal epidermal involvement with regularly distributed single melanocytes and few nests in the basal layer. The thinning of the dermis seen here is sometimes encountered in exophytic, polypoid dermal nevi and it should not be misconstrued as consumption. The moderate variation in size and shape of nuclei and some multinucleation are a common finding in dermal melanocytic nevi (Fig. 7.73c, e, g). The adnexocentric arrangement is typical of a congenital nevus. This lesion comes from an 11-year-old child.

Diagnosis: Dermal nevus, congenital.

7.3.2.4 Example 4: Nodule Arising in a Congenital Nevus in a Newborn (Fig. 7.74)

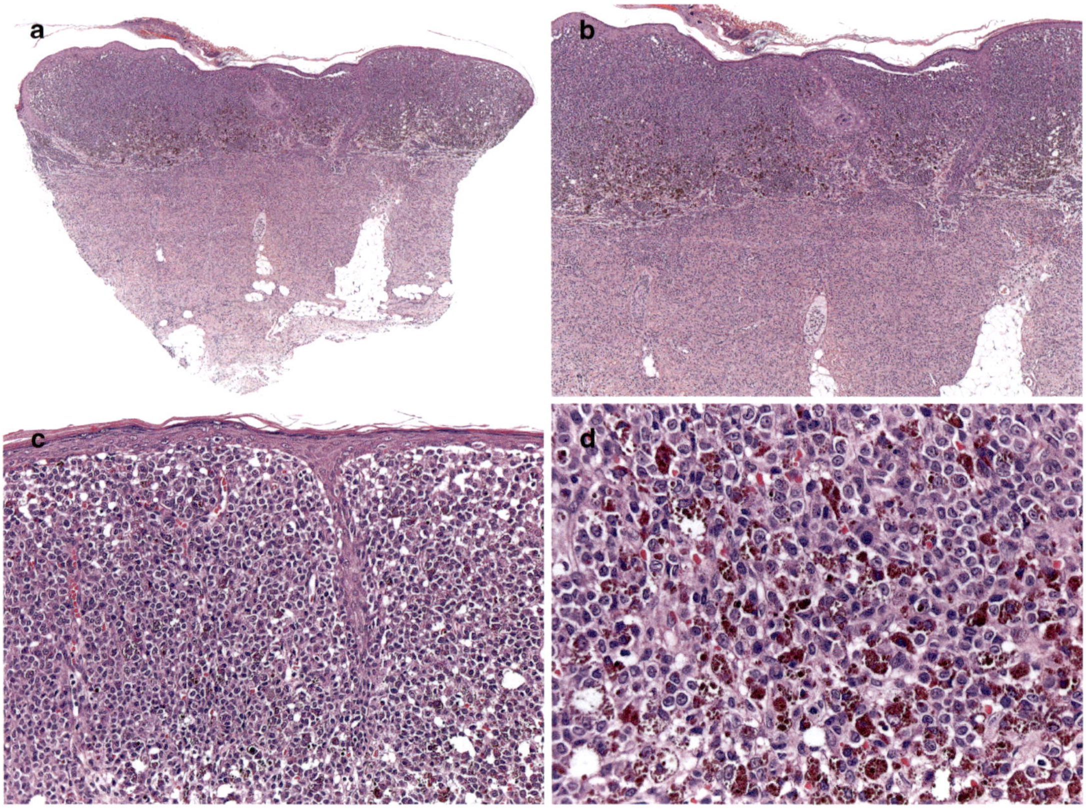

Fig. 7.74 (**a–d**) Newborns, babies, and children, Example 4. (*Images courtesy of Lorenzo Cerroni*. All Rights Reserved)

Overall Pattern: Dermal and Subcutis, Nodules and Sheets

Detailed Description

Silhouette

- Entire dermis and subcutis
- Biopsy

Patterns

Dermis

- Sheets of melanocytes in the upper dermis
- Nests and strands of melanocytes in the deep dermis

Subcutis

- Interstitial strands extending from the deep dermis into subcutaneous septa

Cytology

- Epithelioid melanocytes (upper dermis)
- Monomorphic, lymphocytoid with little cytoplasm and small, roundish nuclei (deeper dermis and subcutis)

Other Changes

- Flattened rete ridges

Integration

Given the clinical description and that the patient is a newborn, the findings are best interpreted as a proliferative nodule in a congenital nevus. The congenital nevus is visible underneath the proliferative nodule (Fig. 7.74a, b). The nodule is typified by sheets of enlarged melanocytes and admixed melanophages (Fig. 7.74c, d).

Diagnosis: Proliferative nodule in a congenital nevus of a newborn.

Bias, Noise, and Error

8

Bias and noise are not the same thing. In colloquial language, the term bias is often used to refer to an unreasonable judgment or prejudice. In the field of statistics, however, bias is a systematic error. For our purposes, it is best to follow the definition of Kahnemann et al. [186]. According to Kahnemann, bias is "the average error in judgments," or put another way, "If you look at many judgments and the errors in those judgments are all in the same direction, that's bias." A dermatopathologist who tends to call Spitz nevi melanomas is biased towards a melanoma diagnosis. Noise, on the other hand, is "random error in any direction," or the variability of error. For example, if five out of ten dermatopathologists refer to the same lesion as a "Spitz nevus" while the other five refer to it as melanoma, this is noise. This type of noise is often referred to as inter-rater variability. Another type of noise, called "occasion noise," occurs when the same observer calls the same lesion a Spitz nevus on one day and a melanoma on another. We refer to this type of noise as intra-rater variability. In general, bias and noise are undesirable, and both lead to errors. However, a certain amount of noise must be accepted and may even be desirable, because if there is no noise at all, the judgments are likely to be extremely biased.

Inter-rater and intra-rater *variability* of pathologists was measured for melanocytic proliferations and was found to be substantial [1]. What is the reason for this large amount of noise? One reason, which hopefully became clear after reading the book, is the large variability in the appearance of melanoma, both clinically and pathologically. No two melanomas look alike, and every melanoma is slightly different. In addition, there is morphologic and biologic overlap between nevi and melanomas, and the expression of features used to distinguish melanomas from nevi is variable. If all melanomas were identical and melanoma and nevi were defined by a single, unambiguous feature, the noise would be low and diagnosis would be as simple as distinguishing between red and blue socks. This intrinsic noise is unavoidable. However, there is also noise that is man-made and avoidable. It is the result of inconsistent definitions, inadequately defined criteria, and overlapping and nonexclusive categories. Following a checklist or algorithm is an easy way to reduce noise, and there is evidence of this within and outside of medicine [186]. Pattern analysis is our version of such a checklist or algorithm. Another measure to reduce noise is to eliminate poorly defined and nonexclusive categories that are too granular. In a recent attempt to simplify the classification of basal cell carcinoma, we found that there was little agreement among experts regarding the subtypes of micronodular, infiltrating, and sclerosing basal cell carcinoma [187]. All three subtypes have a relatively high risk of recurrence. Once we decided to combine all three subtypes into a single class, infiltrative basal cell carcinoma,

A. Böer-Auer et al., *Pattern Analysis for Histopathologic Diagnosis of Melanocytic Lesions*,
https://doi.org/10.1007/978-3-031-07666-4_8

inter-reviewer agreement increased substantially. The resulting classification was easier to use, less noisy, and still conveyed the important distinction between low-risk and high-risk basal cell carcinomas. As indicated in Chap. 3, the currently applied classifications of melanocytic proliferations would benefit from such a revision. Unfortunately, reduction of noise is not usually an important criterion in establishing classifications, although it should be.

Bias is easier to detect than noise. Bias in the form of systematic overdiagnosis of melanoma is common. There may be many reasons for this, including economic incentives and fear of litigation. Diagnosing more melanomas can be profitable for clinicians and pathologists alike. More melanomas mean more excisions, which in turn mean more specimens. We do not mean to imply that this is the main reason for systematic overdiagnosis of melanoma, but it cannot be completely disregarded. Another important reason for bias is fear. In some parts of the world, susceptibility to malpractice suits leads to excessive anxiety, resulting in excessively low thresholds and overdiagnosis [2]. There are other reasons for systematic overdiagnosis or underdiagnosis of melanoma that have to do with specific exposure to ideas and concepts during dermatopathology training. Our mentors shape our thinking, for better or worse. There are several schools of thought in the field of dermatopathology, and some controversies, particularly those surrounding the "dysplastic nevus," "Spitz tumors," and "melanoma in situ" have been long-lasting. Many of these controversies did not lead to a consensus but to the formation of irreconcilable camps with extreme rejection of each other's points of view. Even today there are still after-effects of these trench wars although the main protagonists are long gone. This often leads to distorted opinions. One's own point of view is vigorously defended and the arguments of the opposing side are not taken seriously or are simply ignored. In our opinion, this form of distorted perception is very common and no one is immune to it. The best antidote is openness to the ideas of others and a principled willingness to criticize one's own concepts with the same vigor as the concepts of others.

Apart from noise or bias, errors can result from mishandling or mix-up of specimens, intentional or unintentional deviation from good practice, poor judgment, or incomplete or incorrect information. Mishandling of specimens and mix-ups can occur in the referring physician's office, during transport of the specimen to the laboratory, in the laboratory, in the pathology examination room, or during dictation or writing of the report. Many mix-ups are noticed by pathologists because the diagnosis or the anatomic site indicated on the referral slip does not match the microscopic findings. Sometimes, however, mix-ups go unnoticed. Typically, safety precautions and standard procedures such as dual control (i.e., the requirement that two people approve a particular procedure before it can be performed) are in place in every laboratory to minimize the risk of mix-ups. Sometimes these standard procedures and safeguards are not followed for reasons such as lack of time, incompetence, negligence, or hubris. Poor judgment can occur at any time, and no one is immune, not even experts. Common reasons include distraction and fatigue. Finally, incomplete or incorrect information, such as the referring physician's failure to point out that a particular specimen is only a small part of a clinically larger lesion or the pathologist's failure to examine every piece of tissue on the slide, are common reasons for errors.

The following list is a loose collection of simple rules that should help you to minimize noise, bias, and error:

- Check if the slide number of the specimen matches the slide number on the referral slip.
- Look at the slide unbiased first. Do not let yourself be primed by information on the referral slip or by other opinions.
- Count the number of pieces on the slide and look at all the pieces.
- Look at all parts of the tissue including the subcutaneous fat.
- Use low power first but have at least one look with high power too (blink and think).

- Once you have looked at the slide, check if the information on the referral slip (diagnosis, anatomic site, sampling technique) matches the findings on the slide.
- Do not force an immediate decision. Deeper sections are obligatory if unsure.
- If unsure, use every bit of information you can get, including in vivo images.
- If the referring clinician sent you an image, look at it.
- If the referring clinician does not send you images by default, ask for it.
- Do not force a decision. If you cannot call it, do not call it.
- If you cannot make a decision, sleep over it.
- Discuss difficult cases with colleagues.
- If you read a difficult lesion in the group, everybody should be given an unbiased opportunity to evaluate the lesion independently.
- Be observant if somebody wants to manipulate the group towards a certain decision. If you realize such a situation, speak up and ignore hierarchies (a very hard thing to do).
- Do not rely too much on one piece of information such as molecular aberrations.
- Know your referral physicians. Talk with them if a situation is unclear.
- Use standard protocols, checklists, and a reliable method like pattern analysis.
- Do not base your decision on economic or legal aspects. The most important person is the patient, not you.
- Be aware of reasons for over- and underdiagnosis.
- Be aware of pitfalls.
- Know your weaknesses.
- Employ personal rules such as: if the referral diagnosis is lentigo maligna, perform immunostains—and stick to them.
- If you make a mistake, admit it and do not try to cover it up. Everyone reporting melanocytic skin lesions is making mistakes—constantly.
- Defend your opinion but also listen to others. Embrace the outside view.
- If you are tired, do not continue.
- Seek training in clinical dermatology and dermatoscopy.

8.1 Last Words

Like most scientists, we are critical realists and believe that there is an objective reality out there that can be studied by the human endeavor we call science. However, there is also a certain amount of objective ignorance that will never completely disappear. There are always things we cannot know even if we knew everything. That is, even if we knew every base pair, every epigenetic change, and every function of every molecule in a given melanocytic proliferation, our knowledge will still be incomplete. We will always have to make critical decisions with incomplete information, and despite our best intentions and abilities, we may err. That is only human. However, if we are willing to learn from mistakes instead of hiding them, then the words of Francis Bacon become true: "Truth emerges more readily from error than from confusion."

References

1. Elmore JG, Barnhill RL, Elder DE, Longton GM, Pepe MS, Reisch LM, et al. Pathologists' diagnosis of invasive melanoma and melanocytic proliferations: observer accuracy and reproducibility study. BMJ. 2017;357:j2813.
2. Kittler H. Evolution of the clinical, dermoscopic and pathologic diagnosis of melanoma. Dermatol Pract Concept. 2021;11:e2021163S.
3. Weyers W. Screening for malignant melanoma—a critical assessment in historical perspective. Dermatol Pract Concept. 2018;8:89–103.
4. Ackerman LV. Malignant melanoma of the skin; clinical and pathologic analysis of 75 cases. Am J Clin Pathol. 1948;18:602–24.
5. Allen AC, Spitz S. Malignant melanoma; a clinicopathological analysis of the criteria for diagnosis and prognosis. Cancer. 1953;6:1–45.
6. Clark WH Jr, From L, Bernardino EA, Mihm MC. The histogenesis and biologic behavior of primary human malignant melanomas of the skin. Cancer Res. 1969;29:705–27.
7. Mihm MC, Clark WH, From L. The clinical diagnosis, classification and histogenetic concepts of the early stages of cutaneous malignant melanomas. N Engl J Med. 1971;284:1078–82. https://doi.org/10.1056/NEJM197105132841907.
8. McGovern VJ, Mihm MC Jr, Bailly C, Booth JC, Clark WH Jr, Cochran AJ, et al. The classification of malignant melanoma and its histologic reporting. Cancer. 1973;32:1446–57.
9. Breslow A. Thickness, cross-sectional areas and depth of invasion in the prognosis of cutaneous melanoma. Ann Surg. 1970;172(5):902–8. https://doi.org/10.1097/00000658-197011000-00017.
10. Breslow A. Tumor thickness in evaluating prognosis of cutaneous melanoma. Ann Surg. 1978;187(4):440. https://doi.org/10.1097/00000658-197804000-00020.
11. Price NM, Rywlin AM, Ackerman AB. Histologic criteria for the diagnosis of superficial spreading malignant melanoma: formulated on the basis of proven metastatic lesions. Cancer. 1976;38:2434–41.
12. Goldsmith LA, Askin FB, Chang AE, Cohen C, Dutcher JP, Gilgor RS, et al. Diagnosis and treatment of early melanoma: NIH consensus development panel on early melanoma. JAMA. 1992;268:1314–9.
13. Ferrara G, Argenziano G, Soyer HP, D'Argenio P, Carli P, Cerroni L, et al. Histopathologic interobserver agreement on the diagnosis of melanocytic skin lesions with equivocal dermoscopic features: a pilot study. Tumori. 2000;86:445–9.
14. Lodha S, Saggar S, Celebi JT, Silvers DN. Discordance in the histopathologic diagnosis of difficult melanocytic neoplasms in the clinical setting. J Cutan Pathol. 2008;35:349–52.
15. Shoo BA, Sagebiel RW, Kashani-Sabet M. Discordance in the histopathologic diagnosis of melanoma at a melanoma referral center. J Am Acad Dermatol. 2010;62:751–6.
16. Gerami P, Busam K, Cochran A, Cook MG, Duncan LM, Elder DE, et al. Histomorphologic assessment and interobserver diagnostic reproducibility of atypical spitzoid melanocytic neoplasms with long-term follow-up. Am J Surg Pathol. 2014;38:934–40.
17. Pusiol T, Morichetti D, Piscioli F, Zorzi MG. Theory and practical application of superficial atypical melanocytic proliferations of uncertain significance (SAMPUS) and melanocytic tumours of uncertain malignant potential (MELTUMP) terminology: experience with second opinion consultation. Pathologica. 2012;104:70–7.
18. Gaynor R, Herschman HR, Irie R, Jones P, Morton D, Cochran A. S100 protein: a marker for human malignant melanomas? Lancet. 1981;1:869–71.
19. Nakajima T, Watanabe S, Sato Y, Kameya T. Immunohistochemical demonstration of S100 protein in malignant melanoma and pigmented nevus, and its diagnostic application. Cancer. 1982;50(5):912–8. https://acsjournals.onlinelibrary.wiley.com/doi/abs/10.1002/1097-0142(19820901)50:5%3C912::AID-CNCR2820500519%3E3.0.CO;2-U
20. Springall DR, Gu J, Cocchia D, Michetti F, Levene A, Levene MM, et al. The value of S-100 immunostaining as a diagnostic tool in human malignant melanomas. A comparative study using S-100 and neuron-specific enolase antibodies. Virchows Arch A Pathol Anat Histopathol. 1983;400:331–43.

A. Böer-Auer et al., *Pattern Analysis for Histopathologic Diagnosis of Melanocytic Lesions*, https://doi.org/10.1007/978-3-031-07666-4

21. Davies H, Bignell GR, Cox C, Stephens P, Edkins S, Clegg S, et al. Mutations of the BRAF gene in human cancer. Nature. 2002;417:949–54.
22. Curtin JA, Fridlyand J, Kageshita T, Patel HN, Busam KJ, Kutzner H, et al. Distinct sets of genetic alterations in melanoma. N Engl J Med. 2005;353:2135–47.
23. Hodis E, Watson IR, Kryukov GV, Arold ST, Imielinski M, Theurillat J-P, et al. A landscape of driver mutations in melanoma. Cell. 2012;150:251–63.
24. Hayward NK, Wilmott JS, Waddell N, Johansson PA, Field MA, Nones K, et al. Whole-genome landscapes of major melanoma subtypes. Nature. 2017;545:175–80.
25. Karasarides M, Chiloeches A, Hayward R, Niculescu-Duvaz D, Scanlon I, Friedlos F, et al. B-RAF is a therapeutic target in melanoma. Oncogene. 2004;23:6292–8.
26. Gerami P, Scolyer RA, Xu X, Elder DE, Abraham RM, Fullen D, et al. Risk assessment for atypical spitzoid melanocytic neoplasms using FISH to identify chromosomal copy number aberrations. Am J Surg Pathol. 2013;37:676–84.
27. Miedema J, Andea AA. Through the looking glass and what you find there: making sense of comparative genomic hybridization and fluorescence in situ hybridization for melanoma diagnosis. Mod Pathol. 2020;33:1318–30.
28. Alomari AK, Miedema JR, Carter MD, Harms PW, Lowe L, Durham AB, et al. DNA copy number changes correlate with clinical behavior in melanocytic neoplasms: proposal of an algorithmic approach. Mod Pathol. 2020;33:1307–17.
29. Ferrara G, Argenyi Z, Argenziano G, Cerio R, Cerroni L, Di Blasi A, et al. The influence of clinical information in the histopathologic diagnosis of melanocytic skin neoplasms. PLoS One. 2009;4:e5375.
30. Elder DE, Massi D, Scolyer RA, Willemze R. WHO classification of skin tumours: WHO classification of tumours, vol. 11. Geneva: World Health Organization; 2018.
31. Muse ME, Bergman DT, Salas LA, Tom LN, Tan J-M, Laino A, et al. Genome-scale DNA methylation analysis identifies repeat element alterations that modulate the genomic stability of melanocytic nevi. J Invest Dermatol. 2022;142(7):1893–1902.e7.
32. Cazzato G, Colagrande A, Cimmino A, Arezzo F, Loizzi V, Caporusso C, et al. Artificial intelligence in dermatopathology: new insights and perspectives. Dermatopathology (Basel). 2021;8:418–25.
33. Masson P. Les naevi pigmentaires, tumeurs nerveuses. New York: Masson; 1926.
34. Unna PG. Naevi und Naevocarcinome. Berl Klin Wochenschr. 1893;30:14–6.
35. Bloch B. Das Problem der Pigmentbildung in der Haut. Arch Dermatol Syph. 1917;124:129–208.
36. Kinsler VA, Larue L. The patterns of birthmarks suggest a novel population of melanocyte precursors arising around the time of gastrulation. Pigment Cell Melanoma Res. 2018;31:95–109.
37. Stark MS, Tell-Martí G, Martins da Silva V, Martinez-Barrios E, Calbet-Llopart N, Vicente A, et al. The distinctive genomic landscape of giant congenital melanocytic nevi. J Invest Dermatol. 2021;141:692–695.e2.
38. Tan JM, Tom LN, Jagirdar K, Lambie D, Schaider H, Sturm RA, et al. The BRAF and NRAS mutation prevalence in dermoscopic subtypes of acquired naevi reveals constitutive mitogen-activated protein kinase pathway activation. Br J Dermatol. 2018;178:191–7.
39. Wiesner T, Kutzner H, Cerroni L, Mihm MC Jr, Busam KJ, Murali R. Genomic aberrations in spitzoid melanocytic tumours and their implications for diagnosis, prognosis and therapy. Pathology. 2016;48:113–31.
40. Van Raamsdonk CD, Bezrookove V, Green G, Bauer J, Gaugler L, O'Brien JM, et al. Frequent somatic mutations of GNAQ in uveal melanoma and blue naevi. Nature. 2009;457:599–602.
41. Gruis NA, Sandkuijl LA, van der Velden PA, Bergman W, Frants RR. CDKN2 explains part of the clinical phenotype in Dutch familial atypical multiple-mole melanoma (FAMMM) syndrome families. Melanoma Res. 1995;5:169–77.
42. Christodoulou E, Nell RJ, Verdijk RM, Gruis NA, van der Velden PA, van Doorn R. Loss of wild-type CDKN2A is an early event in the development of melanoma in FAMMM syndrome. J Invest Dermatol. 2020;140:2298–2301.e3.
43. Wiesner T, Obenauf AC, Murali R, Fried I, Griewank KG, Ulz P, et al. Germline mutations in BAP1 predispose to melanocytic tumors. Nat Genet. 2011;43:1018–21.
44. Pampena R, Kyrgidis A, Lallas A, Moscarella E, Argenziano G, Longo C. A meta-analysis of nevus-associated melanoma: prevalence and practical implications. J Am Acad Dermatol. 2017;77:938–945.e4.
45. Tschandl P, Berghoff AS, Preusser M, Burgstaller-Muehlbacher S, Pehamberger H, Okamoto I, et al. NRAS and BRAF mutations in melanoma-associated nevi and uninvolved nevi. PLoS One. 2013;8:e69639.
46. Tschandl P, Hofmann L, Fink C, Kittler H, Haenssle HA. Melanomas vs. nevi in high-risk patients under long-term monitoring with digital dermatoscopy: do melanomas and nevi already differ at baseline? J Eur Acad Dermatol Venereol. 2017;31:972–7.
47. Weyers W. The emperor's new clothes: a critique of the current WHO classification of malignant melanoma. Am J Dermatopathol. 2020;42:989–1002.
48. Mundra PA, Dhomen N, Rodrigues M, Mikkelsen LH, Cassoux N, Brooks K, et al. Ultraviolet radiation drives mutations in a subset of mucosal melanomas. Nat Commun. 2021;12:1–7.
49. Piepkorn MW, Barnhill RL, Elder DE, Knezevich SR, Carney PA, Reisch LM, et al. The MPATH-Dx reporting schema for melanocytic proliferations and melanoma. J Am Acad Dermatol. 2014;70:131–41.
50. Gershenwald JE, Scolyer RA, Hess KR, Sondak VK, Long GV, Ross MI, et al. Melanoma staging: evidence-based changes in the American Joint

Committee on Cancer eighth edition cancer staging manual. CA Cancer J Clin. 2017;67:472–92.
51. Welch HG, Mazer BL, Adamson AS. The rapid rise in cutaneous melanoma diagnoses. N Engl J Med. 2021;384:72–9.
52. Lallas A, Kyrgidis A, Ferrara G, Kittler H, Apalla Z, Castagnetti F, et al. Atypical Spitz tumours and sentinel lymph node biopsy: a systematic review. Lancet Oncol. 2014;15:e178–83.
53. Katz I, O'Brien B, Clark S, Thompson CT, Schapiro B, Azzi A, et al. Assessment of a diagnostic classification system for management of lesions to exclude melanoma. JAMA Netw Open. 2021;4:e2134614.
54. Amin MB, Edge SB, Greene FL, Byrd DR, Brookland RK, Washington MK, et al., editors. AJCC cancer staging manual. 8th ed. Cham: Springer; 2017.
55. Ackerman AB, Boër A, Bennin B, Gottlieb GJ. Histologic diagnosis of inflammatory skin diseases: an algorithmic method based on pattern analysis. New York: Ardor Scribendi; 2005.
56. Ackerman AB, Cerroni L, Kerl H. Pitfalls in histopathologic diagnosis of malignant melanoma. Philadelphia: Lea & Febiger; 1994.
57. Ackerman AB, Massi D, Nielsen TA. Dysplastic nevus: atypical mole or typical myth? New York: Ardor Scribendi; 1999.
58. Massi G, LeBoit PE. Histological diagnosis of nevi and melanoma. New York: Springer; 2013.
59. Barnhill R, Piepkorn M, Bahrami A, Böer-Auer A, Zembowicz A, Wiesner T. Tumors of melanocytes. In: Barnhill R, Neil Crowson A, Magro C, Piepkorn M, Kutzner H, Desman G, editors. Barnhill's dermatopathology. 4th ed. New York: McGraw Hill/Medical; 2019. p. 786–895.
60. Zembowicz A, Kafanas A. Syringotropic melanoma: a variant of melanoma with prominent involvement of eccrine apparatus and risk of deep dermal invasion. Am J Dermatopathol. 2012;34:151–6.
61. Torre-Castro J, Haya-Martínez L, Moya-Martínez C, Núñez-Hipólito L, Mendoza-Cembranos MD, Sabaris MDCF, et al. Syringotropic melanoma: a diagnostic challenge with prognostic implications. Am J Dermatopathol. 2022;44:33–6.
62. Idriss MH, Rizwan L, Sferuzza A, Wasserman E, Kazlouskaya V, Elston DM. Nevoid melanoma: a study of 43 cases with emphasis on growth pattern. J Am Acad Dermatol. 2015;73:836–42.
63. Ackerman AB, Elish D, Shami S. "Spitz's nevus": reassessment critical, revision radical. New York: Ardor Scribendi; 2007.
64. Hu F. Melanocyte cytology in normal skin, melanocytic nevi, and malignant melanomas. Pathology of malignant melanoma. New York: Masson Publications; 1981. p. 1–21.
65. Kerl H, Soyer HP, Cerroni L, Wolf IH, Ackerman AB. Ancient melanocytic nevus. Semin Diagn Pathol. 1998;15:210–5.
66. Ruhoy SM, Kolker SE, Murry TC. Mitotic activity within dermal melanocytes of benign melanocytic nevi: a study of 100 cases with clinical follow-up. Am J Dermatopathol. 2011;33:167–72.
67. Ribero S, Moscarella E, Ferrara G, Piana S, Argenziano G, Longo C. Regression in cutaneous melanoma: a comprehensive review from diagnosis to prognosis. J Eur Acad Dermatol Venereol. 2016;30:2030–7.
68. Kittler H, Tschandl P. Dysplastic nevus: why this term should be abandoned in dermatoscopy. Dermatol Clin. 2013;31:579–88, viii.
69. Clark WH. The dysplastic nevus syndrome. Arch Dermatol. 1988;124(8):1207–10. https://doi.org/10.1001/archderm.124.8.1207.
70. Lynch HT, Shaw TG. Familial atypical multiple mole melanoma (FAMMM) syndrome: history, genetics, and heterogeneity. Fam Cancer. 2016;15:487–91.
71. Ji-Xu A, Dinnes J, Matin RN. Total body photography for the diagnosis of cutaneous melanoma in adults: a systematic review and meta-analysis. Br J Dermatol. 2021;185:302–12.
72. Grob JJ. The "Ugly Duckling" sign: identification of the common characteristics of nevi in an individual as a basis for melanoma screening. Arch Dermatol. 1998;134(1):103–4. https://doi.org/10.1001/archderm.134.1.103-a.
73. Grob JJ, Wazaefi Y, Bruneu Y, Gaudy-Marqueste C, Monestier S, Thomas L, et al. Diagnosis of melanoma: importance of comparative analysis and "ugly duckling" sign. J Clin Oncol. 2012;30:8578. https://doi.org/10.1200/jco.2012.30.15_suppl.8578.
74. Dobrosavljevic D, Brasanac D, Glumac S, Radojevic S, Matija L, Stanisavljevic D. Sensitivity and specificity of ex vivo dermatoscopy: a case series. Int J Dermatol. 2018;57:915–21.
75. Moreno Romero JA, Pérez Muñoz N, Campoy Sánchez A, Urbano Carrillo M, Fernández Figueras MT. Derm dotting: a new technique that improves diagnostic precision in the evaluation of skin lesions. Actas Dermosifiliogr. 2019;110:193–6.
76. Ohsie SJ, Sarantopoulos GP, Cochran AJ, Binder SW. Immunohistochemical characteristics of melanoma. J Cutan Pathol. 2008;35:433–44.
77. Tuna EB, Lebe B, Yörükoğlu K. HMB45 and melan-A expression in renal angiomyolipoma and their significance for the diagnosis. Tumori. 2003;89:46–8.
78. Cassarino DS, Su A, Robbins BA, Altree-Tacha D, Ra S. SOX10 immunohistochemistry in sweat ductal/glandular neoplasms. J Cutan Pathol. 2017;44:544–7.
79. Ramos-Herberth FI, Karamchandani J, Kim J, Dadras SS. SOX10 immunostaining distinguishes desmoplastic melanoma from excision scar. J Cutan Pathol. 2010;37:944–52.
80. Shin J, Vincent JG, Cuda JD, Xu H, Kang S, Kim J, et al. Sox10 is expressed in primary melanocytic neoplasms of various histologies but not in fibrohistiocytic proliferations and histiocytoses. J Am Acad Dermatol. 2012;67:717–26.
81. Behrens EL, Boothe W, D'Silva N, Walterscheid B, Watkins P, Tarbox M. SOX-10 staining in dermal scars. J Cutan Pathol. 2019;46:579–85.

82. May CJ, Piepkorn MW, Knezevich SR, Elder DE, Barnhill RL, Lee AC, et al. Factors associated with use of immunohistochemical markers in the histopathological diagnosis of cutaneous melanocytic lesions. J Cutan Pathol. 2020;47:896–902.
83. Saliba E, Bhawan J. Aberrant expression of immunohistochemical markers in malignant melanoma: a review. Dermatopathology (Basel). 2021;8:359–70.
84. Danga ME, Yaar R, Bhawan J. Melan-A positive dermal cells in malignant melanoma in situ. J Cutan Pathol. 2015;42:388–93.
85. Panse G, McNiff JM. Lichenoid dermatoses with pseudomelanocytic nests vs inflamed melanoma in situ: a comparative study. J Cutan Pathol. 2021;48:745–9.
86. Reed W, Oppedal BR, Eeg LT. Immunohistology is valuable in distinguishing between Paget's disease, Bowen's disease and superficial spreading malignant melanoma. Histopathology. 1990;16:583–8.
87. Palla B, Su A, Binder S, Dry S. SOX10 expression distinguishes desmoplastic melanoma from its histologic mimics. Am J Dermatopathol. 2013;35:576–81.
88. Kanik AB, Yaar M, Bhawan J. p75 nerve growth factor receptor staining helps identify desmoplastic and neurotropic melanoma. J Cutan Pathol. 1996;23:205–10.
89. Radfar A, Stefanato CM, Ghosn S, Bhawan J. NGFR-positive desmoplastic melanomas with focal or absent S-100 staining: further evidence supporting the use of both NGFR and S-100 as a primary immunohistochemical panel for the diagnosis of desmoplastic melanomas. Am J Dermatopathol. 2006;28:162–7.
90. Farah M, Chung HJ. Diagnostic utility of preferentially expressed antigen in melanoma immunohistochemistry in the evaluation of melanomas with a co-existent nevoid melanocytic population: a single-center retrospective cohort study. J Am Acad Dermatol. 2022;87(2):486–8.
91. Vallée A, Denis-Musquer M, Herbreteau G, Théoleyre S, Bossard C, Denis MG. Prospective evaluation of two screening methods for molecular testing of metastatic melanoma: diagnostic performance of BRAF V600E immunohistochemistry and of a NRAS-BRAF fully automated real-time PCR-based assay. PLoS One. 2019;14:e0221123.
92. Juan G, Traganos F, James WM, Ray JM, Roberge M, Sauve DM, et al. Histone H3 phosphorylation and expression of cyclins A and B1 measured in individual cells during their progression through G2 and mitosis. Cytometry. 1998;32:71–7.
93. Gerami P, Yélamos O, Lee CY, Obregon R, Yazdan P, Sholl LM, et al. Multiple cutaneous melanomas and clinically atypical moles in a patient with a novel germline BAP1 mutation. JAMA Dermatol. 2015;151:1235–9.
94. Nielsen PS, Spaun E, Riber-Hansen R, Steiniche T. Automated quantification of MART1-verified Ki-67 indices: useful diagnostic aid in melanocytic lesions. Hum Pathol. 2014;45:1153–61.
95. Oaxaca G, Billings SD, Ko JS. p16 Range of expression in dermal predominant benign epithelioid and spindled nevi and melanoma. J Cutan Pathol. 2020;47:815–23.
96. Uguen A, Talagas M, Costa S, Duigou S, Bouvier S, De Braekeleer M, et al. A p16-Ki-67-HMB45 immunohistochemistry scoring system as an ancillary diagnostic tool in the diagnosis of melanoma. Diagn Pathol. 2015;10:195.
97. Lezcano C, Jungbluth AA, Nehal KS, Hollmann TJ, Busam KJ. PRAME expression in melanocytic tumors. Am J Surg Pathol. 2018;42:1456–65.
98. Koh SS, Cassarino DS. Immunohistochemical expression of p16 in melanocytic lesions: an updated review and meta-analysis. Arch Pathol Lab Med. 2018;142:815–28.
99. See SHC, Finkelman BS, Yeldandi AV. The diagnostic utility of PRAME and p16 in distinguishing nodal nevi from nodal metastatic melanoma. Pathol Res Pract. 2020;216:153105.
100. Gill P, Prieto VG, Austin MT, Giubellino A, Torres-Cabala CA. Diagnostic utility of PRAME in distinguishing proliferative nodules from melanoma in giant congenital melanocytic nevi. J Cutan Pathol. 2021;48:1410–5.
101. LeBlanc RE, Miller DM, Zegans ME. PRAME immunohistochemistry is useful in the evaluation of conjunctival melanomas, nevi, and primary acquired melanosis. J Cutan Pathol. 2021;48:1442–8.
102. Gassenmaier M, Hahn M, Metzler G, Bauer J, Yazdi AS, Keim U, et al. Diffuse PRAME expression is highly specific for thin melanomas in the distinction from severely dysplastic nevi but does not distinguish metastasizing from non-metastasizing thin melanomas. Cancers. 2021;13(15):3864. https://doi.org/10.3390/cancers13153864.
103. McBride JD, McAfee JL, Piliang M, Bergfeld WF, Fernandez AP, Ronen S, et al. PRAME and p16 expression in acral melanocytic neoplasms. J Cutan Pathol. 2022;49(3):220–30.
104. Cesinaro AM, Piana S, Paganelli A, Pedroni G, Santandrea G, Maiorana A. PRAME expression in cellular neurothekeoma: a study of 11 cases. J Cutan Pathol. 2022;49(4):338–42. https://doi.org/10.1111/cup.14163.
105. Raghavan SS, Wang JY, Kwok S, Rieger KE, Novoa RA, Brown RA. PRAME expression in melanocytic proliferations with intermediate histopathologic or spitzoid features. J Cutan Pathol. 2020;47:1123–31.
106. Googe PB, Flanigan KL, Miedema JR. Preferentially expressed antigen in melanoma immunostaining in a series of melanocytic neoplasms. Am J Dermatopathol. 2021;43:794–800.
107. Harvey NT, Peverall J, Acott N, Mesbah Ardakani N, Leecy TN, Iacobelli J, et al. Correlation of FISH and PRAME immunohistochemistry in ambiguous

superficial cutaneous melanocytic proliferations. Am J Dermatopathol. 2021;43:913–20.
108. Straker RJ 3rd, Taylor LA, Neuwirth MG, Sinnamon AJ, Shannon AB, Abbott J, et al. Optimizing detection of lymphatic invasion in primary cutaneous melanoma with the use of D2-40 and a paired melanocytic marker. Am J Dermatopathol. 2022;44:21–7.
109. Conway K, Edmiston SN, Parker JS, Kuan PF, Tsai Y-H, Groben PA, et al. Identification of a robust methylation classifier for cutaneous melanoma diagnosis. J Invest Dermatol. 2019;139:1349–61.
110. Al-Rohil RN, Moore JL, Patterson NH, Nicholson S, Verbeeck N, Claesen M, et al. Diagnosis of melanoma by imaging mass spectrometry: development and validation of a melanoma prediction model. J Cutan Pathol. 2021;48:1455–62.
111. Zarabi SK, Azzato EM, Tu ZJ, Ni Y, Billings SD, Arbesman J, et al. Targeted next generation sequencing (NGS) to classify melanocytic neoplasms. J Cutan Pathol. 2020;47:691–704.
112. Bastian BC, Olshen AB, LeBoit PE, Pinkel D. Classifying melanocytic tumors based on DNA copy number changes. Am J Pathol. 2003;163:1765–70.
113. Emanuel PO, Andea AA, Vidal CI, Missall TA, Novoa RA, Bohlke AK, et al. Evidence behind the use of molecular tests in melanocytic lesions and practice patterns of these tests by dermatopathologists. J Cutan Pathol. 2018;45:839–46.
114. Benton S, Zhao J, Zhang B, Bahrami A, Barnhill RL, Busam K, et al. Impact of next-generation sequencing on interobserver agreement and diagnosis of spitzoid neoplasms. Am J Surg Pathol. 2021;45:1597–605.
115. Sandinha MT, Farquharson MA, McKay IC, Roberts F. Monosomy 3 predicts death but not time until death in choroidal melanoma. Invest Ophthalmol Vis Sci. 2005;46:3497–501.
116. Hotz MJ, O'Halloran EA, Hill MV, Hayden K, Zaladonis AG, Deng M, et al. Tumor mutational burden and somatic mutation status to predict disease recurrence in advanced melanoma. Melanoma Res. 2022;32:112–9.
117. Clarke LE, Warf MB, Flake DD 2nd, Hartman A-R, Tahan S, Shea CR, et al. Clinical validation of a gene expression signature that differentiates benign nevi from malignant melanoma. J Cutan Pathol. 2015;42:244–52.
118. Gerami P, Cook RW, Wilkinson J, Russell MC, Dhillon N, Amaria RN, et al. Development of a prognostic genetic signature to predict the metastatic risk associated with cutaneous melanoma. Clin Cancer Res. 2015;21:175–83.
119. Shain AH, Yeh I, Kovalyshyn I, Sriharan A, Talevich E, Gagnon A, et al. The genetic evolution of melanoma from precursor lesions. N Engl J Med. 2015;373:1926–36.
120. Colebatch AJ, Ferguson P, Newell F, Kazakoff SH, Witkowski T, Dobrovic A, et al. Molecular genomic profiling of melanocytic nevi. J Invest Dermatol. 2019;139:1762–8.
121. van Poppelen NM, van Ipenburg JA, van den Bosch Q, Vaarwater J, Brands T, Eussen B, et al. Molecular genetics of conjunctival melanoma and prognostic value of TERT promoter mutation analysis. Int J Mol Sci. 2021;22(11):5784. https://doi.org/10.3390/ijms22115784.
122. Valiga AA, Fuller CG, Doyle JA, Lee JB. Sarcomatoid dedifferentiated melanoma: the diagnostic role of next-generation sequencing. Am J Dermatopathol. 2022;44(4):282–6. https://doi.org/10.1097/DAD.0000000000002092.
123. Pouryazdanparast P, Newman M, Mafee M, Haghighat Z, Guitart J, Gerami P. Distinguishing epithelioid blue nevus from blue nevus-like cutaneous melanoma metastasis using fluorescence in situ hybridization. Am J Surg Pathol. 2009;33:1396–400.
124. Gerami P, Mafee M, Lurtsbarapa T, Guitart J, Haghighat Z, Newman M. Sensitivity of fluorescence in situ hybridization for melanoma diagnosis using RREB1, MYB, Cep6, and 11q13 probes in melanoma subtypes. Arch Dermatol. 2010;146:273–8.
125. Maize JC Jr, McCalmont TH, Carlson JA, Busam KJ, Kutzner H, Bastian BC. Genomic analysis of blue nevi and related dermal melanocytic proliferations. Am J Surg Pathol. 2005;29:1214–20.
126. Chan MP, Andea AA, Harms PW, Durham AB, Patel RM, Wang M, et al. Genomic copy number analysis of a spectrum of blue nevi identifies recurrent aberrations of entire chromosomal arms in melanoma ex blue nevus. Mod Pathol. 2016;29:227–39.
127. Clayton A. Bernoulli's fallacy: statistical illogic and the crisis of modern science. New York: Columbia University Press; 2021.
128. Zembowicz A. Blue nevi and related tumors. Clin Lab Med. 2017;37:401–15.
129. Massi D, De Giorgi V, Carli P, Santucci M. Diagnostic significance of the blue hue in dermoscopy of melanocytic lesions: a dermoscopic–pathologic study. Am J Dermatopathol. 2001;23:463.
130. Ferrara G, Soyer HP, Malvehy J, Piccolo D, Puig S, Sopena J, et al. The many faces of blue nevus: a clinicopathologic study. J Cutan Pathol. 2007;34:543–51.
131. Zembowicz A, Carney JA, Mihm MC. Pigmented epithelioid melanocytoma: a low-grade melanocytic tumor with metastatic potential indistinguishable from animal-type melanoma and epithelioid blue nevus. Am J Surg Pathol. 2004;28:31.
132. Zembowicz A, Knoepp SM, Bei T, Stergiopoulos S, Eng C, Mihm MC, et al. Loss of expression of protein kinase A regulatory subunit 1α in pigmented epithelioid melanocytoma but not in melanoma or other melanocytic lesions. Am J Surg Pathol. 2007;31:1764.
133. Isales MC, Mohan LS, Quan VL, Garfield EM, Zhang B, Shi K, et al. Distinct genomic patterns in pigmented epithelioid melanocytoma. Am J Surg Pathol. 2019;43:480–8.

134. Zembowicz A, Cohen JN, LeBoit PE. 10—Pigmented epithelioid melanocytoma. In: Busam KJ, Gerami P, Scolyer RA, editors. Pathology of melanocytic tumors. Philadelphia: Elsevier; 2019. p. 124–9.
135. Requena C, Requena L, Kutzner H, Sánchez YE. Spitz nevus: a clinicopathological study of 349 cases. Am J Dermatopathol. 2009;31:107–16.
136. Bastian BC, LeBoit PE, Pinkel D. Mutations and copy number increase of HRAS in Spitz nevi with distinctive histopathological features. Am J Pathol. 2000;157:967–72.
137. Yeh I, de la Fouchardiere A, Pissaloux D, Mully TW, Garrido MC, Vemula SS, et al. Clinical, histopathologic, and genomic features of Spitz tumors with ALK fusions. Am J Surg Pathol. 2015;39:581–91.
138. Yeh I, Busam KJ, McCalmont TH, LeBoit PE, Pissaloux D, Alberti L, et al. Filigree-like rete ridges, lobulated nests, rosette-like structures, and exaggerated maturation characterize spitz tumors with NTRK1 fusion. Am J Surg Pathol. 2019;43:737–46.
139. Houlier A, Pissaloux D, Masse I, Tirode F, Karanian M, Pincus LB, et al. Melanocytic tumors with MAP3K8 fusions: report of 33 cases with morphological-genetic correlations. Mod Pathol. 2020;33:846–57.
140. de la Fouchardière A, Tee MK, Peternel S, Valdebran M, Pissaloux D, Tirode F, et al. Fusion partners of NTRK3 affect subcellular localization of the fusion kinase and cytomorphology of melanocytes. Mod Pathol. 2021;34:735–47.
141. Zembowicz A, McCusker M, Chiarelli C, Dei Tos AP, Granter SR, Calonje E, et al. Morphological analysis of nevoid melanoma: a study of 20 cases with a review of the literature. Am J Dermatopathol. 2001;23:167–75.
142. Mesbah Ardakani N, Singh S, Thomas C, Van Vliet C, Harvey NT, Calonje JE, et al. Mitotically active nevus and nevoid melanoma: a clinicopathological and molecular study. Am J Dermatopathol. 2021;43:182.
143. Pennacchia I, Garcovich S, Gasbarra R, Leone A, Arena V, Massi G. Morphological and molecular characteristics of nested melanoma of the elderly (evolved lentiginous melanoma). Virchows Arch. 2012;461:433–9.
144. Jegou M-H, Huet P, Penchet I. Mélanome en thèques. Annales de Dermatologie et de Vénéréologie. 2017;144:60–4.
145. Kornberg R, Ackerman AB. Pseudomelanoma: recurrent melanocytic nevus following partial surgical removal. Arch Dermatol. 1975;111:1588–90.
146. Sommer LL, Barcia SM, Clarke LE, Helm KF. Persistent melanocytic nevi: a review and analysis of 205 cases. J Cutan Pathol. 2011;38:503–7.
147. Leleux TM, Prieto VG, Diwan AH. Aberrant expression of HMB-45 in traumatized melanocytic nevi. J Am Acad Dermatol. 2012;67:446–50.
148. Böer A, Wolter M, Kaufmann R. [Pseudomelanoma following laser treatment or laser-treated melanoma?]. J Dtsch Dermatol Ges. 2003;1:47–50.
149. Selim MA, Vollmer RT, Herman CM, Pham TTN, Turner JW. Melanocytic nevi with non-surgical trauma: a histopathologic study. Am J Dermatopathol. 2007;29:134–6.
150. Blum A, Hofmann-Wellenhof R, Marghoob AA, Argenziano G, Cabo H, Carrera C, et al. Recurrent melanocytic nevi and melanomas in dermoscopy: results of a multicenter study of the International Dermoscopy Society. JAMA Dermatol. 2014;150:138–45.
151. Vilain RE, McCarthy SW, Scolyer RA. The regenerating naevus. Pathology. 2016;48:108–12.
152. Requena C, Botella-Estrada R, Traves V, Nagore E, Almenar S, Guillén C. [Problems in defining melanoma regression and prognostic implication]. Actas Dermosifiliogr. 2009;100:759–66.
153. Cartron AM, Aldana PC, Khachemoune A. Reporting regression in primary cutaneous melanoma. Part 1: history, histological criteria and pathogenesis. Clin Exp Dermatol. 2021;46:28–33.
154. Ribero S, Galli F, Osella-Abate S, Bertero L, Cattaneo L, Merelli B, et al. Prognostic impact of regression in patients with primary cutaneous melanoma >1 mm in thickness. J Am Acad Dermatol. 2019;80:99–105.e5.
155. Cartron AM, Aldana PC, Khachemoune A. Reporting regression in primary cutaneous melanoma. Part 2: prognosis, evaluation and management. Clin Exp Dermatol. 2020;45:818–23.
156. El Sharouni M-A, Aivazian K, Witkamp AJ, Sigurdsson V, van Gils CH, Scolyer RA, et al. Association of histologic regression with a favorable outcome in patients with stage 1 and stage 2 cutaneous melanoma. JAMA Dermatol. 2021;157:166–73.
157. Tas F, Erturk K. Coexistence of regression and tumor infiltrating lymphocytes is associated with more favorable survival in melanoma. J Cancer Res Clin Oncol. 2021;147:2721–9.
158. Aouthmany M, Weinstein M, Zirwas MJ, Brodell RT. The natural history of halo nevi: a retrospective case series. J Am Acad Dermatol. 2012;67:582–6.
159. Miyazaki A, Saida T, Koga H, Oguchi S, Suzuki T, Tsuchida T. Anatomical and histopathological correlates of the dermoscopic patterns seen in melanocytic nevi on the sole: a retrospective study. J Am Acad Dermatol. 2005;53:230–6.
160. Saida T, Koga H, Goto Y, Uhara H. Characteristic distribution of melanin columns in the cornified layer of acquired acral nevus: an important clue for histopathologic differentiation from early acral melanoma. Am J Dermatopathol. 2011;33:468.
161. Tschandl P, Rosendahl C, Kittler H. Dermatoscopy of flat pigmented facial lesions. J Eur Acad Dermatol Venereol. 2014;29:120–7.
162. Tschandl P, Gambardella A, Boespflug A, Deinlein T, de Giorgi V, Kittler H, et al. Seven non-melanoma

features to rule out facial melanoma. Acta Derm Venereol. 2017;97:1219–24.
163. El Shabrawi-Caelen L, Kerl H, Cerroni L. Melan-A: not a helpful marker in distinction between melanoma in situ on sun-damaged skin and pigmented actinic keratosis. Am J Dermatopathol. 2004;26:364–6.
164. Guitera P, Pellacani G, Crotty KA, Scolyer RA, Li L-XL, Bassoli S, et al. The Impact of in vivo reflectance confocal microscopy on the diagnostic accuracy of lentigo maligna and equivocal pigmented and nonpigmented macules of the face. J Invest Dermatol. 2010;130:2080–91.
165. Scope A, Mahmood U, Gareau DS, Kenkre M, Lieb JA, Nehal KS, et al. In vivo reflectance confocal microscopy of shave biopsy wounds: feasibility of intraoperative mapping of cancer margins. Br J Dermatol. 2010;163:1218–28.
166. Guitera P, Moloney FJ, Menzies SW, Stretch JR, Quinn MJ, Hong A, et al. Improving management and patient care in lentigo maligna by mapping with in vivo confocal microscopy. JAMA Dermatol. 2013;149:692–8.
167. Alarcon I, Carrera C, Alos L, Palou J, Malvehy J, Puig S. In vivo reflectance confocal microscopy to monitor the response of lentigo maligna to imiquimod. J Am Acad Dermatol. 2014;71:49–55.
168. Schiffner R, Schiffner-Rohe J, Vogt T, Landthaler M, Wlotzke U, Cognetta AB, et al. Improvement of early recognition of lentigo maligna using dermatoscopy. J Am Acad Dermatol. 2000;42:25–32.
169. Lieberherr S, Cazzaniga S, Haneke E, Hunger RE, Seyed Jafari SM. Melanoma of the nail apparatus: a systematic review and meta-analysis of current challenges and prognosis. J Eur Acad Dermatol Venereol. 2020;34:967–76.
170. Benati E, Ribero S, Longo C, Piana S, Puig S, Carrera C, et al. Clinical and dermoscopic clues to differentiate pigmented nail bands: an International Dermoscopy Society study. J Eur Acad Dermatol Venereol. 2017;31:732–6.
171. Ruben BS. Pigmented lesions of the nail unit: clinical and histopathologic features. Semin Cutan Med Surg. 2010;29:148–58.
172. Shin H-T, Jang K-T, Mun G-H, Lee D-Y, Lee JB. Histopathological analysis of the progression pattern of subungual melanoma: late tendency of dermal invasion in the nail matrix area. Mod Pathol. 2014;27:1461–7.
173. High WA, Quirey RA, Guillén DR, Munõz G, Taylor RS. Presentation, histopathologic findings, and clinical outcomes in 7 cases of melanoma in situ of the nail unit. Arch Dermatol. 2004;140:1102–6.
174. Ren M, Ren J, Cai X, Shen X-X, Kong J-C, Dai B, et al. Clinicopathological, immunohistochemical and fluorescence in-situ hybridisation features of early subungual melanoma: an analysis of 65 cases. Histopathology. 2021;78:717–26.
175. Parra O, Linos K, Li Z, Yan S. PRAME expression in melanocytic lesions of the nail. J Cutan Pathol. 2022;49(7):610–7.
176. Hosler GA, Moresi JM, Barrett TL. Nevi with site-related atypia: a review of melanocytic nevi with atypical histologic features based on anatomic site. J Cutan Pathol. 2008;35:889–98.
177. Ahn CS, Guerra A, Sangüeza OP. Melanocytic nevi of special sites. Am J Dermatopathol. 2016;38:867–81.
178. El Shabrawi-Caelen L, Soyer HP, Schaeppi H, Cerroni L, Schirren CG, Rudolph C, et al. Genital lentigines and melanocytic nevi with superimposed lichen sclerosus: a diagnostic challenge. J Am Acad Dermatol. 2004;50:690–4.
179. Pinto A, Mclaren SH, Poppas DP, Magro CM. Genital melanocytic nevus arising in a background of lichen sclerosus in a 7-year-old female: the diagnostic pitfall with malignant melanoma. A literature review. Am J Dermatopathol. 2012;34:838.
180. Furusato E, Hidayat AA, Man Y-G, Auerbach A, Furusato B, Rushing EJ. WT1 and Bcl2 expression in melanocytic lesions of the conjunctiva: an immunohistochemical study of 123 cases. Arch Ophthalmol. 2009;127:964–9.
181. Busam KJ, Fang Y, Jhanwar SC, Pulitzer MP, Marr B, Abramson DH. Distinction of conjunctival melanocytic nevi from melanomas by fluorescence in situ hybridization. J Cutan Pathol. 2010;37:196–203.
182. Grimes JM, Shah NV, Samie FH, Carvajal RD, Marr BP. Conjunctival melanoma: current treatments and future options. Am J Clin Dermatol. 2020;21:371–81.
183. van Poppelen NM, de Bruyn DP, Bicer T, Verdijk R, Naus N, Mensink H, et al. Genetics of ocular melanoma: insights into genetics, inheritance and testing. Int J Mol Sci. 2020;22(1):336. https://doi.org/10.3390/ijms22010336.
184. Virgili G, Parravano M, Gatta G, Capocaccia R, Mazzini C, Mallone S, et al. Incidence and survival of patients with conjunctival melanoma in Europe. JAMA Ophthalmol. 2020;138:601–8.
185. Soto H, Bowen RC, Raval V, Yeaney G, Singh A. Primary acquired melanosis/melanoma: utility of conjunctival map biopsy. Br J Ophthalmol. 2022;106(5):605–9. https://doi.org/10.1136/bjophthalmol-2020-317772.
186. Kahneman D, Sibony O, Sunstein CR. Noise: a flaw in human judgment. New York: Little, Brown Spark; 2021.
187. Fernández-Figueras MT, Malvehi J, Tschandl P, Rutten A, Rongioletti F, Requena L, et al. Position paper on a simplified histopathological classification of basal cell carcinoma: results of the European Consensus Project. J Eur Acad Dermatol Venereol. 2022;36(3):351–9. https://doi.org/10.1111/jdv.17849.

Index

A. Böer-Auer et al., *Pattern Analysis for Histopathologic Diagnosis of Melanocytic Lesions*, https://doi.org/10.1007/978-3-031-07666-4

GPSR Compliance

The European Union's (EU) General Product Safety Regulation (GPSR) is a set of rules that requires consumer products to be safe and our obligations to ensure this.

If you have any concerns about our products, you can contact us on ProductSafety@springernature.com

In case Publisher is established outside the EU, the EU authorized representative is:

Springer Nature Customer Service Center GmbH
Europaplatz 3
69115 Heidelberg, Germany

Batch number: 10732801

Printed by Printforce, the Netherlands